Understanding and Managing Oncologic Emergencies

A Resource for Nurses

Editor

Marcelle Kaplan, RN, MS, OCN®, AOCN®

ONCOLOGY NURSING SOCIETY

PITTSBURGH, PENNSYLVANIA

ONS Publishing Division
Publisher: Leonard Mafrica, MBA, CAE
Director of Commercial Publishing: Barbara Sigler, RN, MNEd
Production Manager: Lisa M. George, BA
Technical Editor: Angela D. Klimaszewski, RN, MSN
Staff Editor: Lori Wilson, BA
Copy Editor: Amy Nicoletti, BA
Graphic Designer: Dany Sjoen

Understanding and Managing Oncologic Emergencies: A Resource for Nurses

Library of Congress Control Number: 2006931073

ISBN-13: 978-1-890504-62-5
ISBN-10: 1-890504-62-9

Publisher's Note
This book is published by the Oncology Nursing Society (ONS). ONS neither represents nor guarantees that the practices described herein will, if followed, ensure
safe and effective patient care. The recommendations contained in this book reflect
ONS's judgment regarding the state of general knowledge and practice in the field
as of the date of publication. The recommendations may not be appropriate for use
in all circumstances. Those who use this book should make their own determinations
regarding specific safe and appropriate patient-care practices, taking into account
the personnel, equipment, and practices available at the hospital or other facility at
which they are located. The editors and publisher cannot be held responsible for any
liability incurred as a consequence from the use or application of any of the contents
of this book. Figures and tables are used as examples only. They are not meant to be
all-inclusive, nor do they represent endorsement of any particular institution by ONS.
Mention of specific products and opinions related to those products do not indicate
or imply endorsement by ONS.

ONS publications are originally published in English. Permission has been granted
by the ONS Board of Directors for foreign translation. (Individual tables and figures
that are reprinted or adapted require additional permission from the original source.)
However, because translations from English may not always be accurate or precise,
ONS disclaims any responsibility for inaccuracies in words or meaning that may occur
as a result of the translation. Readers relying on precise information should check the
original English version.

Printed in the United States of America

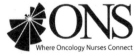

Oncology Nursing Society
Integrity • Innovation • Stewardship • Advocacy • Excellence • Inclusiveness

Contributors

Editor

Marcelle Kaplan, RN, MS, OCN®, AOCN®
Clinical Nurse Specialist, Breast Oncology
Department of Medical/Surgical Nursing
New York-Presbyterian Hospital, Weill Cornell Medical Center
New York, New York
Chapter 3. Hypercalcemia of Malignancy; Chapter 8. Spinal Cord Compression

Authors

Jeanne K. Clancey, RN, MSN, CNRN
Education and Development Specialist
Neuroscience Clinical Nurse Specialist
Western Pennsylvania Hospital
Pittsburgh, Pennsylvania
Chapter 4. Increased Intracranial Pressure; Chapter 7. Syndrome of Inappropriate Antidiuretic Hormone Secretion

Susan A. Ezzone, MS, RN, CNP
Nurse Practitioner, Blood and Marrow Stem Cell Transplant
Arthur G. James Cancer Hospital and Solove Research Institute
The Ohio State University Medical Center
Columbus, Ohio
Chapter 2. Disseminated Intravascular Coagulation

Barbara Holmes Gobel, RN, MS, AOCN®
Oncology Nurse Specialist
Northwestern Memorial Hospital
Adjunct Faculty
Rush University Medical Center
Chicago, Illinois
Chapter 6. Sepsis and Septic Shock; Chapter 10. Tumor Lysis Syndrome

Elena Kuzin, RN, MSN, APRN,BC, AOCN®
Geriatric and Adult Nurse Practitioner in Radiation Oncology
Continuum Cancer Centers of New York—Beth Israel Cancer Center
New York, New York
Chapter 9. Superior Vena Cava Syndrome

Glen J. Peterson, RN, OCN®, ACNP
Nurse Practitioner
Hematological Malignancies and Blood and Marrow Transplant
University of Colorado Hospital and Health Sciences Center
Aurora, Colorado
Chapter 6. Sepsis and Septic Shock

Kristine Turner Story, RN, MSN, APRN
Nurse Practitioner
Internal Medicine Health West
Omaha, Nebraska
Chapter 1. Cardiac Tamponade; Chapter 5. Malignant Pleural Effusion

Table of Contents

Chapter 6. Sepsis and Septic Shock 159

Chapter 7. Syndrome of Inappropriate Antidiuretic Hormone Secretion.. 197

Chapter 8. Spinal Cord Compression 219

Foreword

The overall relative five-year survival rate for cancer is now 65%, and more than 10.5 million individuals in the United States are cancer survivors, representing 3.5% of the U.S. population. Although these figures have improved dramatically over the last 30 years, many survivors continue to have a burden of illness long after their initial diagnosis and treatment. Oncologic emergencies pose such a burden and can contribute to poorer outcomes in both quality *and* quantity of life. Oncologic emergencies may signal the presence of a malignancy, develop as a result of ablative therapies, or arise years after all treatments have been completed.

I once had a patient with lung cancer who was experiencing fatigue. On more careful assessment, I learned that he also had constipation with some back pain. Any one of those symptoms may occur in a person with cancer. The constellation, however, raised a red flag regarding the possibility of a spinal cord compression; a focused evaluation revealed that this, indeed, was the case. Treatment began promptly and prevented him from becoming a paraplegic. As a result of the rapid diagnosis and intervention, he was able to remain mobile and independent the last few months of his life.

Understanding and Managing Oncologic Emergencies: A Resource for Nurses provides nurses and other healthcare providers with a comprehensive resource on the epidemiology, pathophysiology, assessment, and management of common oncologic emergencies. The tables and figures also make it useful as a quick reference when immediate information is needed. By keeping alert clinically to the possibility that an emergency may occur in high-risk individuals, we use this resource to help to prevent, recognize, and effectively manage an oncologic emergency. These efforts will help us to make the lives we save worth living.

Deborah K. Mayer, PhD, RN, AOCN®, FAAN
Assistant Professor
Tufts School of Medicine
Boston, Massachusetts

Preface

The impetus for the development of this book was the need for a nursing reference dedicated solely to oncologic emergencies, a subject that is critical to the quality of life and survival of individuals with a history of cancer. This book is designed to be the definitive, practical, one-stop guide to understanding and managing oncologic emergencies from a nursing perspective.

As cancer survival intervals increase, early recognition of and prompt intervention for disease- or treatment-related oncologic complications are becoming more important than ever. Nurses are key to improving patient outcomes when an oncologic emergency occurs. Devastating functional losses may be limited, a reasonable quality and length of life maintained, and the progression to a life-threatening emergency prevented by the actions of alert nurses.

Nurses involved in the care of patients with a history of cancer—whether the patients are newly diagnosed, are in the process of being treated, or have completed treatment years ago—will find up-to-date, comprehensive information within this book regarding the 10 most common oncologic emergencies. *Understanding and Managing Oncologic Emergencies: A Resource for Nurses* provides complete information in a user-friendly format that will help readers to

- Identify which patients are at increased risk for oncologic emergencies.
- Recognize the signs and symptoms associated with the complications.
- Understand the underlying pathophysiologic processes.
- Learn pertinent diagnostic evaluations and therapeutic interventions.
- Assess patients appropriately.
- Apply nursing management strategies across a continuum from acute through chronic care.

Chapters are presented alphabetically for easy location of topics of interest, and each follows a consistent structure to facilitate information gathering. Tables, figures, and boxes are liberally incorporated throughout the text to summarize or emphasize detailed information and to make the book a quick reference.

Each in-depth chapter begins with an overview of the epidemiology of the oncologic emergency, followed by discussion of the associated pathophysiologic mechanisms, clinical manifestations, patient assessments, diagnostic evaluations, and therapeutic management modalities. Nursing management strategies, including prevention and early detection measures, ongoing patient assessments and symptom management, treatment and side effect management, rehabilitation and palliative care, and patient and caregiver education recommendations are presented in detail. Terms or concepts that may be unfamiliar are explained throughout, and an extensive reference list concludes each chapter, guiding readers to additional resources on each topic.

Oncology nurses are the natural audience for this book, but others practicing in a variety of patient care settings—ambulatory care, medical-surgical hospital units, home care, palliative care, critical care, emergency departments, and physician offices—as well as nurse educators and those preparing for oncology nursing certifications or advanced practice roles in oncology also will find valuable information within this clinical reference.

It is my hope that this book has met the goal of being the definitive nursing resource for complete, detailed information regarding all aspects of understanding and managing the care of patients experiencing oncologic emergencies.

Thanks are due to many people who were essential to the creation of this comprehensive nursing resource. I gratefully acknowledge the contributions of the chapter authors who shared their knowledge and expertise. Their dedication to creating a quality reference book is apparent in their chapters. I commend the editorial staff of the ONS Publishing Division for their expert guidance and expertise in shaping the manuscript into a quality book.

I am also fortunate to have had the resources of two highly regarded medical libraries literally at my fingertips, both physically and electronically: the libraries of the Weill Medical College of Cornell University and Memorial Sloan-Kettering Cancer Center. Their staffs were unfailingly helpful. I also thank the Department of Medical-Surgical Nursing at Weill Cornell Medical Center of New York-Presbyterian Hospital for supporting my work on this book over a long period of time.

I send my love to my children, Andrea Kaplan and Richard Kaplan, and Richard's wife, Lydie, for their enthusiasm and encouragement along every step of the way. We all take great pride in each other. Lastly, I acknowledge the contributions of my husband, Jack Lubowsky, PhD, whose unstinting love and support encouraged me to take on this challenge and shepherd it through to completion. He patiently worked on table layouts for my chapters and created several figures for the book. To him I dedicate this book.

Marcelle Kaplan, RN, MS, OCN®, AOCN®
Editor

Kristine Turner Story, RN, MSN, APRN

⊃Chapter 1

Cardiac Tamponade

Introduction

Cardiac tamponade is a life-threatening oncologic emergency. It occurs when excessive fluid accumulates in the pericardial sac surrounding the heart and exerts extrinsic pressure on the cardiac chambers. This causes obstruction to the inflow of blood to the ventricles, interfering with cardiac function and resulting in decreased cardiac output (Braunwald, 2001; Flounders, 2003). The buildup of fluid in the pericardial sac is known as pericardial effusion and precedes tamponade in most cases. It is important to distinguish between pericardial effusion and cardiac tamponade. *Pericardial effusion* is the presence of abnormal pericardial fluid that often has no hemodynamic consequence, whereas *cardiac tamponade* causes increased pericardial pressure with resultant hemodynamic consequence. Cardiac tamponade exists when the pericardial pressure is 30 mm Hg or greater (Shabetai, 2004). It occurs when fluid accumulates faster than the pericardium can stretch. The heart becomes compressed by the accumulation of pericardial fluid, blood, clots, or pus (Hawley, Dreher, & Vasso, 2003). Tamponade can occur from as little as 50–80 ml of fluid collection (Humphreys, 2003; Merrill, 2000; Shelton, 2000). If left untreated, cardiac tamponade ultimately will result in cardiovascular collapse, shock, and death.

Incidence

The exact incidence of cardiac tamponade in malignancy is unknown. Some authors report the incidence of pericardial effusion, a risk factor for tamponade, as occurring in 5%–50% of all malignancies (Grannis, Wagman, Lai, & Curcio, 2002; Myers, 2001; Warren, 2000), but it is likely underreported as symptoms may be vague, undiagnosed, or attributed to other cardiac conditions. Autopsy studies have reported pericardial malignancies in 7% of patients with lung cancer, 7% of patients with esophageal cancer, and 3% of patients with breast cancer (Warren). Rarely, a pericardial effusion may be the initial manifestation of malignancy (Grannis et al.; Schrump & Nguyen, 2001). Only a small percentage of patients with cancer and effusions are thought to develop clinical tamponade (Read & Denes, 2002). Effusions caused by cancer more often progress to cardiac tamponade than nonmalignant effusions, primarily because of bleeding in the pericardial sac, and may occur in as many as 5%–15% of patients with a neoplasm that involves the heart (Keefe, 2000; Myers). Mean life expectancy after diagnosis of malignant pericardial effusion is two to five months and is greatly influenced by the success of controlling the underlying malignancy (Read & Denes; Shelton, 2000). Approximately 25% of selected patients treated surgically for cardiac tamponade have a one-year survival rate (Grannis et al.).

Risk Factors

Malignancies and their treatments are the major causes of pericardial effusions and cardiac tamponade in medical patients (Keefe, 2000). Primary tumors of the pericardium, although rare, account for a significant number of cases of malignant pericardial effusion and subsequent tamponade. Malignant mesothelioma is the most common primary tumor of the heart. Much less common are malignant fibrous histiocytoma, rhabdomyosarcoma, and angiosarcoma. Often, primary tumors may present a clinical picture similar to cardiac tamponade when, in fact, the symptoms are caused by constrictive pericarditis attributable to diffuse thickening of the pericardium by the tumor (Warren, 2000). Invasion of the myocardium by metastatic disease is most common in lung and breast cancers and lymphoma. Malignant thymoma, esophageal tumors, sarcomas, melanoma, gastrointestinal tumors, and liver, pancreatic, ovarian, and cervical cancers are much less common sources (Flounders, 2003; Grannis et al., 2002; Read & Denes, 2002; Warren). Hematogenous spread of tumor to the pericardium is most common with lymphoma, melanoma, and leukemia, especially acute myeloid leukemia, lymphoblastic leukemia, and chronic myeloid leukemia in blast crisis. Effusions with negative cytology are more common in mediastinal lymphoma, Hodgkin disease, and breast cancer (Grannis et al.). Extension of the tumor into the pericardium may cause cardiac herniation, leading to rapid effusion and tamponade. Metastasis also may cause obstruction of mediastinal lymph nodes, interfering with lymph drainage in the pericardial space, and is considered to be the most common cause of pericardial effusion in malignancy (Schrump & Nguyen, 2001; Warren). Table 1-1 provides an overview of the risk factors associated with the development of cardiac tamponade.

Chest radiation therapy of 4,000 centigray (cGy) delivered to more than 33% of the heart in fraction sizes greater than 300 cGy per day increases the risk of developing a pericardial effusion (Flounders, 2003; Loerzel & Dow, 2003). Approximately 5% of patients who receive 4,000 cGy or more of radiation to the mediastinum develop acute pericarditis with or without pericardial effu-

Table 1-1. Risk Factors for Development of Cardiac Tamponade	
Cause	**Risk Factors**
Disease related	• Primary tumors of the heart • Direct tumor extension to the heart • Obstruction of mediastinal lymph nodes

Treatment related	• Chest radiation therapy
	• Chemotherapy
	  − Anthracyclines
	  − Cytosine arabinoside
	  − Cyclophosphamide
	• Biotherapy
	  − Interferon
	  − Interleukin-2
	  − Interleukin 11
	  − Granulocyte macrophage–colony-stimulating factor
	• Improper central line or pacemaker insertion

Other	• Medications
	  − Anticoagulants
	  − Hydralazine
	  − Procainamide
	• Coexisting heart disease
	• Connective tissue disorders
	• Myxedema
	• Tuberculosis
	• Bacterial endocarditis
	• Pericarditis
	• Trauma
	• Aneurysms
	• Cardiac surgery, particularly valve surgery

Note. Based on information from Braunwald, 2001; Flounders, 2003; Loerzel & Dow, 2003; Miaskowski, 1999; Myers, 2001; Schrump & Nguyen, 2001; Shelton, 2000.

sion during treatment or chronic constrictive pericarditis for up to 20 years after treatment. The majority of cases occur in the first year after radiation treatment (Miaskowski, 1999; Myers, 2001).

Chemotherapy and biotherapy agents that increase capillary permeability also increase risk of effusion. These include anthracyclines (doxorubicin, daunorubicin, and others), cytosine arabinoside, cyclophosphamide, interferon, interleukin-2 and interleukin 11, and granulocyte macrophage–colony-stimulating factor. Generally, the risk is greater in higher dose regimens containing these products or with combinations of chemotherapy and radiation therapy (Loerzel & Dow, 2003; Myers, 2001; Shelton, 2000). Other drugs that may cause cardiac tamponade include anticoagulants (heparin, sodium warfarin), hydralazine (Apresoline®, Novartis Pharmaceuticals Corp., East Hanover, NJ), and procainamide (procaine SR, Pronestyl® [Apothecon, Inc., Princeton, NJ]) (Myers).

Other risk factors for cardiac tamponade include coexisting heart disease, systemic lupus erythematosus, rheumatoid arthritis, scleroderma, myxedema, tuberculosis, bacterial endocarditis, and pericarditis (Braunwald, 2001; Flounders, 2003). Hemorrhagic tamponade may occur as the result of direct trauma to the chest, aneurysmal leakage, improper insertion of a central line or pacemaker, or as an adverse event following cardiac surgery, particularly valvular surgery. An estimated 3%–7% of patients experience tamponade after cardiac surgery (Hawley et al., 2003).

An infectious etiology occasionally can be the cause of pericardial effusion and tamponade. Hypoproteinemia and the presence of a coexisting infection may exacerbate an existing effusion, increasing the risk of tamponade (Ruckdeschel & Jablons, 2001). The presence of a coagulopathy or the use of anticoagulation therapy increases the risk, particularly if patients with acute pericarditis receive this treatment (Braunwald, 2001; Hawley et al., 2003). End-stage renal failure also can result in significant effusion leading to tamponade.

Pathophysiology

The pericardium is a sac-like membrane that surrounds the heart and great vessels. It consists of two layers—the visceral layer, a thin, elastic serous membrane that lies on the surface of the heart, and the thick, stiff parietal layer, which comprises the outer layer. The parietal layer provides strength and protection for the heart. Between these two layers is the pericardial space, which normally contains approximately 10–50 ml of fluid. The mesothelial cells of the visceral pericardium produce this fluid, which prevents friction between the membranes during contraction and relaxation of the heart. The lymph channels reabsorb and drain the fluid into the mediastinum and right heart (Flounders, 2003; Hawley et al., 2003) (see Figure 1-1).

The pericardium has several functions. One function is to provide stability of the heart muscle. The pericardium is not directly attached to the heart at any point; rather, ligaments attach the pericardium to the diaphragm and mediastinum, providing structural support for the heart and limiting excessive cardiac motion, especially with changes in body position (Goldstein, 2004). Other functions attributed to the pericardium are equalizing right and left ventricular output, buffering changes in ventricular filling pressure and output with position change, limiting acute dilatation of the heart, and providing immune effects, primarily by limiting the spread of infection from contiguous structures (Goldstein). However, the presence of an intact pericardium is not essential for normal cardiac function.

The most important role of the pericardium is its mechanical interactions with the cardiac chambers. Under normal physiologic conditions, the pericardium is a relatively fixed and inelastic sac with stiff, noncompliant pressure-volume characteristics. It acts as a hydrostatic system, equally distributing forces

Figure 1-1. Anatomy of the Pericardial Space

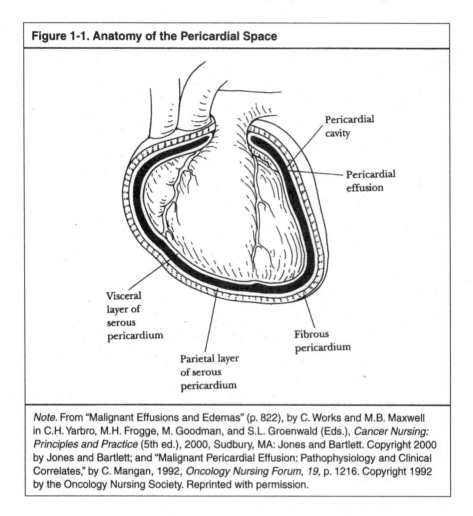

Note. From "Malignant Effusions and Edemas" (p. 822), by C. Works and M.B. Maxwell in C.H. Yarbro, M.H. Frogge, M. Goodman, and S.L. Groenwald (Eds.), *Cancer Nursing: Principles and Practice* (5th ed.), 2000, Sudbury, MA: Jones and Bartlett. Copyright 2000 by Jones and Bartlett; and "Malignant Pericardial Effusion: Pathophysiology and Clinical Correlates," by C. Mangan, 1992, *Oncology Nursing Forum, 19,* p. 1216. Copyright 1992 by the Oncology Nursing Society. Reprinted with permission.

over the surface of the cardiac chambers, which helps to maintain equality of end-diastolic pressures in the ventricles, uniform stretch of cardiac muscle fibers, and a normal cardiac shape (Goldstein, 2004).

Normal cardiac pressures are subatmospheric, which allows for an inflow of venous blood to the right side of the heart. An imbalance among the pressure, production, and clearance of normal fluid in the pericardial space results in the development of an effusion. The primary pathology causing effusion is obstruction of the venous and lymphatic drainage of the heart, thus preventing reabsorption of fluid (Shelton, 2000; Works & Maxwell, 2000). The presence of cancer cells stimulates the pericardium to produce excessive fluid. In addition, invasive tumors may bleed into the pericardial space. Blood accumulates more rapidly than fluid, thereby increasing the risk of tamponade (Flounders, 2003).

Because the pericardial sac is stiff and noncompliant, increases in fluid volume can have adverse hemodynamic consequences. The normal pericardium has a small reserve volume, so small increases in fluid result in only trivial increases in intrapericardial pressure. Slow increases in fluid volume may be asymptomatic to as much as 2,000 ml of fluid, whereas rapid increases in fluid generally cause rapid hemodynamic collapse (Flounders, 2003; Hawley et al., 2003). Increases in fluid volume may elevate the pressure in the pericardial space to such an extent that the heart is prevented from relaxing completely between beats. When ventricular filling is restricted by fluid in the pericardial sac, cardiac output decreases. Decreased stroke volume and cardiac output cause hypotension and compensatory tachycardia (Goldstein, 2004; Shelton, 2000).

Pericardial effusions are classified by exudative type. Transudative effusions are low in protein and are the result of abnormal capillary permeability caused by nonmalignant mechanical factors, such as cirrhosis. Analysis of transudative fluid will demonstrate lactate dehydrogenase (LDH) levels less than 200 IU/L and protein levels less than 35 g/dl. Exudative effusions are rich in protein and are caused by leakage from blood vessels with increased permeability. Exudates will reveal LDH levels greater than 200 IU/L and protein levels greater than 35 g/dl (Shelton, 2000). Most malignant pericardial effusions are exudates that contain cellular debris caused by irritation of the serous membrane by cancer cells or tumor implants (Flounders, 2003; Myers, 2001; Ruckdeschel & Jablons, 2001).

Factors that determine whether an effusion is symptomatic include the volume of fluid, the rate at which the fluid accumulates, and the compliance characteristics of the pericardium. Although slowly developing effusions may be asymptomatic until large volumes of fluid are present, a critical point is eventually reached where additional fluid accumulation will quickly outpace any remaining compensatory mechanisms, and a dramatic increase in pressure occurs. At that point, even a small increase in fluid can cause a large compressive force on the heart, especially if the pericardium is stiff and noncompliant, resulting in cardiac tamponade (Hawley et al., 2003; Shabetai, 2004; Shelton, 2000).

Surgical tamponade occurs when the intrapericardiac pressure rises quickly, usually within a matter of hours, and generally is a result of hemorrhage from trauma. *Medical* tamponade occurs when a slow buildup of fluid accrues over days to weeks before tamponade occurs. This most likely is caused by a low-intensity inflammatory process and is more consistent with the course of most malignant effusions (Maisch et al., 2004). The steep rise in pressure makes tamponade a "last-drop" phenomenon; the final addition of fluid produces critical cardiac compression, and the first decrease in volume during drainage produces the largest relative decompression (Spodick, 2003).

In tamponade, the right atrium and right ventricle initially are compressed, leading to decreased right atrial filling during diastole. When the normally low pericardial pressure rises to the level of normal right atrial pressure, cardiac tamponade is trivial. When it equals normal left atrial pressure, tamponade is mild. When pericardial pressure exceeds 10–12 mm Hg, moderate tamponade is present. Pressure in the venous circulation becomes elevated as evidenced by increased jugular venous distention, increased diastolic pressure, hepatomegaly, and edema. At this point, the blood pressure and cardiac output usually are only slightly lowered. When pericardial pressure is greater than 25 mm Hg, then tamponade becomes severe, pulsus paradoxus may be present, blood pressure and stroke volume are decreased, and tachycardia is present. Continued compression causes decreased ventricular filling, leading to decreased stroke volume, decreased cardiac output, and decreased tissue perfusion (Flounders, 2003; Ruckdeschel & Jablons, 2001; Shabetai, 2004). Death in patients with tamponade usually is heralded by pulseless electrical activity, in which the electrocardiogram (EKG) continues to register complexes in the absence of blood flow or pressure (Spodick, 2003). Figure 1-2 presents a linear depiction of the pathologic events resulting from cardiac tamponade.

A variety of cardiac compensatory mechanisms attempt to correct tamponade. Fluid loading of the ventricles can temporarily counteract intrapericardiac pressure. Reciprocal filling of right and left chambers with inspiration and expiration from paradoxical movement of the septum of the ventricle is the last mechanism to maintain blood flow until cardiovascular collapse and death occur (Grannis et al., 2002). The sympathetic nervous system attempts to compensate with cardiac stimulation, resulting in tachycardia and vasoconstriction. Given sufficient time, blood volume will expand. Decreased tissue perfusion also causes activation of the renin-angiotensin-aldosterone system to increase blood volume and stroke volume. Over time, these compensatory mechanisms increase the workload of the heart. Without intervention, the heart eventually will fail, leading to shock, cardiac arrest, and subsequent death (Flounders, 2003; Spodick, 2003) (see Figure 1-2).

Clinical Manifestations

Patients with pericardial effusions and cardiac tamponade experience a wide variety of signs and symptoms that are related to the amount of fluid and rapidity of onset and subsequent impact on hemodynamic status (see Table 1-2). Early signs and symptoms may be subtle and may not correlate with the amount of pericardial fluid present. Many developing effusions may be asymptomatic or attributed to other causes. Often, the patient is thought to have right heart failure, and diuretics are administered, which may worsen tamponade (Works & Maxwell, 2000). Symptoms increase in severity as small effusions become larger or if fluid accumulates rapidly. Patients may deteriorate rapidly, and if tamponade goes unrecognized, the mortality rate rises to 65% (Miaskowski, 1999).

Figure 1-2. Pathophysiologic Processes in Cardiac Tamponade

Fluid accumulates in the pericardial sac.
↓
Increase in intrapericardial pressure from subatmospheric pressure
to positive pressure surrounding the heart
↓
Decreased venous return to the right atrium
↓
Decreased stroke volume
↓
Decreased cardiac output
↓
Compensatory mechanisms are triggered.
↓
Increased heart rate
Stretching of the pericardial sac
Increased peripheral vasoconstriction
↓
Increased vascular volume
↓
Pericardial effusion worsens.
↓
Further increase in pericardial pressure
↓
Compensatory mechanisms fail.
↓
Decreased cardiac output
↓
Severe hypotension
↓
Circulatory collapse

Note. From "Oncologic Emergencies" (p. 228), by C. Miaskowski in C. Miaskowski and P. Buchsel (Eds.), *Oncology Nursing Assessment and Clinical Care,* 1999, St. Louis, MO: Mosby. Copyright 1999 by Mosby. Reprinted with permission.

Patients may complain of fatigue, malaise, dyspnea at rest, and orthopnea. Dyspnea on exertion that progresses to air hunger is a common initial presentation. Patients may complain of dull, diffuse, nonpositional chest pain and a nonproductive cough and may appear anxious or restless (Flounders, 2003; Myers, 2001; Ruckdeschel & Jablons, 2001; Spodick, 2003).

Patients may describe chest pain as "heaviness," or it may disappear with tamponade (Shelton, 2000). As tamponade progresses, patients will have increased shortness of breath, cold sweats, and confusion. They may find relief of their symptoms by sitting up and leaning forward. Late symptoms include hoarseness, coughing, hiccups, or dysphagia because of compression of extracardiac structures. Patients may feel dizzy, lightheaded, or agitated if hypoxic and may have vague gastrointestinal complaints, such as anorexia,

---

Table 1-2. Signs and Symptoms of Pericardial Effusion/Cardiac Tamponade

Onset	Symptoms	Signs
Earlier	May be asymptomatic	Tachycardia = 100 bpm
	Fatigue	Mild peripheral edema
	Malaise	Mild abdominal distention
	Light-headedness	Decreased peripheral pulses
	Dyspnea on exertion	Mild JVD
	Dull, diffuse, nonpositional chest pain	Muffled heart sounds
	Vague abdominal distress	PMI shifted
	Palpitations	Increased CVP, 8–13 mm Hg
		Low-voltage QRS complex
		Oliguria
Later	Dyspnea at rest	Tachycardia > 100 bpm
	Orthopnea	Increased JVD
	Increased retrosternal chest pain	Hepatojugular reflex
	Chest pain heavier or may disappear	Muffled or absent heart sounds
	Cold sweats	Friction rub
	Mental status changes	Narrowed pulse pressure
	Hoarseness	Pulsus paradoxus
	Coughing	PMI shifted or barely palpable
	Hiccups	Decreased carotid pulse
	Dysphagia	Increased CVP, 12–22 mm Hg
	Anxiety	Massive edema, ascites—may be absent if rapidly developing
	Apprehension	Electrical alternans
		Anuria

bpm—beats per minute; CVP—central venous pressure; JVD—jugular venous distention; PMI—point of maximal impulse

Note. Based on information from Flounders, 2003; Myers, 2001; Shelton, 2000; Works & Maxwell, 2000.

---

nausea, and vomiting caused by visceral venous congestion. Patients also may present with mental status changes, including lethargy, restlessness, confusion, decreased level of consciousness, and seizures because of increasing hypoxia (Flounders, 2003; Grannis et al., 2002; Hawley et al., 2003; Kaplow, 2000; Loerzel & Dow, 2003).

Patient Assessment

History

Identification of cardiac tamponade relies on a detailed history and thorough physical assessment. Healthcare professionals should note a current or past history of cancer, particularly cancers with the highest risk of cardiac tamponade. They also should note prior treatment with chemotherapy or other agents that have known cardiac toxicities or history of radiation therapy to the mediastinum. Assessing for other medical conditions, medications, or recent procedures that can cause cardiac tamponade may rule out malignancy as the cause of the tamponade (Flounders, 2003; Humphreys, 2003; Myers, 2001; Shelton, 2000).

Physical Assessment

Objective patient findings include nonpulsatile jugular venous distention or distention of superficial veins in the face, scalp, and ocular fundi, although jugular venous distention may be absent if patients are dehydrated or hypovolemic (Read & Denes, 2002; Warren, 2000). Rapid tamponade may cause exaggerated jugular pulsations with distention if there is insufficient time for blood volume expansion (Spodick, 2003). Patients may have a positive *hepatojugular reflex,* which is defined as an elevation in jugular venous pressure by 1 cm or more because of venous congestion in the liver. It is elicited by elevating the head of the bed to 30°–45° and slowly applying pressure over the right upper quadrant of the abdomen for 30–60 seconds (Flounders, 2003; Myers, 2001; Spodick). See Table 1-3 for a description of the signs associated with cardiac tamponade.

As the effusion worsens, patients will be tachycardic, tachypneic, hypotensive, and diaphoretic. Fever and a pericardial friction rub are more likely with radiation-induced or nonmalignant effusions (Spodick, 2003; Warren, 2000). A previously heard friction rub may disappear as an enlarging effusion separates the inflamed layers of the pericardium (Braunwald, 2001; Humphreys, 2003). The point of maximal impulse in the apex of the heart may be shifted to the left and downward. Distant or muffled heart sounds with a weak or undetectable apical pulse, because of fluid accumulation, is generally a later finding (Flounders, 2003). *Ewart sign,* dullness to percussion of the left lung over the angle of the scapula, may occur because of compressive collapse of the pericardial sac (Braunwald; Humphreys). The lungs usually are clear, but crackles in the bases may be present with coexisting pulmonary disease (Hawley et al., 2003; Kaplow, 2000). Peripheral pulses may be decreased, while a moderate increase may occur in central venous pressure to 15–18 cm H_2O from the normal pressure of 5–10 cm H_2O. Patients with slowly developing effusions may exhibit pedal edema, whereas none may be present with rapid effusions (Ruckdeschel & Jablons, 2001). Prolonged periods of hypotension may cause decreased perfusion to the kidneys, resulting in oliguria or anuria (Kaplow). Ascites is a less frequent finding and is associated with significant right heart failure (Flounders; Merrill, 2000). Cyanosis is uncommon, as is *Kussmaul sign,* a narrow pulse pressure, which is a late sign and indicates potential for rapid deterioration (Ruckdeschel & Jablons).

The combination of distant heart sounds, hypotension and a narrow pulse pressure, and jugular venous distention in conjunction with head and neck edema is known as the *Beck triad* and is associated with cardiac tamponade (Hawley et al., 2003; Kaplow, 2000). Tamponade without two or more inflammatory signs (pleuritic-type pain, pericardial friction rub, fever, diffuse ST segment elevation) usually is associated with a malignant effusion (Maisch et al., 2004).

Pulsus paradoxus is considered a hallmark sign of cardiac tamponade but actually is an infrequent finding (Hawley et al., 2003; Keefe, 2000; Merrill, 2000). Pulsus paradoxus is defined as a greater than 10 mm Hg difference in systolic blood pressure between expiration and inspiration. It represents the decreased cardiac output associated with decreased left ventricular filling that varies with respiration (Braunwald, 2001; Flounders, 2003). It occurs when negative pressure in the thorax during inspiration limits cardiac filling, decreases cardiac output, and causes a weak pulse (Kaplow, 2000; Merrill). Pulsus paradoxus is a late finding more commonly associated with nonma-

Table 1-3. Physical Findings in Cardiac Tamponade

Sign	Physical Finding
Beck triad	Distant heart sounds, hypotension, and narrowed pulse pressure, combined with jugular venous distention and head and neck edema, associated with cardiac tamponade
Ewart sign	Dullness to percussion of the left lung over the angle of the scapula because of collapse of the pericardial sac
Hepatojugular reflex	Elevation in jugular venous pressure by 1 cm or more because of venous congestion in the liver, elicited by putting slow pressure on the liver and observing for increased jugular venous pressure
Korotkoff sounds	Sounds heard over an artery when pressure is reduced below systolic arterial pressure, as when determining blood pressure by auscultation
Kussmaul sign	Narrowed pulse pressure caused by a paradoxical increase in venous distention and pressure during inspiration
Pulsus paradoxus	Greater than 10 mm Hg difference in systolic blood pressure between expiration and inspiration because of decreased cardiac output

Note. Based on information from Braunwald, 2001; Flounders, 2003; Hawley et al., 2003; Humphreys, 2003; Kaplow, 2000; Keefe, 2000; Merrill, 2000; Myers, 2001; Ruckdeschel & Jablons, 2001; Spodick, 2003.

lignant effusions, particularly constrictive pericarditis, in only approximately one-third of the cases (Braunwald). Pulmonary disease, labored respirations, pulmonary embolism, asthma, right ventricular infarction, extreme obesity, and tense ascites also can cause pulsus paradoxus, so it is not necessarily diagnostic of cardiac tamponade (Hawley et al.; Jay et al., 2000; Keefe). Mechanical ventilation can artificially mimic pulsus paradoxus. It may be undetectable in certain coexisting conditions, even if tamponade is present. These include extreme hypotension, acute left ventricular myocardial infarction, pericardial adhesions, pulmonary fibrosis, right ventricular hypertrophy, severe aortic regurgitation, atrial septal defects, severe renal failure, and some cases of low-pressure tamponade (Myers, 2001; Shabetai, 2004; Spodick, 2003).

Healthcare providers can measure pulsus paradoxus by auscultating with a sphygmomanometer for respiratory variation in systolic blood pressure or on an arterial line tracing. When cardiac tamponade is severe, palpating a weakness or absence of the arterial pulse during inspiration may detect paradoxus (Braunwald, 2001). More beats also may be palpated on expiration than inspiration (Hawley et al., 2003). Obtaining an accurate pulsus paradoxus measurement is technically challenging, and even in model situations, many skilled clinicians are unable to obtain accurate readings (Jay et al., 2000).

To auscultate pulsus paradoxus, determine the systolic blood pressure first. Then, starting 10–20 mm Hg above this point, slowly deflate the sphygmomanometer to the point when *Korotkoff sounds* are heard during expiration, and note this point. Then slowly deflate the cuff until Korotkoff sounds are heard throughout the respiratory cycle. The difference between the pressures at which Korotkoff sounds are first heard and when they are heard continuously during respiration is the pulsus (Merrill, 2000). Korotkoff sounds may completely disappear during inspiration in severe cases of tamponade (Flounders, 2003; Warren, 2000).

Another method to determine the pulsus on an arterial tracing is to calculate the difference between the highest and lowest systolic blood pressure during the respiratory cycle (Hawley et al., 2003; Keefe, 2000). In very low cardiac output, this may be the only means to detect pulsus paradoxus (Spodick, 2003). The "rule of 20," which represents a decrease in pulse pressure of more than 20 mm Hg, pulsus paradoxus greater than 20 mm Hg, and central venous pressure greater than 20 cm H_2O, is an indicator of impending tamponade and a signal for aggressive intervention (Myers, 2001).

Diagnostic Evaluation

A variety of diagnostic modalities exist to assess the presence and extent of cardiac tamponade. A chest x-ray (CXR) will demonstrate an enlarged cardiac silhouette, but only when an effusion has reached a volume of at least 250 ml (Hawley et al., 2003; Shatzer & Castor, 2004) (see Figure 1-3). Lung fields usually are clear on CXR (Kaplow, 2000). Patients may have a widened

Figure 1-3. Chest X-Ray Findings in Chronic Pericardial Effusion

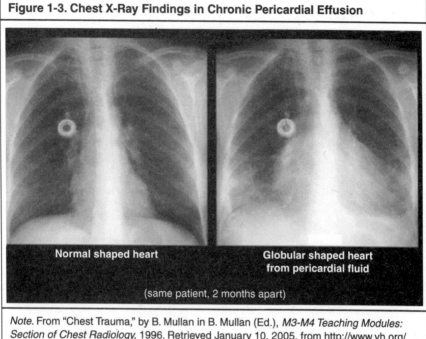

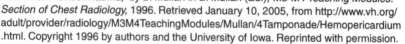

Normal shaped heart

Globular shaped heart from pericardial fluid

(same patient, 2 months apart)

Note. From "Chest Trauma," by B. Mullan in B. Mullan (Ed.), *M3-M4 Teaching Modules: Section of Chest Radiology,* 1996. Retrieved January 10, 2005, from http://www.vh.org/ adult/provider/radiology/M3M4TeachingModules/Mullan/4Tamponade/Hemopericardium .html. Copyright 1996 by authors and the University of Iowa. Reprinted with permission.

mediastinum and an irregular, nodular contour of the cardiac shadow, and the heart may have a classic "water bottle" shape. Any significant change in the cardiac width greater than 2 cm from a prior CXR is diagnostic of effusion and requires further evaluation (Kaplow; Ruckdeschel & Jablons, 2001). Up to 50% of patients may have a coexisting pleural effusion, and up to 35% have lung involvement by the tumor, obscuring the heart silhouette (Warren, 2000). A CXR cannot differentiate the cause of an enlarged heart and does not provide conclusive evidence of effusion. A negative CXR does not preclude the diagnosis, however, and if symptomatic, other tests should be performed.

EKG changes include a low-voltage QRS complex, tachycardia, nonspecific ST-T changes, and premature atrial or ventricular contractions. Bradycardia, unexplained atrial fibrillation, or heart block may indicate impending tamponade (Shelton, 2000; Warren, 2000). Electrical alternans is a rare EKG finding that occurs when the heart swings freely in the pericardial sac, causing a constantly changing electrical axis. The EKG tracing will show variations in the height of the P wave and QRS complex from beat to beat (Humphreys, 2003). Electrical alternans is an unreliable indicator of tamponade, however, as only a small percentage of patients will exhibit this finding (Merrill, 2000) (see Figure 1-4).

Figure 1-4. Twelve-Lead Electrocardiogram Showing Electrical Alternans

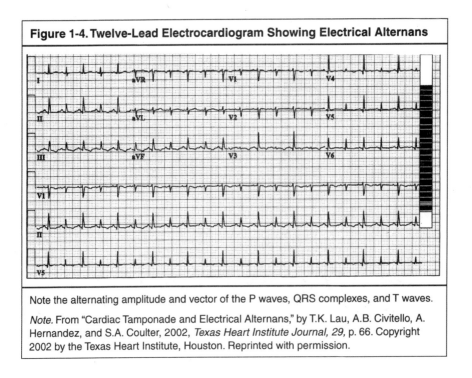

Note the alternating amplitude and vector of the P waves, QRS complexes, and T waves.

Note. From "Cardiac Tamponade and Electrical Alternans," by T.K. Lau, A.B. Civitello, A. Hernandez, and S.A. Coulter, 2002, *Texas Heart Institute Journal, 29*, p. 66. Copyright 2002 by the Texas Heart Institute, Houston. Reprinted with permission.

A two-dimensional echocardiogram is the diagnostic modality of choice. It is painless and noninvasive and can be performed at the bedside. This test will assess for the presence, location, and approximate quantity of pericardial fluid accumulation in the pericardial sac and will assess overall cardiac function. Echo-free spaces that separate the moving walls from the pericardium indicate that fluid is present. The spaces generally occur posteriorly and then anteriorly. Absence of pericardial fluid rules out cardiac tamponade (Kaplow, 2000; Myers, 2001).

The size of effusions can be graded with compression of the heart as small (echo-free space in diastole is less than 10 mm), medium (10–20 mm), large (greater than 20 mm), or very large (greater than 30 mm) (Maisch et al., 2004). In large pericardial effusions, the heart may move freely in the pericardial cavity ("swinging heart") (Flounders, 2003; Maisch et al.; Shatzer & Castor, 2004).

An echocardiogram also will demonstrate the key findings compatible with the diagnosis of tamponade: diastolic collapse of the right ventricle, notching of the right ventricular wall in systole, and inversion of the right atrium. These findings are diagnostic of tamponade and do not occur in pericardial effusion (Shatzer & Castor, 2004; Warren, 2000). In approximately 25% of patients, the left atrium also collapses, and this finding is highly specific for tamponade (Spodick, 2003). Echocardiography is operator dependent, however, and some studies have shown its sensitivity and specificity to be as low as 38% in correctly identifying right ventricular diastolic collapse (Cooper, Oliver, Currie, Walker, & Swanton, 1995). Because the echocardiogram is done at rest and some patients are only symptomatic with exertion, the diagnosis may be delayed (Ruckdeschel & Jablons, 2001).

Healthcare providers may perform a transesophageal echocardiogram (TEE) to clarify findings or if the diagnosis is in question. It is particularly helpful in critically ill patients who are hypotensive, in cases of bleeding with clot formation, and in identifying metastases and pericardial thickening (Maisch et al., 2004; Myers, 2001). The TEE scope, a modification of an endoscope, is placed in the esophagus at the level of the heart and allows high-resolution images of the heart from a variety of positions. It can be done at the bedside, in the operating room, or as an outpatient procedure (Myers).

A computed tomography (CT) scan of the chest may be ordered if the diagnosis is in question or if the pericardium is caked with tumor. Images obtained by CT may be as good as or better than an echocardiogram, can detect as little as 50 ml of pericardial fluid, and are less operator dependent. Magnetic resonance imaging (MRI) also may be useful in confirming the diagnosis, with resolution superior to echocardiogram in some cases (Warren, 2000). CT and MRI may be particularly useful in differentiating constrictive pericarditis with effusion versus radiation fibrosis (Myers, 2001). These tests are not the diagnostic modalities of choice, however, as they are time consuming, expensive, and no more accurate than echocardiogram (Schrump & Nguyen, 2001).

Cardiac catheterization may be indicated to assess for cardiac function or if the diagnosis is in question. Cardiac catheterization will show equalization of diastolic pressures and elevated right heart pressures to 15–30 mm Hg. Reciprocation of pressures during respiration may be present, with an inspiratory increase on the right side of the heart accompanied by a concomitant decrease on the left, the cause of pulsus paradoxus (Spodick, 2003). If right atrial pressure exceeds 20 mm Hg, hemodynamic compromise is severe (Keefe, 2000). Cardiac catheterization also may be useful to rule out superior vena caval obstruction, to identify microvascular tumor spread to the lungs with secondary pulmonary hypertension, and to document constrictive pericarditis (Grannis et al., 2002). An endomyocardial biopsy may be performed to rule out cardiomyopathy from prior anthracycline use (Warren, 2000).

Video-assisted pericardioscopy may be done if the diagnosis is in question. This allows for confirmation of the diagnosis, biopsy of cardiac tissues if appropriate, and immediate drainage of fluid (Ruckdeschel & Jablons, 2001). Pericardial biopsy is frequently nondiagnostic and may have little value (Schrump & Nguyen, 2001). Pericardial fluid may be evaluated for LDH and protein to determine whether the effusion is a transudate or an exudate. Other fluid studies include specific gravity, cell counts, stains, cultures, and cytologic analysis. Serum LDH, protein, and glucose levels may be obtained to compare to pericardial fluid (Myers, 2001; Shelton, 2000). Malignant effusions may appear bloody, serosanguineous, or serous (Kaplow, 2000).

Treatment Modalities

Cardiac tamponade is a life-threatening emergency. The immediate goal of treatment for tamponade is the removal of pericardial fluid to restore hemodynamic stability. Additional treatment varies based on the life expectancy and comorbidities of patients. The primary purpose of treatment is palliation of symptoms. Withholding treatment may be appropriate in rapidly progressing or critically ill patients. Needle aspiration of the pericardial fluid may be used for immediate relief of symptoms, but it is associated with rapid reaccumulation of fluid and has little long-term benefit. If asymptomatic, an aggressive approach in patients with a life expectancy of three to four months or more probably will prolong palliation. The presence of an exudative effusion can increase the risk of constrictive changes, resulting in the need for a more extensive surgical procedure later (Flounders, 2003; Maisch et al., 2004; Ruckdeschel & Jablons, 2001). Table 1-4 presents an overview of the more common treatment modalities used in managing cardiac tamponade.

Healthcare providers should systematically evaluate all patients with pericardial effusions before determining utility of treatment. Both the management and natural course of an effusion depend on the status of the patients, extent of clinical symptoms, and type and extent of the underlying malignancy. The availability of facilities and the experience of the medical and nursing staff also are important factors in determining a course of therapy (Warren, 2000). Evaluation of existing treatments is difficult because of the many patient variables and comorbidities, lack of prospective data for each treatment option, and the relative rarity of the condition. In general, close monitoring and treatment of the underlying disease may manage asymptomatic, small effusions. Symptomatic, moderate-to-large effusions that are not an emergency require treatment aimed at relieving symptoms and preventing recurrence of the effusion. Cardiac tamponade is a true emergency and requires immediate pericardiocentesis. Without additional definitive treatment, however, the effusion will recur rapidly (Grannis et al., 2002; Maisch et al., 2004).

Two theoretical mechanisms for the control of pericardial effusion exist, and these provide the basis for treatment. The first involves creating a permanent defect in the pericardium, which allows for fluid to drain out and be absorbed by surrounding tissues, negating any impact on cardiac function. The second involves injuring the mesothelium of the pericardial space with the use of sclerosing agents. This mechanism stimulates formation of fibrous tissue that obliterates the pericardial cavity, preventing reaccumulation of fluid (Grannis et al., 2002).

Pericardiocentesis

Pericardiocentesis is an initial treatment for rapidly advancing effusion and cardiac tamponade that involves draining the fluid from the pericardium to relieve symptoms and to further evaluate the effusion. The benefit of peri-

Table 1-4. Treatment of Neoplastic Cardiac Tamponade

Treatment	Indications	Methodology
Pericardiocentesis	Life-threatening cardiac tamponade in the presence of moderate-to-large pericardial effusions when open procedure cannot be performed quickly	Fluid is removed by an emergency bedside insertion of a needle into the pericardial sac. Needle is inserted into the subxiphoid and pointed toward the left shoulder. Needle is backed off, and fluid is aspirated.
Pericardial catheter—may use to drain, then remove, or may leave in for several days	Short-term emergent removal of slowly or rapidly developing effusions	Fluoroscopic-directed pericardial catheter is used with drainage and/or sclerosis (bleomycin, doxycycline, talc, thiotepa).
Balloon pericardiotomy	Short-term emergent removal of slowly or rapidly developing effusions	Catheter is inserted into the pericardial sac, and a balloon is inflated to open a hole in the pericardial sac; catheter is immediately removed, and pericardial fluid drains into mediastinum.
Pericardioperitoneal shunt	Palliative management of recurrent malignant effusions, particularly with limited life expectancy	Local anesthesia is used for percutaneous subxiphoid insertion of a Denver shunt that drains pericardial fluid into the abdomen.
Pericardial window	Chronic, severe effusions in patients with otherwise good performance status; must be able to tolerate a thoracoscopic procedure	Thoracotomy with resection of the lower section of the pericardial sac; screen-like grid is placed to allow pericardial drainage into the mediastinum.
Pericardiectomy	Chronic, severe effusions in patients with otherwise good performance status; must be able to tolerate a thoracoscopic procedure. Used only after catheter or balloon fluid removal and pericardial window have failed.	Pericardial sac is resected or stripped so that there is no place for pericardial fluid to accumulate.

Note. From "Pericarditis/Pericardial Effusion/Cardiac Tamponade" (pp. 393–395), by B. Shelton in C.A. Ziegfeld, B.G. Lubejko, and B.K. Shelton (Eds.), *Oncology Fact Finder: Manual of Clinical Oncology,* 1998, Philadelphia: Lippincott Williams & Wilkins. Copyright 1998 by Lippincott Williams & Wilkins. Adapted with permission.

cardiocentesis is that it quickly relieves tamponade, but the complication rate ranges from 10%–25% and can include puncture of the cardiac muscle or arteries, accidental introduction of air into the heart chambers, dysrhythmia, vasovagal reaction with bradycardia, infection, and abscess formation (Flounders, 2003; Myers, 2001).

Pericardial fluid is usually serous or serosanguineous but may be frankly bloody in up to one-third of cases. Malignant cells may be found on cytologic exam, but even in patients with biopsy-proven cardiac malignancy, cytology is positive in only 79% of cases. This is especially true with mesothelioma and lymphoma. The use of image DNA cytometric analysis has higher sensitivity than routine cytology. In general, if the effusion has characteristics of an exudate, clinicians should strongly suspect malignancy (Flounders, 2003; Warren, 2000).

Pericardiocentesis is done most safely by a subxiphoid approach (see Figure 1-5). In a truly emergent situation, it can be done without benefit of echocardiogram or fluoroscopy, but the use of some imaging modality is preferable to identify the optimal point to penetrate the pericardial space (Grannis et al., 2002; Maisch et al., 2004). The patient is placed in a semi-upright position, and the anterior chest wall and upper abdomen are prepped and draped. Lidocaine is placed at the entry site 2 cm below the xiphoid and to the left of the midline. A 21-gauge spinal needle is advanced at a 45° angle toward the left shoulder. An EKG lead may be attached to the needle, which will demonstrate EKG changes if the needle comes into contact with the epicardium (Warren, 2000). The use of echocardiogram or fluoroscopy is optimal because the use of an EKG electrode may provide misleading results (Spodick, 2003). Once fluid is encountered, it is continuously aspirated while the needle is advanced. If previously clear fluid becomes bloody, clinicians should suspect a puncture of the right ventricle. Pericardial fluid does not clot, which will differentiate it from blood (Warren). When effusions are drained, they must be decompressed slowly over several minutes to avoid acute right heart ventricular distention and failure (Ruckdeschel & Jablons, 2001). Once the needle is in the proper position and the patient is stable, a catheter can be left in place to allow drainage over several days and to serve as a route for the instillation of a sclerosing agent. The catheter is drained each shift and may be irrigated daily with a small volume of saline or heparinized saline. Bleeding is the most serious complication of pericardiocentesis, and this procedure is relatively contraindicated in patients with thrombocytopenia or coagulopathy. Surgical back-up should be available while it is being performed (Myers, 2001; Warren).

Based on a retrospective review of 275 patients treated for cardiac tamponade, the Mayo Clinic recommends percutaneous pericardiocentesis with extended catheter drainage as initial therapy. Recurrences then are treated surgically (Tsang et al., 2000). Up to one-third of patients do not have recurrent effusions after 30 days. It is theorized that the mere presence of a drainage catheter in the pericardial space may be enough to cause adhesion formation without the need for further intervention (Warren, 2000). A subsequent long-term analysis of these data showed that extended pericardial catheter

Figure 1-5. Needle Pericardiocentesis by the Subxiphoid Approach

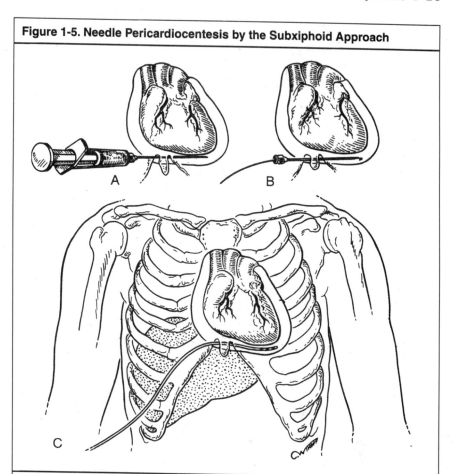

(A). Guide wire introduced through needle into the pericardial space (B). Percutaneous catheter drainage of the pericardial space (C).

Note. From "Pericardial Drainage Procedures," by D.W.O. Moores and S.W. Dziuban, 1995, *Chest Surgery Clinics of North America, 5,* p. 361. Copyright 1995 by Elsevier. Reprinted with permission.

drainage over one to three days was associated with a lower recurrence rate (6% versus 23%) than in those without catheter drainage (Tsang et al., 2002). Placement of long-term drainage catheters can be done via a pericardioperitoneal shunt. In this procedure, a catheter is inserted into the pericardial space and into the peritoneum to allow continuous drainage of pericardial fluid. Alternatively, a Pleurx® (Denver Biomedical, Inc., Denver, CO) catheter may be inserted percutaneously directly in the pericardial sac and the pericardial fluid drained into vacuum bottles. Once drainage subsides, sclerosing agents seal the pericardial space (Warren).

Pericardiocentesis With Sclerosis

Pericardial sclerosis involves the instillation of an agent into the pericardial sac to create inflammation of the pericardial space, thereby obliterating the space and preventing reaccumulation of fluid. This should be performed only after the pericardium is fully drained. The best outcomes have occurred when sclerosing agents were used at the time of initial drainage rather than at the time of recurrence. Most agents are instilled over several days rather than in single-dose boluses (Warren, 2000). Sclerosis is considered successful when no drainage occurs for a 24-hour period (Myers, 2001).

In the past, tetracycline was the sclerosing agent of choice, but the powdered form is no longer available in North America. The use of this agent has an excellent track record, but significant problems with pain, fever, and arrhythmias during sclerosis have occurred (Grannis et al., 2002; Warren, 2000). The use of tetracycline derivatives such as doxycycline, oxytetracycline, and minocycline appears to be safe with no long-term side effects, but results have been mixed (Keefe, 2000; Warren). Instilling talc is an option, but it is associated with a high incidence of severe pain, fever, and a high probability of constrictive pericarditis (Keefe). A variety of chemotherapeutic agents have been tried in the past as sclerosing agents with varied effect. Nitrogen mustard, doxorubicin, quinacrine chloride, methotrexate, and 5-fluorouracil have resulted in considerable chest pain and bone marrow suppression caused by systemic absorption. Several studies have shown bleomycin and thiotepa to be safe and effective (Warren).

A prospective study comparing bleomycin to doxycycline found both agents to be equally efficacious, but bleomycin was associated with less pain and a shorter time to achieve sclerosis (Liu, Grump, Goss, Dancey, & Shepherd, 1996). Another prospective study of bleomycin in 22 patients with non-small cell lung cancer and pericardial effusion reported no adverse events and no recurrent pericardial effusions over a mean survival time of 15 weeks (Seto, Nagashina, Yoshino, Semba, & Ichinose, 2001).

Thiotepa also is gaining favor as a sclerosing agent, especially in cases of pericardial effusion caused by breast cancer. It has a low incidence of side effects and has the advantage of being both a sclerosing and antineoplastic agent. In a study of 33 patients with malignant pericardial effusion and poor performance status, 15 mg of thiotepa was instilled into the pericardium on days 1, 3, and 5 after pericardiocentesis. No procedure-related complications or side effects occurred, and researchers noted no recurrent effusions in the first month. The median survival was 115 days in the overall population and 272 days in patients with breast cancer (Martinoni et al., 2004). Other nonrandomized studies have reported similar results (Bishiniotis et al., 2000; Girardi, Ginsberg, & Burt, 1997), suggesting that aggressive treatment with thiotepa may be considered a first-choice treatment for patients with malignant pericardial effusion (Martinoni et al.).

Radioisotopes also have been used as sclerosing agents, but they are expensive and require isolation of patients, thus limiting their use. A study of the efficacy of ^{32}P radioactive colloid in 36 patients with malignant pericardial effusion revealed that 94% had complete resolution and died of aggressive disease at other sites. Toxicity was minimal, with only one case of transient tachycardia (Dempke & Firusian, 1999). Intrapericardial instillation of OK-432, an immunomodulator, resulted in excellent control of effusion in 10 patients, with little toxicity (Imamura et al., 1991). Administration of the biologic response modifier interleukin-2 controlled recurrence of effusion in 67% of cases in one study (Lissoni, Barni, & Ardizzoia, 1992). Most studies of sclerosing agents are nonrandomized and have small sample sizes, making interpretation and application difficult.

Surgical Options

Multiple surgical options are available for the management of pericardial effusion, but little consensus exists on which is the preferred modality. Variables to consider when choosing which surgical intervention to use include patient characteristics, comorbidities, and feasibility. A history of prior pleurodesis for malignant pleural effusion may limit options (Grannis et al., 2002). In general, a surgical procedure is reserved for those with good performance status, patients with a longer life expectancy, or those who have failed pericardiocentesis with sclerosis.

According to some authors, the treatment of choice is subxiphoid pericardiotomy. It is associated with lower morbidity and mortality than other procedures and may be performed under local anesthesia (Ruckdeschel & Jablons, 2001; Schrump & Nguyen, 2001; Warren, 2000). In this procedure, the patient is placed in a supine position and prepped and draped, and then local anesthesia is administered in the subxiphoid region. The pericardium is exposed through an external midline incision of 3–8 cm, a small incision is made in the pericardium, and fluid is removed for cytology, culture, and chemistry analysis. At this point, a pericardial window may be created. This involves removing a small "button" of the pericardium with a diameter of approximately 3 cm, which allows pericardial fluid to drain into surrounding tissues. Tube drainage or sclerosis also may be combined with this procedure. Patients generally will have one or more chest tubes in place for several days following subxiphoid pericardiotomy (Schrump & Nguyen; Warren). In a series of 654 patients undergoing this procedure, researchers reported an overall mortality rate of 0.46%, an overall morbidity rate of 1.53%, and a recurrence rate of 3.52% (Schrump & Nguyen).

Another surgical method involves creating a subxiphoid pericardioperitoneal window through the diaphragm to allow continued drainage of pericardial fluid into the peritoneum. There may be less recurrence with this approach, but experience is limited, and the procedure may not be possible in patients with a prior median sternotomy (Grannis et al., 2002). Placement of a pleuroperitoneal shunt has had success in draining the pericardial fluid into the peritoneal cavity, but further evaluation of this approach is necessary (Schrump & Nguyen, 2001; Wang, Feikes, Morgensen, Vyhmeister, & Bailey, 1994).

A pericardial window also can be performed via an anterior thoracotomy. It is associated with a small risk of recurrence and lower morbidity than a subtotal pericardial resection, but recovery may be slower than with pericardiocentesis. Cardiac herniation is possible if the size of the pericardial window is too large. In addition, if the effusion is drained too quickly, there is a risk that the heart will dilate to fill the pericardial space, causing right heart failure. Use of catheter drainage before a window is created may prevent this complication, and it is managed with aggressive diuresis should it occur (Keefe, 2000).

In a study comparing subxiphoid pericardiostomy to pericardiocentesis with catheter drainage, no operative deaths occurred among the 94 patients who underwent the open technique, and one operative death occurred among the 23 patients who underwent the percutaneous approach. The complication rate was higher with the percutaneous approach, 17% versus 1.1% for the open approach (Allen, Faber, Warren, & Shaar, 1999). In a long-term follow-up study of patients who underwent subxiphoid pericardiostomy for both benign and malignant effusions, ultrasound studies demonstrated that only 18% had recurrence, half of which were symptomatic. Only one of the patients with malignant effusion died from reaccumulation of the effusion; all others died from distant disease (Mueller et al., 1997).

The definitive treatment for pericardial effusion is a subtotal pericardial resection (pericardiectomy), which involves complete or partial removal of the pericardial sac, allowing continuous fluid drainage into the pleural space. Almost no chance exists of recurrence or constriction following this procedure, but it requires general anesthesia, and cardiopulmonary bypass usually is required when a complete pericardiectomy is performed (Kaplow, 2000). Pericardiectomy carries a higher morbidity rate and a longer recovery than other procedures, so it is undesirable for patients with a short life expectancy. It generally is restricted to patients with recurrent effusions who are expected to live more than one year (Grannis et al., 2002; Myers, 2001; Warren, 2000). The procedure also is used to treat patients with radiation-induced constrictive pericarditis (Flounders, 2003). A limited lateral or video-assisted thoracoscopic pericardial resection technique is gaining favor because of its lower morbidity and mortality rates versus open procedures. General anesthesia still is required, however, which may limit its use in patients with major airway obstruction (Grannis et al.; Schrump & Nguyen, 2001; Warren).

Another procedure whose role has yet to be fully assessed is a percutaneous balloon pericardiotomy. With this technique, a balloon-dilating catheter is placed across the pericardium under fluoroscopic guidance. Inflation of the balloon creates a window by tearing the pericardium. Often, more than one pericardial site is dilated. No tissue is resected, so scarring and closure of the site is possible. Because this is a closed procedure, it is not possible to obtain a biopsy with this technique. Complications of percutaneous balloon pericardiotomy have included febrile episodes, bleeding, and pneumothorax (Flounders, 2003; Warren, 2000). In one series, the technique was effective in

46 of 50 patients, and the incidence of recurrent effusions or tamponade was at least 4% (Ziskind et al., 1993). The procedure is technically feasible but requires special equipment and the presence of an interventional cardiologist or radiologist to perform the procedure. It has been used in limited situations, but long-term results are not known at this time (Grannis et al., 2002; Ruckdeschel & Jablons, 2001; Schrump & Nguyen, 2001; Spodick, 2003).

Other Treatment Options

Radiation therapy has a limited role in the treatment of pericardial effusion and tamponade but may be useful in patients with radiosensitive tumors who have not had prior radiation therapy. Radiation therapy is delivered to an area that includes the heart, pericardial structures, and mediastinum to a total dose of 2,000–4,000 cGy. Cardiac tolerance is 3,500–4,000 cGy; higher doses increase the risk of pericarditis (Myers, 2001). Studies have shown response rates of 66%–93%, depending on the type of tumor, with best success in leukemia, lymphoma, and breast cancer (Flounders, 2003; Grannis et al., 2002; Schrump & Nguyen, 2001; Shelton, 2000).

Chemotherapy is effective in treating pericardial effusions in patients with breast cancer, hematologic malignancies, and lymphoma (Grannis et al., 2002). Chemotherapy may be the initial treatment of a pericardial effusion if the patient is asymptomatic and the effusion is slowly developing (Myers, 2001). A retrospective review of 82 patients with non-small cell lung cancer and pericardial tamponade showed a significant increase in survival in those who received local treatment of their tamponade plus systemic chemotherapy versus those who received local treatment alone. Median survival was 74 days, with one-year survival rates of 7% (Wang et al., 2000). Vaitkus, Herrmann, and LeWinter (1994) studied 46 patients with breast cancer, lymphoma, or other solid tumors. Recurrence of effusion was prevented in 31 patients (67%) who had combined pericardiocentesis and systemic chemotherapy.

Additional Medical Management

Additional medical management of patients with pericardial effusion is relatively controversial and has been based on the results of animal studies, which have yielded conflicting results (Spodick, 2003). Traditional medical treatment includes ongoing pharmacologic therapy to maintain blood pressure and optimal cardiac function. Mild effusions initially may be cautiously treated with diuretics such as furosemide (Lasix®, Aventis Pharmaceuticals Inc., Bridgewater, NJ) or spironolactone (Aldactone®, G.D. Searle LLC, Chicago, IL), observing for fluid volume compromise. High-dose steroids or nonsteroidal anti-inflammatory drugs also may be administered, particularly in the case of constrictive pericarditis associated with radiation therapy (Flounders, 2003; Myers, 2001). When these drugs are discontinued, the pericarditis usually recurs.

Saline, plasma, and blood products may be administered to expand circulatory volume but must be closely monitored. Volume expansion may increase intracardiac pressures as well as heart size, increasing pericardial pressure, which also may precipitate tamponade (Kaplow, 2000; Spodick, 2003). Other interventions include the use of vasoactive drugs to maintain cardiac perfusion, low-dose dopamine to improve cardiac contractility, and isoproterenol to increase heart rate (Flounders, 2003; Myers, 2001). Nitroprusside, an arterial vasodilator, may be given to decrease the work of the heart and to help increase blood pressure, but beta blockers should be avoided because beta-stimulation of the heart is already maximal, and the addition of pharmacologic agents may provide no benefit (Kaplow; Spodick).

Avoid mechanical ventilation with positive airway pressure in patients with tamponade, because this further decreases cardiac output. In the event of cardiac arrest, external compression has little value because there is little room for additional filling; if systolic pressure rises, diastolic pressure falls, resulting in decreased coronary perfusion pressure (Kaplow, 2000; Spodick, 2003).

Nursing Management

Nursing management of patients with cardiac tamponade is multifaceted and complex (see Figure 1-6). Astute observation and assessment are critical as patients may develop tamponade slowly or quite rapidly. Physical findings may be confused with other conditions, so knowledge of the course of these conditions as well as a high degree of suspicion is necessary to correctly identify patients at risk or those who are experiencing pericardial effusions or tamponade.

Frequent assessment of cardiopulmonary status is paramount to identification and early intervention in cardiac tamponade. Assessment of cardiac status includes frequent monitoring of patients' blood pressure, pulse, cardiac rhythm, heart sounds, pulse pressures, and cardiac output. If irregularities in cardiac rhythm are detected, place a cardiac monitor and check the readings for findings associated with cardiac tamponade: ST segment elevation, T-wave inversion, onset of atrial fibrillation or heart block, or electrical alternans. Auscultate heart sounds for onset of murmurs, gallops, or rubs. If suspicious of developing tamponade, assess for pulsus paradoxus, noting any difference greater than 10 mm Hg. Healthcare providers also should monitor arterial and central venous pressures and pulmonary capillary wedge pressures if using these devices (Warren, 2000). Observe jugular venous pulses for increased jugular venous pressure. The effectiveness of cardiac output is monitored, noting skin color, temperature, turgor, capillary refill, peripheral pulses, and changes in mental status and level of consciousness related to hypoxia. Notify the physician immediately if the patient's status changes. In addition, nurses should monitor laboratory and test results, paying close attention to

---

Figure 1-6. Nursing Management of Patients With Cardiac Tamponade

- Frequent assessment of cardiac, respiratory, and nervous systems
  - Monitor vital signs and pulse oximetry.
  - Auscultate heart and lung sounds.
  - Assess for cough, dyspnea, Kussmaul sign, air hunger, and cyanosis.
  - Assess for chest pain, arrhythmias, electrocardiogram changes, pulsus paradoxus, jugular venous distention, decreased activity tolerance, and clubbing.
  - Monitor arterial, central venous, and pulmonary capillary wedge pressures if indicated.
  - Assess for headache, change in mental status, and level of consciousness.
- Maintenance of optimal pulmonary status
  - Administer oxygen to keep saturation > 92%.
  - Position patients with head of bed up or in forward-leaning position.
  - Encourage energy conservation/frequent rest periods.
  - Include deep breathing, coughing, pursed-lip breathing, postural drainage, and suctioning.
- Maintenance of optimal cardiac status
  - Administer IV fluids, vasopressors, and blood products as ordered.
  - Prepare for cardiac arrest and resuscitation in acute tamponade.
  - Provide comfort measures.
  - Administer analgesics as ordered.
  - Administer antianxiety medications as ordered.
  - Encourage relaxation techniques.
- Preparation for invasive procedures
- Care of drainage tubes and other devices as indicated
- Patient and caregiver education
- Discharge planning

Note. Based on information from Hawley et al., 2003; Kaplow, 2000; Miaskowski, 1999; Myers, 2001; Warren, 2000; Works & Maxwell, 2000.

---

electrolytes, as abnormalities may affect cardiac rhythm (Miaskowski, 1999; Myers, 2001).

Measures to maintain optimal cardiac output in patients experiencing acute tamponade are implemented as ordered. Administer vasoactive drugs to increase cardiac output, improve contractility, and improve preload. IV fluids, typically normal saline or lactated ringers, are infused to increase filling pressure in acute tamponade (Warren, 2000). Blood products may be given to maintain volume. Diuretics will likely be avoided in acute tamponade. Nurses should be prepared for cardiac arrest and resuscitation (Kaplow, 2000; Myers, 2001).

The patient's respiratory status also provides important information. Nurses should observe for any abnormalities associated with tamponade, including dyspnea, tachypnea, Kussmaul sign, air hunger, and hypoxemia; auscultate breath sounds; and check oximetry levels. If necessary, healthcare providers should initiate oxygen therapy to keep saturation levels greater than 92% and make preparations for mechanical ventilation. Positioning patients with the head of the bed elevated or in a forward-leaning position, if this is more comfortable, may help to ease air hunger. The nurse should encourage frequent deep breathing and coughing, provide frequent mouth care and suctioning, if necessary, and give patients frequent rest periods and assistance with all activities to help them to conserve energy. The use of analgesics, antianxiety medications, comfort measures, and relaxation techniques may help to decrease the workload on the heart and lungs. However, nurses should observe and report any adverse effects of analgesics on respiratory function and adjust the dose as ordered (Hawley et al., 2003; Kaplow, 2000; Myers, 2001).

Preparing patients and caregivers for all invasive procedures or transfers to the operating room is an important part of the nurses' role. Provide education to patients and caregivers regarding each procedure, including sensations that might be experienced, the type of equipment that may be used, and expected outcomes of each procedure. Try to allay patients' anxiety by providing simple explanations, and allow patients to discuss concerns. This will help to reduce psychosocial distress and also may decrease workload on the heart (Kaplow, 2000). Prior to all procedures, ensure that informed consent is obtained, that all equipment is procured as needed, including emergency resuscitation equipment, and that IV access is established and sedation is administered as ordered. Position the patient appropriately, and verify that all necessary monitoring equipment is present and in working order. During the procedure, monitor cardiac rhythm, vital signs, and hemodynamic status. Observe for complications, and monitor the amount and characteristics of any drainage obtained, ensuring that all specimens are sent to the laboratory for analysis as ordered. Maintain aseptic technique throughout (Kaplow; Miaskowski, 1999; Works & Maxwell, 2000).

Once the procedure is completed, assess for complications, including bleeding, signs of infection, increasing dyspnea, absent or decreased breath sounds, which may indicate pneumothorax or pleural effusion, and evidence of reaccumulation of pericardial fluid as evidenced by worsening of hemodynamic status. Perform pulmonary toilet to prevent atelectasis and pneumonia. Monitor the amount and characteristics of any drainage, and provide care for drainage tubes and chest tubes if present. Perform postprocedure wound assessment and wound care using sterile technique (Kaplow, 2000; Works & Maxwell, 2000).

Patient and Caregiver Education

Once the patient is stabilized and ready for discharge, provide patient and caregiver education regarding the signs and symptoms of an effusion recurrence and the importance of prompt reporting. Some patients may be asymptomatic and only require periodic office visits to monitor their status. Healthcare providers should stress the importance of adequate hydration and nutrition, scheduled rest periods, and measures to decrease anxiety. If patients have an indwelling drainage tube, catheter care and maintenance must be taught. A home healthcare referral also should be made for those patients. Other patients may require short-term or long-term care in an extended care facility or a hospice referral. Patients and their caregivers should be informed of the prognosis associated with pericardial effusion and tamponade, be encouraged to identify plans and goals in the event of recurrence, and be provided with emotional support and referrals to social services if necessary.

Conclusion

Cardiac tamponade is a life-threatening oncologic emergency that requires rapid identification and intervention to avoid cardiovascular collapse and death. Malignancies and their treatments are the major causes of pericardial effusions and cardiac tamponade in medical patients, and these conditions may occur in up to 50% of patients with cancer. Symptoms often are vague, and inexperienced clinicians may overlook them or attribute them to other causes. The aim of treatment is rapid drainage of excessive pericardial fluid to improve cardiac output. Patients may require additional treatment depending on their status and goals of therapy. Nurses should possess knowledge of who is at risk and the signs and symptoms associated with this serious oncologic emergency. This, coupled with a high degree of suspicion and astute assessment, will lead to successful identification, earlier intervention, and improved outcomes.

References

Allen, K.B., Faber, L.P., Warren, W.H., & Shaar, C.J. (1999). Pericardial effusion: Subxiphoid pericardiostomy versus percutaneous catheter drainage. *Annals of Thoracic Surgery, 67,* 437–440.

Bishiniotis, T.S., Antoniadou, S., Katseas, G., Mouratidou, D., Litos, A.G., & Balamoutsos, N. (2000). Malignant cardiac tamponade in women with breast cancer treated by pericardiocentesis and intrapericardial administration of triethylenethiophosphoramide (thiotepa). *American Journal of Cardiology, 86,* 362–364.

Braunwald, E. (2001). Pericardial disease. In E. Braunwald, A.S. Fauci, D.L. Kasper, S.L. Hauser, D.L. Longo, & J.L. Jameson (Eds.), *Harrison's principles of internal medicine* (5th ed., pp. 1365–1372). New York: McGraw-Hill.

Cooper, J.P., Oliver, R.M., Currie, P., Walker, J.M., & Swanton, R.H. (1995). How do the clinical findings in patients with pericardial effusions influence the success of aspiration? *British Heart Journal, 73,* 351–354.

Dempke, W., & Firusian, N. (1999). Treatment of malignant pericardial effusion with 32P-colloid. *British Journal of Cancer, 80,* 1955–1957.

Flounders, J.A. (2003). Cardiovascular emergencies: Pericardial effusion and cardiac tamponade [Online exclusive]. *Oncology Nursing Forum, 30,* E48–E55.

Girardi, L.N., Ginsberg, R.J., & Burt, M.E. (1997). Pericardiocentesis and intrapericardial sclerosis: Effective therapy for malignant pericardial effusions. *Annals of Thoracic Surgery, 64,* 1422–1428.

Goldstein, J.A. (2004). Cardiac tamponade, constrictive pericarditis, and restrictive cardio-myopathy. *Current Problems in Cardiology, 29,* 503–567.

Grannis, F.W., Wagman, L.D., Lai, L., & Curcio, L.D. (2002). Fluid complications. In R. Pazdur, L.R. Coia, W.J. Hoskins, & L.D. Wagman (Eds.), *Cancer management: A multidisciplinary approach* (pp. 943–958). Melville, NY: PRR.

Hawley, J., Dreher, H.M., & Vasso, M. (2003). Under pressure: Treating cardiac tamponade. *Nursing Management, 34*(2), 44D–44H.

Humphreys, M. (2003). Conditions affecting the pericardium. *Connect, The World of Critical Care Nursing, 2,* 80–84.

Imamura, T., Tamura, K., Takenaga, M., Nagatomo, Y., Ishikawa, T., & Nakagawa, S. (1991). Intrapericardial OK-432 instillation for the management of malignant pericardial effusion. *Cancer, 68,* 259–263.

Jay, G.D., Onuma, K., Davis, R., Chen, M.H., Mansell, A., & Steele, D. (2000). Analysis of physician ability in the measurement of pulsus paradoxus by sphygmomanometry. *Chest, 118,* 348–352.

Kaplow, R. (2000). Cardiac tamponade. In C.H. Yarbro, M.H. Frogge, M. Goodman, & S.L. Groenwald (Eds.), *Cancer nursing: Principles and practice* (5th ed., pp. 857–868). Sudbury, MA: Jones and Bartlett.

Keefe, D.L. (2000). Cardiovascular emergencies in the cancer patient. *Seminars in Oncology, 27,* 244–255.

Lissoni, P., Barni, S., & Ardizzoia, A. (1992). Intracavity administration of interleukin-2 as a palliative therapy for neoplastic effusions. *Tumori, 78,* 118–120.

Liu, G., Grump, M., Goss, P.E., Dancey, J., & Shepherd, F.A. (1996). A prospective comparison of the sclerosing agents doxycycline and bleomycin for the primary management of malignant pericardial effusion and cardiac tamponade. *Journal of Clinical Oncology, 14,* 3141–3147.

Loerzel, V.W., & Dow, K.H. (2003). Cardiac toxicity related to cancer treatment. *Clinical Journal of Oncology Nursing, 7,* 557–562.

Maisch, B., Seferovic, P.M., Ristic, A.D., Erbel, R., Rienmuller, R., Adler, Y., et al. (2004). Guidelines on the management of pericardial diseases executive summary. *European Heart Journal, 25,* 587–610.

Martinoni, A., Cipolla, C.M., Cardinale, D., Civelli, M., Lamantia, G., Colleoni, M., et al. (2004). Long-term results of intrapericardial chemotherapeutic treatment of malignant pericardial effusions with thiotepa. *Chest, 126,* 1412–1416.

Merrill, P. (2000). Oncologic emergencies. *Lippincott's Primary Care Practice, 4,* 400–409.

Miaskowski, C. (1999). Oncologic emergencies. In C. Miaskowski & P. Buchsel (Eds.), *Oncology nursing assessment and clinical care* (pp. 221–243). St. Louis, MO: Mosby.

Mueller, X.M., Tevaearai, H.T., Hurni, M., Ruchat, P., Fischer, A.P., Stumpe, F., et al. (1997). Long-term results of surgical subxiphoid pericardial drainage. *Thoracic and Cardiovascular Surgeon, 45,* 65–69.

Myers, J.S. (2001). Oncologic complications. In S.E. Otto (Ed.), *Oncology nursing* (4th ed., pp. 498–581). St. Louis, MO: Mosby.

Read, W., & Denes, A. (2002). Oncologic emergencies. In R. Govindan (Ed.), *Washington manual of oncology* (pp. 465–466). Philadelphia: Lippincott Williams & Wilkins.

Ruckdeschel, J.C., & Jablons, D. (2001). Malignant effusions in the chest. In J.M. Kirkwood, M.T. Lotze, & J.M. Yasko (Eds.), *Current cancer therapeutics* (4th ed., pp. 334–339). Philadelphia: Current Medicine.

Schrump, D.S., & Nguyen, D.M. (2001). Malignant pleural and pericardial effusions. In V.T. DeVita, S. Hellman, & S.A. Rosenberg (Eds.), *Cancer: Principles and practice of oncology* (6th ed., pp. 2729–2744). Philadelphia: Lippincott Williams & Wilkins.

Seto, T., Nagashina, S., Yoshino, I., Semba, H., & Ichinose, Y. (2001). The effect of pericardial drainage and the intrapericardial instillation of bleomycin in patients with carcinomatous pericarditis associated with non-small cell lung cancer: A phase II study [Abstract]. *Proceedings of the American Society of Clinical Oncology, 20,* 2466.

Shabetai, R. (2004). Pericardial effusion: Haemodynamic spectrum. *Heart, 90,* 255–256.

Shatzer, M., & Castor, A. (2004). How transthoracic echocardiography detects cardiac tamponade. *Nursing 2004, 34*(3), 73–74.

Shelton, B.K. (2000). Pericarditis/pericardial effusion/cardiac tamponade. In D. Camp-Sorrell & R.A. Hawkins (Eds.), *Clinical manual for the oncology advanced practice nurse* (pp. 307–326). Pittsburgh, PA: Oncology Nursing Society.

Spodick, D.H. (2003). Acute cardiac tamponade. *New England Journal of Medicine, 349,* 684–690.

Tsang, T.S., Enriquez-Sarano, M., Freeman, W.K., Barnes, M.E., Sinak, L.J., Gersh, B.J., et al. (2002). Consecutive 1127 therapeutic echocardiographically guided pericardiocenteses: Clinical profile, practice patterns, and outcomes spanning 21 years. *Mayo Clinic Proceedings, 77,* 429–436.

Tsang, T.S., Seward, J.B., Barnes, M.E., Bailey, K.R., Sinak, L.J., Urban, L.H., et al. (2000). Outcomes of primary and secondary treatment of pericardial effusion in patients with malignancy. *Mayo Clinic Proceedings, 75,* 248–253.

Vaitkus, P.T., Herrmann, H.C., & LeWinter, M.M. (1994). Treatment of malignant pericardial effusion. *JAMA, 272,* 59–64.

Wang, N., Feikes, J.R., Morgensen, T., Vyhmeister, E.E., & Bailey, L.L. (1994). Pericardio-peritoneal shunt: An alternative treatment for malignant pericardial effusion. *Annals of Thoracic Surgery, 57,* 289–292.

Wang, P., Yang, K.Y., Chao, J.Y., Liu, J.M., Perng, R.P., & Yen, S.H. (2000). Prognostic role of pericardial fluid cytology in cardiac tamponade associated with non-small cell lung cancer. *Chest, 118,* 744–749.

Warren, W.H. (2000). Malignancies involving the pericardium. *Seminars in Thoracic and Cardiovascular Surgery, 12,* 119–129.

Works, C., & Maxwell, M.B. (2000). Malignant effusions and edemas. In C.H. Yarbro, M.H. Frogge, M. Goodman, & S.L. Groenwald (Eds.), *Cancer nursing: Principles and practice* (5th ed., pp. 813–830). Sudbury, MA: Jones and Bartlett.

Ziskind, A.A., Pearce, A.C., Lemmon, C.C., Burstein, S., Gimple, L.W., Herrmann, H.C., et al. (1993). Percutaneous balloon pericardiotomy for the treatment of cardiac tamponade and large pericardial effusions: Description of technique and report of the first 50 cases. *Journal of the American College of Cardiology, 21,* 1–5.

Susan A. Ezzone, MS, RN, CNP

⮕ **Chapter** *2*

Disseminated Intravascular Coagulation

Introduction

Disseminated intravascular coagulation (DIC) is a complex disorder characterized by microvascular dysfunction resulting in activation of coagulation pathways, leading to thrombotic events and bleeding. During the 1950s, early reports existed of patients experiencing clinical sequelae that clinicians now refer to as DIC (Ratnoff, Pritchard, & Colopy, 1955). Recently, Levi (2004) reported that from 1966–2003, approximately 10,000 articles were published on DIC, mostly as case reports. Over the years, much of the literature describes DIC as a syndrome that is poorly understood and has varied interpretations of the contributing pathophysiology.

The contribution of DIC to morbidity and risk of mortality varies depending on the underlying clinical condition and the intensity of the coagulation disorder. DIC can present as an acute, subacute, or chronic condition. Acute DIC is associated with systemic bleeding and life-threatening hemorrhagic events, whereas subacute or chronic forms usually are associated with thrombus formation rather than hemorrhage (Furlong & Furlong, 2005; Schmaier, 2004). Although bleeding is often a presenting symptom of DIC, thrombosis may occur first, followed by hemorrhage. The hypercoagulation that develops with DIC causes small clot formation in the microcirculation of many organs and an associated depletion of platelets and coagulation factors (Gobel, 2005a). Bleeding occurs, thus complicating decisions about treatment options. Several reports indicate that DIC increases the risk of organ failure and death. In a large number of clinical studies, the occurrence of DIC appeared to be associated with an unfavorable outcome and was an independent predictor of mortality (Levi & Ten Cate, 1999). The sequelae of DIC can be devastating, so early recognition, evaluation, and treatment are critical.

Incidence

DIC is an acquired disorder that occurs in a wide variety of clinical conditions. Table 2-1 lists the most common clinical conditions and the mechanisms for triggering DIC. The incidence of DIC is difficult to determine and has not been reported for many of the clinical conditions associated with its development. In 1994, the number of cases of DIC was estimated at 18,000 in the United States (Furlong & Furlong, 2005).

Infection, particularly of bacterial origin, is the most common clinical condition leading to the development of acute DIC. Septicemia is the most common clinical condition associated with DIC and occurs in 30%–50% of patients with gram-negative sepsis. Other infectious organisms that may lead to DIC include gram-positive bacteria, viruses (e.g., HIV, cytomegalovirus, varicella, hepatitis), protozoa (malaria), and fungi (histoplasma) (Furlong & Furlong, 2005; Levi, de Jonge, van der Poll, & Ten Cate, 2001). Infection may induce a generalized inflammatory response and activation of the cytokine network, subsequently resulting in hypercoagulation and DIC.

The malignancy most frequently associated with the development of acute DIC is acute promyelocytic leukemia (APL). Solid tumors, especially metastatic mucin-secreting adenocarcinomas (prostate, lung, breast, pancreas, stomach), may be underlying disorders of chronic DIC (Friend & Pruett, 2004; Schmaier, 2004). The incidence of DIC in patients with cancer has been reported as 10% for those with solid tumors and 85% for those with APL (Gouin-Thibault, Achkar, & Samama, 2001; Levi & Ten Cate, 1999; Messmore & Wehrmacher, 2002). It has been estimated that 10%–15% of patients with metastatic tumors and 15% of patients with acute leukemia have evidence of DIC. The mechanism of the derangement of the coagulation system in patients with cancer is not clear. Several studies have indicated that tissue factor, which is expressed on the surface of tumor cells, is involved in the development of DIC. Patients with APL develop a hyperfibrinolytic state as well as activation of the coagulation system, leading to DIC. Some reports describe the use of all-trans-retinoic acid in patients with APL to reduce the incidence of severe DIC (Levi & Ten Cate).

Researchers have linked many other clinical conditions with a risk for DIC development (see Table 2-1). Severe trauma, especially to the brain, may lead to acute DIC caused by a systemic inflammatory response and activation of cytokines in 50%–70% of patients (Levi & Ten Cate, 1999). DIC may occur as an acute complication of obstetrical disorders, such as abruptio placentae and amniotic fluid embolism. It has been reported that DIC may occur in more than 50% of women with these clinical conditions and 7% of women with preeclampsia (Levi et al., 2001; Levi & Ten Cate). Widespread burns, incompatible blood transfusions, snakebites, acute hepatic failure, and transplant rejection also may lead to the development of acute DIC (Furlong & Furlong, 2005; Schmaier, 2004).

Table 2-1. Clinical Conditions and Mechanisms Associated With Development of Disseminated Intravascular Coagulation

Clinical Condition	Mechanisms
Sepsis/severe infection • Bacterial infections (gram-negative or gram-positive organisms) • Viral infections (varicella, hepatitis, cytomegalovirus) • Parasitic infections	Endotoxins activate factor XII to factor XIIa. Platelet release reaction Induce release of tumor necrosis factor-alpha (TNF-α), interleukin (IL)-1, and complement activation. Lipopolysaccharides Inflammatory response Proinflammatory cytokines Result in endothelial damage, endothelial permeability, and multiorgan damage
Trauma • Polytrauma • Neurotrauma • Fat embolism	Activation of coagulation Release of tissue material such as fat, phospholipids, and enzymes into circulation Hemolysis Endothelial damage Cytokine release
Burns	Microhemolysis Release of red cell membrane phospholipids or red cell adenosine diphosphate (ADP) Release of tissue materials or cellular enzymes into systemic circulation
Solid tumors: Mucin-secreting adenocarcinomas • Prostate • Lung • Breast • Stomach	Activation of coagulation Tumor cells may express procoagulant materials (e.g., tissue factor, cysteine protease with factor X activating properties). Severe hyperfibrinolysis
Hematologic malignances • Acute promyelocytic leukemia • Myeloproliferative diseases • Lymphoproliferative disease	Severe hyperfibrinolysis Activation of coagulation Bleeding and thrombosis
Hematologic disease • Polycythemia rubra vera • Paroxysmal nocturnal hemoglobinuria	Underlying compensated disseminated intravascular coagulation process Thrombosis Thromboembolism
Obstetrical conditions • Placental abruption • Amniotic fluid emboli • Preeclampsia	Amniotic fluid activates coagulation. Placental separation Leakage of thromboplastin-like material from the placenta Activation of coagulation in preeclampsia

(Continued on next page)

Table 2-1. Clinical Conditions and Mechanisms Associated With Development of Disseminated Intravascular Coagulation *(Continued)*

Clinical Condition	Mechanisms
Intravascular hemolysis • Any etiology • Transfusion reaction	Trigger intravascular coagulation Activation of coagulation Release of red cell ADP Release of red cell membrane phospholipoprotein
Vascular disorders • Aortic aneurysms • Hemangiomas • Kasabach-Merritt syndrome	Activation of coagulation Consumption of coagulation proteins and platelets Overflow of coagulation factors to systemic circulation
Microangiopathic hemolytic anemias	Thrombocytopenic thrombotic purpura Hemolytic uremic syndrome Chemotherapy-induced microangiopathic hemolytic anemia Malignant hypertension HELLP syndrome (hemolysis, elevated liver-enzyme levels, and a low platelet count occurring in association with preeclampsia) Endothelial damage Platelet aggregation Thrombin formation Impaired fibrinolysis
Severe hepatic failure	Intrahepatic or extrahepatic cholestasis
Metabolic acidosis	Endothelial sloughing Activation of factor XII to XIIa Activation of factor XI to XIa Platelet release Clinical circumstances of acidosis Cytokine release of TNF, IL-1, IL-6, and interferon-gamma activates the coagulation pathway with eventual fibrin deposition. Decreased thrombomodulin associated with increased TNF-α Inhibition of thrombin-mediated activities Activation of protein C and S system is antithrombotic. Thrombus formation End-organ damage
Severe toxic or immunologic reactions • Snakebites • Recreational drugs • Transfusion reactions • Transplant rejection	Endothelial damage Circulating antigen-antibody complexes Endotoxemia Tissue damage Platelet or red cell damage

Note. Based on information from Bick, 2003; Furlong & Furlong, 2005; Levi, 2004.

Chronic types of DIC may occur in conjunction with a variety of hematologic, vascular, and inflammatory conditions, such as myeloproliferative disorders and paroxysmal nocturnal hemoglobinuria; rheumatoid arthritis and Raynaud disease; and ulcerative colitis, Crohn disease, and sarcoidosis (Furlong & Furlong, 2005). Localized DIC may occur in association with several conditions. The presence of giant hemangiomas (Kasabach-Merritt syndrome) and large aortic aneurysms may lead to DIC because of local activation of coagulation and increased thrombin formation (Furlong & Furlong; Schmaier, 2004). The incidence of DIC in patients with giant hemangiomas has been reported as 25% and with large aortic aneurysms as 0.5%–1% (Levi & Ten Cate, 1999).

The microangiopathic hemolytic anemias are syndromes that may lead to organ failure and mimic the clinical picture of DIC. Disorders that comprise the microangiopathic hemolytic anemias include thrombocytopenic thrombotic purpura, hemolytic uremic syndrome, chemotherapy-induced microangiopathic hemolytic anemia, malignant hypertension, and HELLP syndrome (hemolysis, elevated liver-enzyme levels, and a low platelet count occurring in association with preeclampsia). The common pathologic feature is endothelial damage and related platelet adhesion and aggregation, thrombin formation, and impaired fibrinolysis. Thrombosis develops, causing occlusion of small and mid-sized vessels. These clinical conditions are distinct disease entities that are not clearly described as DIC (Levi et al., 2001).

Risk Factors

The triggering mechanisms leading to DIC are associated with either a systemic inflammatory response or the presence of a procoagulant substance in the bloodstream. Researchers have associated numerous clinical conditions with the risk of developing DIC (see Table 2-1). Systemic infections such as sepsis cause an inflammatory response that leads to activation of a cytokine network and coagulation pathways. Release of bacterial endotoxins or the presence of cell membrane components, such as lipopolysaccharides or endotoxins, stimulates the inflammatory response (Levi, 2004). Solid tumors and hematologic malignancies have been associated with the development of DIC because of both the expression of procoagulant substances and severe hyperfibrinolysis.

Other clinical conditions that may cause DIC include aortic aneurysms and giant hemangiomas because of activation of coagulation. Obstetrical complications may lead to activation of coagulation and development of DIC because of the release of thromboplastin into the uterine and maternal circulation. Each clinical condition is thought to have specific mechanisms responsible for causing DIC, but all are commonly associated with activation of the coagulation system and fibrin deposition. Figure 2-1 illustrates triggering mechanisms for DIC development.

Figure 2-1. Triggering Mechanisms for Disseminated Intravascular Coagulation

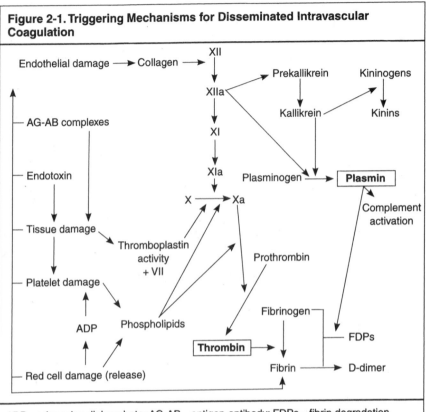

ADP—adenosine diphosphate; AG-AB—antigen-antibody; FDPs—fibrin degradation products

Note. From "Disseminated Intravascular Coagulation: Current Concepts of Etiology, Pathophysiology, Diagnosis, and Treatment," by R.L. Bick, 2003, *Hematology/Oncology Clinics of North America, 17,* p. 155. Copyright 2003 by Elsevier. Reprinted with permission.

Pathophysiology

A brief overview of the normal coagulation process is useful for understanding the underlying pathophysiologic mechanisms that lead to DIC. Normal hemostasis, the control of bleeding following vascular or tissue injury, is the result of a fine balance between blood clot formation (coagulation) and blood clot dissolution (fibrinolysis). In general, all the substances necessary for clotting to occur are in circulation within the bloodstream in soluble, inactive form. A stimulus, such as injury to small blood vessels or endothelial tissue injury, triggers a series of events, called the coagulation cascade, in which each clotting factor is activated sequentially until a stable, insoluble fibrin clot forms to control the bleeding. When the coagulation cascade is triggered, opposing fibrinolytic pathways also are activated to defend against excessive clot formation and ultimately dissolve the clot and restore normal blood flow (Gobel, 2005a).

In DIC, an inappropriate activation of the coagulation system disrupts the balance between coagulation and fibrinolysis, which then leads to thrombi formation and consumption of coagulation proteins and platelets (Levi, 2004). DIC is a systemic thrombohemorrhagic disorder that occurs secondary to several underlying conditions and results in laboratory evidence of procoagulant activation, fibrinolytic activation, inhibitor consumption, cytokine release, cellular activation, and biochemical evidence of end-organ damage (Bick, 2003; Levi, 2004). A systemic intravascular activation of the coagulation cascade results in fibrin formation and deposition in the microvasculature of various organs, leading to multiorgan failure (see Figure 2-2). Because of consumption of coagulation proteins and platelets, hemorrhagic events occur simultaneously with thrombi formation (Levi, 2004).

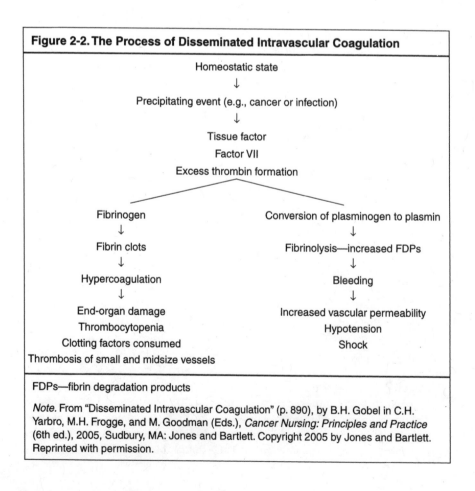

Figure 2-2. The Process of Disseminated Intravascular Coagulation

Homeostatic state
↓
Precipitating event (e.g., cancer or infection)
↓
Tissue factor
Factor VII
Excess thrombin formation

Fibrinogen	Conversion of plasminogen to plasmin
↓	↓
Fibrin clots	Fibrinolysis—increased FDPs
↓	↓
Hypercoagulation	Bleeding
↓	↓
End-organ damage	Increased vascular permeability
Thrombocytopenia	Hypotension
Clotting factors consumed	Shock
Thrombosis of small and midsize vessels	

FDPs—fibrin degradation products

Note. From "Disseminated Intravascular Coagulation" (p. 890), by B.H. Gobel in C.H. Yarbro, M.H. Frogge, and M. Goodman (Eds.), *Cancer Nursing: Principles and Practice* (6th ed.), 2005, Sudbury, MA: Jones and Bartlett. Copyright 2005 by Jones and Bartlett. Reprinted with permission.

Production of thrombin occurs approximately three to five hours after an event such as bacteremia or release of endotoxins and may be initiated by expression of tissue factor and activation of factor VIIa (FVIIa). Tissue factor, which is expressed on mononuclear cells and endothelial cells, has a role in the activation of coagulation, but researchers do not clearly understand its role in the pathogenesis of DIC. It is hypothesized that tissue factor may be expressed on leukocytes and transferred to activated platelets by mononuclear cells. Activation of coagulation occurs with formation of intravascular fibrin and fibrin deposition (Levi, 2004). Impairment of physiologic mechanisms of anticoagulation pathways may be associated with formation of thrombin and fibrin, leading to DIC. Anticoagulation mechanisms that inhibit the coagulation cascade, such as tissue factor pathway inhibitor (TFPI), activated protein C, and antithrombin III (AT III), are largely defective (Furlong & Furlong, 2005; Levi, 2004).

AT III acts to inhibit thrombin formation and is a potent inhibitor of the coagulation cascade under normal circumstances. During DIC, plasma levels of AT III decrease because of its consumption; degradation by elastase, a substance released from activated neutrophils; and impaired synthesis (Levi, 2001). In addition, suppression of the protein C system pathway, which normally acts to inhibit clotting, promotes a procoagulant state resulting in increased morbidity and mortality (Levi, 2004). Protein C deficiency occurs with sepsis, promotes thrombin formation in the microvasculature, and may augment inflammation and endothelial cell dysfunction. Circulating thrombin leads to the formation of fibrin and microvascular and macrovascular thrombosis. Thrombin release leads to thrombosis, vascular occlusion, and end-organ damage or failure through induction of monocyte release of tumor necrosis factor (TNF), interleukin (IL)-1, and IL-6. Plasmin, a component of the fibrinolytic system, is a proteolytic enzyme that degrades fibrin, leading to an appearance of fibrin degradation products (FDPs), such as D-dimer, in the circulation. The presence of plasmin and TNF activates the complement pathway in the circulation and induces platelet lysis, causing thrombocytopenia. The complement pathway leads to the lysis of red blood cells and platelets, which provides more procoagulant material.

Following the development of thrombi, blood flow is interrupted, thus leading to the development of peripheral ischemia and end-organ damage. Fibrin is deposited in the circulation and results in trapping of platelets and thrombocytopenia. In addition, plasmin circulates systemically and causes cleavage of fibrinogen and release of FDPs. The presence of circulating FDPs interferes with hemostasis, leading to platelet dysfunction and hemorrhage. Induction of synthesis of several cytokines, including IL-1, IL-6, and plasminogen activator inhibitor type 1, by FDPs and D-dimer results in vascular endothelial and end-organ damage (Bick, 2003).

Another important mechanism in DIC is the generation of factor XII and eventual conversion of kininogen into circulating kinins. Clinically, activation of the complement system and kinin system in DIC leads to increased vascular permeability, hypotension, and shock (Bick, 2003). Many of the consequences of DIC are a result of thrombin-activated systems, release of cytokines, circulation of plasmin, and endothelial disruption or damage.

Proinflammatory cytokines, neutrophil activation, and endothelial cell injury have been associated with development of DIC and organ dysfunction. Activation of the coagulation pathway has been found to perpetuate the inflammatory response through a thrombin/receptor interaction (Gando, 2001). In trauma patients, multiorgan dysfunction syndrome and acute respiratory distress occur because of tissue hypoxia, which results from the production of microvascular thrombosis in DIC.

The pathophysiology of DIC is complex, and multiple factors contribute to the risk of its development in a variety of clinical conditions. Several mechanisms that were previously described may trigger the procoagulant state, which may result in consumption of coagulation proteins, bleeding, and thrombosis. As healthcare providers gain a better understanding of the pathophysiology of DIC, they will improve recognition of the risks of developing this complication.

Clinical Manifestations

DIC may be silent and undetected or acute and severe in onset. It may present as an acute life-threatening complication or as a subacute or chronic condition. Clinical manifestations of DIC may not occur until late in the disease process. Signs and symptoms of DIC are most commonly based on the underlying etiologic factor that has led to the activation of the coagulation system (Bick, 2003; Levi, 2004). Evidence of both bleeding and thrombosis may occur. Acute DIC is characterized by generalized bleeding; subacute bleeding and diffuse thrombosis characterize chronic DIC (Furlong & Furlong, 2005). Signs of bleeding are more common, may occur at any site, and may be subtle or obvious, ranging from oozing to uncontrolled hemorrhage. Common sites of bleeding include surgical sites, venipuncture sites, wound sites, and mucous membranes. Symptoms of bleeding may include petechiae, purpura (bruising), hematomas, acral cyanosis (intense, painful erythema of palms and soles), wound bleeding, and blood oozing at a venipuncture site. In severe cases, patients may develop fever and hypovolemic shock–like features, such as tachycardia, hypotension, acidosis, and hypoxia (Bick; Furlong & Furlong). Bleeding may occur from any body orifice. Signs of bleeding may be evident in the urine, stool, or emesis, and all specimens should be evaluated for the presence of blood. The possibility of occult internal or intracerebral bleeding also exists. Patients may experience abdominal fullness and tenderness as symptoms of gastrointestinal bleeding. Mental status changes may include headache, papillary changes, confusion, disorientation, and irritability if a central nervous system bleed has occurred.

Thrombus formation usually does not occur until later in the stages of the DIC process. Clinical manifestations of thrombus formation may be subtle and clinically undetectable (Gobel, 2005a). Symptoms associated with thrombosis at any organ site develop as a result of hypoperfusion, ischemia, infarction, necrosis, and organ failure.

Patient Assessment

History

DIC may be fulminant or low grade, depending on the disease associated with triggering the syndrome (Bick, 2003; Toh & Dennis, 2003). A thorough history to determine risk factors should include ascertaining the presence of conditions that may increase the risk of DIC (see Table 2-1) and previous episodes and symptoms of bleeding or clotting, such as gastrointestinal bleeding or deep vein thrombosis. Additional information obtained may include the patient's history of bleeding tendencies; nutritional status to evaluate for vitamin K deficiency; medications, including over-the-counter drugs; and previous transfusions (Friend & Pruett, 2004). A history of bleeding from at least three unrelated sites raises suspicion for DIC (Furlong & Furlong, 2005).

Physical Assessment

Assessment of patients at risk for developing DIC should include evaluation of clinical manifestations that may occur as a result of bleeding or thrombosis (see Table 2-2). Healthcare providers should assess each organ system to evaluate for risk or presence of bleeding. The central nervous system can be assessed by determining the presence of any symptoms commonly associated with an intracranial bleed, such as headache, nausea, and visual disturbances. Presence of gastrointestinal bleeding should be considered if patients complain of abdominal pain, hematemesis, and change in color of or frank blood in stool. Common signs of sinopulmonary bleeding include epistaxis, blood-tinged nasal drainage or sputum, cough, abnormal breath sounds, tachypnea, dyspnea, and airway compromise. Presence of blood in the urine, change in urinary frequency, painful urination, and passage of blood clots in the urine may indicate hemorrhagic cystitis. Cardiovascular signs of bleeding include tachycardia, hypotension, and change in color and temperature of skin and extremities. A thorough multiorgan system assessment is important when evaluating patients for risk or presence of bleeding.

Diagnostic Evaluation

The diagnosis of DIC is based on clinical evidence and laboratory findings that support the diagnosis and provide evidence of activation of coagulation

Table 2-2. Physical Assessment for Patients at Risk for Bleeding or Thrombosis

Organ	Assessment
CNS: Symptoms dependent on site and size of bleeding or clot	Headache, nausea/vomiting, retching, mental status changes (restlessness, confusion, lethargy, obtundation, coma), vertigo, seizures, changes in pupil size and reactivity; eye deviations, sensory or motor strength alterations, speech alterations, paralysis
Eyes	Visual disturbances—blurring, diplopia, absent or altered fields of vision, nystagmus, increased injections in sclera, conjunctival hemorrhage, periorbital edema; note if sclera are icteric.
Nose	Petechiae, blood-tinged drainage, epistaxis
Mouth	Petechiae of oral mucosa, pain, dysphagia, hematemesis, bleeding gums/mucosa, blood-tinged secretions, ulcerations with frank bleeding
Upper gastrointestinal: Esophagus/stomach	Dysphagia, hematemesis, blood-tinged secretions, substernal burning and pain, epigastric discomfort (burning, tenderness, or cramping), coffee ground emesis, nausea, vomiting, fever, weakness, anorexia, melena, hyperactive bowel sounds
Lower gastrointestinal: Duodenum/anus	Pain (location, occurrence, duration, quality), nausea, vomiting, tarry stools, diarrhea, bowel sounds (hyper- or hypoactive), cramping, occult blood in stools, frank blood in stools (rectum or lower), blood around anus, frequency and quantity of stools, pain with bowel movements (hemorrhoids)
Lungs	Tachypnea, dyspnea, air hunger, respiration rate, depth, and exertion Crackles, rubs, wheezing, diminished breath sounds, hemoptysis (frothy bright red blood sputum—major airway bleeding), stridor, tickling in throat or chest with desire to cough
Cardiovascular	Tachycardia and hypotension (characteristic of anemia and acute blood loss) Changes in VS, color and temperature of extremities, peripheral pulses (present, quality), and changes in peripheral perfusion Pericardial effusions: Dyspnea, cough, pain, orthopnea, venous distension, tamponade (muted heart sounds, hypotension, pulsus paradoxus, angina, palpitations)

(Continued on next page)

Table 2-2. Physical Assessment for Patients at Risk for Bleeding or Thrombosis *(Continued)*	
Organ	**Assessment**
Abdomen	Hepatomegaly (liver disease—possible coagulation disorder), RUQ pain, abdominal distension Splenomegaly (increased risk for bleeding): Assess for any history of trauma; if spleen ruptures, rapid hypovolemic shock ensues; left flank or shoulder pain Retroperitoneal bleeding: Vague abdominal complaints, ecchymoses over flank, occasional bulging flanks and tenderness; associated with hypovolemia
Genitourinary	Decreased urinary output due to massive bleeding is associated with hypovolemia and shock. Hematuria: Dysuria, burning, frequency, pain on urination, suprapubic pain and cramping, gross blood in urine, clots Menorrhagia: Suprapubic pain and cramping, gross blood in urine, clots (may need to straight catheterize female patients to distinguish between urinary or vaginal bleeding) Frequency and size of clots, number of sanitary napkins used, and color of urine are important in measuring bleeding.
Musculoskeletal	Bleeding into joints is usually associated with alterations in coagulation; swollen, warm, sore joint with decreased mobility (active and passive ROM); usually unilateral; tapping the joint's synovial fluid is frequently required to distinguish infection from bleeding.
Skin	Petechiae, ecchymosis, purpura, hematoma; oozing from venipuncture sites, central lines, catheters, injection sites, incisional sounds, nasogastric tubes Gangrene, alterations in skin color (e.g., pallor, cyanosis), alterations in skin temperature

CNS—central nervous system; ROM—range of motion; RUQ—right upper quadrant; VS—vital signs

Note. From "Bleeding and Thrombotic Complications" (p. 238), by P.H. Friend and J. Pruett in C.H. Yarbro, M.H. Frogge, and M. Goodman (Eds.), *Cancer Symptom Management* (3rd ed.), 2004, Sudbury, MA: Jones and Bartlett. Copyright 2004 by Jones and Bartlett. Reprinted with permission.

and fibrinolysis, consumption of clot inhibitors, and biochemical evidence of end-organ damage or failure (Furlong & Furlong, 2005). Interpretation of laboratory data is difficult because a variety of clinical conditions may be associated with the abnormalities. Table 2-3 describes common laboratory abnormalities. Laboratory tests screen for abnormalities along a specific coagulation pathway that reflect a deficiency of coagulation factors. When the extrinsic or common pathway is affected, the prothrombin time (PT)

Table 2-3. Laboratory Data in Disseminated Intravascular Coagulation (DIC)

Laboratory Test	Result	Comments
Prothrombin time varies: Compare with normal control.	Prolonged	Prolonged, shortened, or normal in DIC Coagulation deficiency of the extrinsic and common pathway May be prolonged because of several coagulation factors May be the result of liver disease, deficiency of vitamin K, obstructive biliary disease, or warfarin therapy
Partial thromboplastin time varies: Compare with normal control.	Prolonged	Prolonged, shortened, or normal in DIC Deficiency of intrinsic and common pathways Decreased quantity of any coagulation factor, except VII or XIII May be caused by heparin therapy, increased fibrin degradation products, and consumption of clotting factors
International normalized ratio	Prolonged	Prolonged, shortened, or normal in DIC Evaluates overall coagulation
Fibrin degradation products	Elevated	Measures the breakdown of fibrin and fibrinogen Elevated level may occur with surgery, obstetric complication, various medical problems, and DIC.
D-dimer	Elevated	Elevated levels indicate hyperfibrinolysis. Common in DIC, pulmonary and cerebral embolism, phlebitis, thrombosis, and postoperative prothrombotic risks
Antithrombin III level	Decreased	Accelerated coagulation
Activated partial thromboplastin time	Prolonged, shortened, or normal	Nonspecific in DIC
Thrombin time	Elevated	Estimate of plasma fibrinogen Prolonged because of heparin, streptokinase, or urokinase therapy Prolonged in DIC, liver disease, or fibrinogen deficiency
Fibrinogen	Decreased	Nonspecific in DIC Plasma concentration of fibrinogen Low because of congenital or acquired hypofibrinogenemia, DIC, fibrinolysis, severe liver disease, malignant processes, or obstetrical trauma Elevated in some malignancies or inflammatory conditions

(Continued on next page)

Table 2-3. Laboratory Data in Disseminated Intravascular Coagulation (DIC) *(Continued)*

Laboratory Test	Result	Comments
Platelet count	Decreased	Nonspecific finding in DIC
Peripheral smear	Schistocytes present	Nonspecific finding in DIC
Plasminogen levels	Decreased	Hyperfibrinolysis
Alpha-1 antiplasmin levels	Decreased	Hyperfibrinolysis
Fibrinopeptide A level	Elevated	Indicates accelerated coagulation and fibrin formation

Note. Based on information from Friend & Pruett, 2004; Gobel, 2005a, 2005b.

may be prolonged. Likewise, when the intrinsic and common pathway is affected, the partial thromboplastin time (PTT) may be prolonged. The common pathway is considered to be defective if both the PT and PTT are prolonged. The international normalized ratio is considered to be a more standardized test that screens for status of overall coagulation and is prolonged, shortened, or normal in DIC (Friend & Pruett, 2004; Gobel, 2005a). Other laboratory data common in DIC include D-dimer, FDPs, thrombin time, and fibrinogen levels.

Diagnostic studies to determine the presence of bleeding are helpful in evaluating the severity of DIC. Bedside testing of hemoccult of stools, emesis, and nasogastric output, as well as urinalysis or urine dipstick, is important to determine the presence of bleeding. Radiologic studies such as computed tomography scans, magnetic resonance imaging, x-rays, or ultrasounds to evaluate the presence of internal bleeding or thrombosis may be ordered. Clinicians may perform endoscopic examinations to determine the presence of bleeding in the upper or lower gastrointestinal tract. Angiography may determine the presence of bleeding or thrombosis. Invasive procedures are done with caution because of the potential for bleeding and should be preceded by the administration of clotting factor and platelet repletion (Furlong & Furlong, 2005).

The International Society on Thrombosis and Haemostasis (ISTH) (Taylor, Toh, Hoots, Wada, & Levi, 2001) published a uniform definition and diagnostic criteria for DIC in an attempt to facilitate basic and clinical research as well as lead to progress in clinical management. Its proposed definition of DIC is: "DIC is an acquired syndrome characterized by the intravascular activation of coagulation with loss of localization arising from different causes. It can originate from and cause damage to the microvasculature, which if sufficiently severe, can produce organ dysfunction" (Taylor et al.). Criteria for overt and nonovert DIC were developed using a diagnostic algorithm and scoring system. The diagnostic algorithm is based on risk assessment and evaluation of coagulation test results. Usefulness of the ISTH DIC scoring system has been evaluated in clinical practice (Bakhtiari, Miejers, de Jonge, & Levi, 2004; Sivula, Tallgren, & Pettila, 2004; Toh & Downey, 2005). Although the ISTH criteria and scoring system assist in the diagnosis of DIC, additional factors may facilitate use of the scoring system as a predictor of mortality. Further investigations are needed to determine whether the definition, algorithm, and scoring system are applicable and predictable in practice.

Treatment Modalities

The goals of management of patients with DIC are to correct coagulation abnormalities and minimize the risk of bleeding and thrombosis. Management of DIC focuses on removing the causative agent, providing supportive care, and administering agents to slow the coagulation process and prevent thrombosis. The clinical course of DIC is somewhat unpredictable. DIC may resolve after correction of the underlying condition, or it may progress even after initiation of treatment. Therapy is based on the clinical and laboratory evaluation of hemostasis and should be as aggressive as the patient's age, disease, and severity of hemorrhage and thrombosis warrant (Furlong & Furlong, 2005). Supportive care measures implemented to minimize the effects of DIC may reduce morbidity and mortality (Levi, 2004).

Treatment for acute DIC incorporates the use of anticoagulants, blood components, and antifibrinolytic agents. Therapy aimed at anticoagulation is indicated in patients with DIC who manifest evidence of thromboembolism or fibrin deposition. Administering heparin may accomplish inhibition of coagulation pathways. The goals of heparin therapy are to inhibit intravascular fibrin formation, prevent thrombus formation, and reduce the consumption of platelets and clotting factors (Barbui & Falanga, 2001). Heparin cannot lyse existing clots but acts to prevent the conversion of fibrinogen to fibrin and also potentiates the anticoagulation effects of AT III, thus preventing further clot formation after fibrinolysis (Schmaier, 2004). Although the intention is to reduce the risk of bleeding, heparin therapy should be used with caution in patients who have a known risk of bleeding. Clinicians must consider the risks versus the benefits of heparin therapy prior to initiating treatment. It is debatable whether heparin therapy is safe in patients who are at increased risk of bleeding, such as patients with APL. In patients who have central nervous system disorders, open wounds, or recent surgery, heparin therapy is contraindicated because of the risk of hemorrhage. Heparin therapy is intended to maintain the activated PTT at one to two times the normal levels (Gobel, 2005b). Ongoing laboratory and clinical monitoring is mandatory during heparin therapy.

Other anticoagulant agents directed against the action of tissue factor, such as inactivated FVIIa, recombinant nematode anticoagulant protein c2, and TFPI, are theoretically expected to provide benefit in treating DIC, but the results have been mixed (Levi, 2004).

Researchers have investigated therapy with human recombinant TFPI in the treatment of DIC associated with sepsis for its potential to reduce endotoxin-induced activation of coagulation (Levi, 2001). The expression and release of tissue factor are major triggers for the activation of coagulation in patients with sepsis. The administration of recombinant TFPI to septic animals has demonstrated survival benefit, and it is associated with anti-inflammatory activity represented by decreased levels of IL-6 and IL-8. Tissue factor on the surface of endothelial cells binds with circulating clotting factor VII to create a complex (TF/FVIIa) that promotes formation of a fibrin clot. TFPI is the major physiologic inhibitor of the extrinsic coagulation pathway and binds with TF/FVIIa to form a stable complex, preventing further thrombin generation and fibrin formation. In addition, recent studies have shown that the TF/FVIIa complex is implicated in promoting tumor growth and angiogenesis and may stimulate the formation of tumor cell/platelet/fibrin complexes, facilitating the spread of metastatic disease (Hembrough et al., 2004). An increased risk of bleeding has occurred in patients receiving TFPI, so it must be used with caution (Levi, 2001).

AT III is a protease that is a potent inhibitor of thrombin and other procoagulant factors, such as factor Xa (Harper, 2005). Low levels of AT III have been identified in patients with septic shock and are associated with increased mortality in patients with DIC (Levi, 2004). An AT III replacement product, alpha-2 globulin, is derived from pooled human plasma and is heat-treated for viral inactivation (Harper). It may be used in the treatment of moderately severe to severe DIC or when natural levels are markedly decreased (Furlong & Furlong, 2005). Reports have shown that AT III supplementation has reduced the duration of DIC associated with septic shock. Evidence indicates that AT III acts as an anti-inflammatory agent, thus preventing endothelial cell injury and a procoagulant state (Levi, 2001). Clinical trials using AT III supplementation have shown improvement in laboratory parameters, shortened duration of DIC, and improved organ function (Levi, 2004).

The main effect of protein C is to reduce the production of thrombin, which has proinflammatory, procoagulant, and antifibrinolytic actions. Protein C also inhibits the influence of tissue factors in stimulating the clotting system and has anti-inflammatory properties. It is theorized that the suppression of the protein C system and its anticoagulant functions is associated with the development of DIC. Protein C acts to inhibit the production of thrombin, which has procoagulant and antifibrinolytic properties, and is consumed in states of sepsis and systemic inflammation. Protein C supplementation with drotrecogin alfa, a recombinant form of human activated protein C (APC), has been used in the treatment of DIC associated with sepsis. Drotrecogin alfa acts directly by deactivating clotting factors V and

VIII and indirectly by inhibiting the profibrinolytic activity of plasminogen activator inhibitor (PAI-1). The beneficial effects of APC supplementation are primarily to limit the development of coagulation abnormalities and lessen organ failure. Drotrecogin alfa may exert an anti-inflammatory effect by inhibiting the production of TNF by monocytes and limiting thrombin-induced inflammatory responses within the microvascular endothelium (Furlong & Furlong, 2005). It has anti-inflammatory, anticoagulation, and antiapoptotic properties. The drug is used cautiously and is administered as a 96-hour infusion (Toh & Dennis, 2003).

Healthcare providers may administer transfusion of platelets, cryoprecipitate, and plasma during episodes of DIC in patients who show evidence of active bleeding, require an invasive procedure, or are at increased risk of bleeding. Patients may receive coagulation factor concentrates to correct specific factor deficiencies such as fibrinogen (Levi, 2004). It is recommended that transfusion of platelets and coagulation factors should not be based only on laboratory results but also on the presence of clinical indications that may increase the risk of bleeding (Levi, 2004). Considerations for platelet transfusions include maintaining a platelet count of more than 20×10^9/L if active bleeding is not present and maintaining platelets above 50×10^9/L if active bleeding is present (Barbui & Falanga, 2001). If the patient is symptomatic or if active bleeding occurs, transfusion of packed red blood cells may maintain the hemoglobin at > 8 g/dl. Clinicians may consider transfusion of fresh frozen plasma or cryoprecipitate to infuse clotting factors and fibrinogen (Gobel, 2005a; Levi, 2004).

Nursing Management

An important role of nurses in the management of DIC includes recognizing which patients may be at increased risk for developing this complication. Nurses have a key role in the early recognition of signs and symptoms of DIC as well as in the administration of pharmaceutical agents and transfusion of blood components to correct coagulation abnormalities. Careful physical assessment of patients at risk for DIC is essential to recognize subtle symptoms of bleeding or thrombosis and to determine treatment effectiveness.

Nursing care of patients at risk for DIC includes astutely monitoring vital signs, hemodynamic status, oxygenation, and fluid status. Tachycardia and hypotension may indicate acute blood loss requiring urgent interventions. Signs of bleeding may be evident in multiple organ systems as described in Table 2-2 and the previous sections on clinical manifestations and physical assessment. Routine physical assessments should focus on signs of bleeding or thrombosis. Strict monitoring of patients' daily weight, as well as their intake and output, is important to avoid dehydration or fluid overload.

During the clinical course of DIC, nurses are responsible for administration of anticoagulant therapy and other medications, blood products, and IV fluids. Monitoring of coagulation studies during heparin therapy is important to titrate infusion rates to maintain a therapeutic range. Blood component therapy may include transfusion of red blood cells, platelets, fresh frozen plasma, and cryoprecipitate as indicated. Nurses also have a significant role in providing patient education regarding the risks of bleeding and thrombosis as well as the management of DIC. Collaboration among the healthcare team members is imperative to minimize the risk of clinical sequelae of DIC.

Patient and Caregiver Education

DIC is a complex syndrome that can be frightening to patients and caregivers because of the potential or actual risk of bleeding or thrombosis. Nurses have a key role in providing patient and caregiver education for those patients who are considered to be at risk for developing DIC. Nurses should review with patients and caregivers the measures to prevent consequences of DIC such as bleeding. Strategies to prevent or minimize the risk of bleeding should be reviewed and may include, but are not limited to, avoiding sharp objects, razors, operating heavy equipment, contact sports, and strenuous activities. In addition, patients are instructed to avoid taking medications that interfere with platelet function (e.g., aspirin-containing products, nonsteroidal anti-inflammatory drugs).

Conclusion

DIC is a complex syndrome characterized by disruption of hemostasis through activation of the coagulation system, thrombus formation, and overwhelming depletion of coagulation factors resulting in hemorrhage. The ISTH (Taylor et al., 2001) published a definition and diagnostic criteria for DIC in its attempt to facilitate basic and clinical research into this condition. The goal of the ISTH was to develop diagnostic criteria and a scoring system that would assist in the clinical management of DIC. Medical practice patterns for the management of DIC remain somewhat inconsistent because of the variety of patient-specific clinical conditions and risk factors. Further research is needed in the diagnosis and management of DIC.

References

Bakhtiari, K., Miejers, J.C.M., de Jonge, E., & Levi, M. (2004). Prospective validation of the International Society of Thrombosis and Haemostasis scoring system for disseminated intravascular coagulation. *Critical Care Medicine, 32,* 2416–2421.

Barbui, T., & Falanga, A. (2001). Disseminated intravascular coagulation in acute leukemia. *Seminars in Thrombosis and Hemostasis, 27,* 593–604.

Bick, R.L. (2003). Disseminated intravascular coagulation: Current concepts of etiology, pathophysiology, diagnosis, and treatment. *Hematology/Oncology Clinics of North America, 17,* 149–176.

Friend, P.H., & Pruett, J. (2004). Bleeding and thrombotic complications. In C.H. Yarbro, M.H. Frogge, & M. Goodman (Eds.), *Cancer symptom management* (3rd ed., pp. 233–251). Sudbury, MA: Jones and Bartlett.

Furlong, M.A., & Furlong, B.R. (2005, March). *Disseminated intravascular coagulation.* Retrieved September 18, 2005, from http://www.emedicine.com/emerg/topic150.htm

Gando, S. (2001). Disseminated intravascular coagulation in trauma patients. *Seminars in Thrombosis and Hemostasis, 27,* 585–592.

Gobel, B.H. (2005a). Disseminated intravascular coagulation. In C.H. Yarbro, M.H. Frogge, & M. Goodman (Eds.), *Cancer nursing: Principles and practice* (6th ed., pp. 887–894). Sudbury, MA: Jones and Bartlett.

Gobel, B.H. (2005b). Metabolic emergencies. In J.K. Itano & K.N. Taoka (Eds.), *Core curriculum for oncology nurses* (4th ed., pp. 383–388). St. Louis, MO: Elsevier.

Gouin-Thibault, I., Achkar, A., & Samama, M.M. (2001). The thrombophilic state in cancer patients. *Acta Haematologica, 106,* 33–42.

Harper, J.L. (2005, June). *Antithrombin III deficiency.* Retrieved September 20, 2005, from http://www.emedicine.com/ped/topic119.htm

Hembrough, T.A., Ruiz, J.R., Swerdlow, B.M., Swartz, G., Hammers, H.J., Zhang, L., et al. (2004). Identification and characterization of a very low density lipoprotein receptor-binding peptide from tissue factor pathway inhibitor that has antitumor and antiangiogenetic activity. *Blood, 103,* 3374–3380.

Levi, M. (2001). Pathogenesis and treatment of disseminated intravascular coagulation in the septic patient. *Journal of Critical Care, 16,* 167–177.

Levi, M. (2004). Current understanding of disseminated intravascular coagulation. *British Journal of Haematology, 124,* 567–576.

Levi, M., de Jonge, E., van der Poll, R., & Ten Cate, H. (2001). Advances in the understanding of the pathogenic pathways of disseminated intravascular coagulation result in more insight in the clinical picture and better management strategies. *Seminars in Thrombosis and Hemostasis, 27,* 569–575.

Levi, M., & Ten Cate, H. (1999). Disseminated intravascular coagulation. *New England Journal of Medicine, 341,* 586–592.

Messmore, H.L., Jr., & Wehrmacher, W.H. (2002, March). Disseminated intravascular coagulation: A primer for primary care physicians [Web exclusive]. *Postgraduate Medicine, 111*(3). Retrieved June 25, 2005, from http://www.postgradmed.com/issues/2002/03_02/messmore.htm

Ratnoff, O.D., Pritchard, J.A., & Colopy, J.E. (1955). Hemorrhagic states during pregnancy. *New England Journal of Medicine, 250,* 89–95.

Schmaier, A.H. (2004, August). *Disseminated intravascular coagulation.* Retrieved September 18, 2005, from http://www.emedicine.com/med/topic577.htm

Sivula, M., Tallgren, M., & Pettila, V. (2004). Impact of scoring system for DIC in the critically ill [Abstract]. *Critical Care Medicine, 32*(Suppl. 12), A78.

Taylor, F.B., Jr., Toh, C.H., Hoots, W.K., Wada, H., & Levi, M. (2001, August). *Scientific and Standardization Committee Communications: Towards a definition, clinical and laboratory criteria, and a scoring system for disseminated intravascular coagulation.* Retrieved September 1, 2005, from http://www.med.unc.edu/isth/SSC/communications/dic/definitionofdic.pdf

Toh, C.H., & Dennis, M. (2003). Disseminated intravascular coagulation: Old disease, new hope. *BMJ, 327,* 974–977.

Toh, C.H., & Downey, C. (2005). Performance and prognostic importance of a new clinical and laboratory scoring system for identifying non-overt disseminated intravascular coagulation. *Blood Coagulation and Fibrinolysis, 16,* 69–74.

Marcelle Kaplan, RN, MS, OCN®, AOCN®

⊃ **Chapter 3**

Hypercalcemia of Malignancy

Introduction

Hypercalcemia is a complex metabolic disorder and one of the most common life-threatening complications of malignancy. It occurs in up to 30% of all people with cancer at some point in the course of their disease (Solimando, 2001) but occurs most often in the advanced stages. The appearance of hypercalcemia is considered a marker for increased mortality, with median survival measured in weeks to months. Survival beyond six months is uncommon (Guise & Mundy, 1998; Wimalawansa, 1995). Pathologically increased destruction of bone is the most common mechanism contributing to the development of malignancy-associated hypercalcemia, but greatly elevated renal reabsorption of calcium also occurs in at least 50% of patients. In some cancers, tumor-induced synthesis of vitamin D plays an important role (Wimalawansa). Recognition of the specific events involved in the pathogenesis of hypercalcemia of malignancy (HCM) can indicate prognosis and can help healthcare providers in selecting the most effective therapy.

In recent years, effective preventive methods and early initiation of treatment, coupled with newer, more potent drugs, have led to the successful management of HCM. However, diagnosis still may be delayed or go unrecognized, even in the hospital setting, because of the nonspecificity of most symptoms and confusion with a wide variety of other conditions (Lamy, Jenzer-Closut, & Burckhardt, 2001; National Cancer Institute [NCI], 2004). Oncology nurses need to be aware of which patients are at risk and be alert for the early manifestations of hypercalcemia. Appropriate management and palliative measures may increase survival and enhance end-of-life quality.

Incidence

HCM occurs mostly in the setting of solid tumors, especially breast cancer and squamous cell lung cancer, which together represent more than half of

51

all HCM cases (Block, 2001). Multiple myeloma accounts for the third-highest incidence. Other hematologic malignancies associated with hypercalcemia include adult T-cell lymphoma, Hodgkin disease, and non-Hodgkin lymphoma (Heys, Smith, & Eremin, 1998; Ikeda et al., 1994; Richerson, 2004). Squamous cell carcinomas of the kidney, head, neck, and esophagus and some uncommon tumors, such as small cell carcinoma of the ovary and cholangiocarcinoma, frequently are associated with HCM (Block; Tummula, 1997). Interestingly, HCM rarely occurs with small cell lung cancer, adenocarcinoma of the lung, or prostate cancer, all of which frequently metastasize to bone, nor with primary bone cancers, such as osteogenic sarcoma. It also is rare with colon and stomach cancers (Grill & Martin, 2000; Kovacs, MacDonald, Chik, & Bruera, 1995). Table 3-1 lists the incidence and etiologies commonly associated with HCM.

Risk Factors

The primary mechanism contributing to the development of HCM is increased bone breakdown (resorption). The excess calcium released into the circulation overwhelms the renal mechanisms responsible for calcium excretion (Meriney & Reeder, 1998). In the pathogenesis of HCM, the malignant process stimulates the secretion or activation of a variety of humoral factors that act on the target organs of bone and kidney and disrupt normal calcium homeostasis. Eventually, compensatory mechanisms are overwhelmed, and hypercalcemia develops. Renal function status also plays a critical role in the etiology of HCM. Any disease-related or treatment-related condition that causes or increases dehydration or depletion of fluid volume can potentiate or exacerbate the development of HCM in at-risk patients. Anorexia, nausea, vomiting, mucositis, dysphagia, fever, the use of thiazide diuretics, and renal failure all can have a negative effect on calcium excretion through the kidney (Coward, 1986; Kaplan, 1994). Immobility also may be a rare contributing factor because of increased bone loss from prolonged lack of weight-bearing activity (Richerson, 2004; Wimalawansa, 1995).

Normal Calcium Homeostasis

Calcium is an inorganic element that plays a vital role in many fundamental metabolic processes in the body. Calcium is required for the formation and maintenance of bones and teeth; contractility of cardiac, smooth, and skeletal muscle; transmission of nerve impulses; normal clotting mechanisms; hormone secretion; and cellular permeability (Meriney & Reeder, 1998). The distribution of calcium within the body is dependent on the balance between calcium intake and calcium loss (Morton & Lipton,

Table 3-1. Incidence and Suggested Etiology of Hypercalcemia of Malignancy (HCM)

Malignancy	Incidence of HCM	Incidence of Bone Metastases	Suggested Etiology of Hypercalcemia

Breast cancer with bone metastases	30%–40%	65%–75%	Both humoral and local osteolytic mechanisms are important:
			• PTHrP is the major humoral mediator and stimulates:
			  – Osteoclastic bone resorption
			  – TGF-β release from bone; also acts to accelerate growth of breast cancer in bone
			  – Increased renal tubular calcium reabsorption
			  – Enhanced RANKL/OPG ratio in bone.*
			• Local mediators:
			  – RANKL secreted by metastatic cells in bone
			  – TGF-α
			  – IL-6, IL 11
			  – Prostaglandin E
			  – PDGF
			  – IGF-1
			  – Procathepsin D—enzyme associated with TGF-β activation
			Hormonal therapy (estrogens and antiestrogens) leads to increased synthesis of prostaglandin E.
			Direct resorption of bone by metastatic tumor cells is minor contribution.

Multiple myeloma	20%–40%	70%–90%	Local osteolytic bone resorbing mechanisms predominate:
			• Osteoclast activation mediated by
			  – Osteoblasts increase RANKL expression and suppress OPG production in response to myeloma cells.
			  – RANKL expressed directly by myeloma cells
			  – OPG degradation by myeloma cells
			  – IL-1
			  – IL-6—growth and survival factor for myeloma cells
			  – TNF-β (lymphotoxin)—produced by myeloma cells
			Renal insufficiency leads to decreased GFR and impaired renal excretion of calcium.
			Direct invasion by tumor is minor contribution.

*See page 62 for discussion.

(Continued on next page)

Table 3-1. Incidence and Suggested Etiology of Hypercalcemia of Malignancy (HCM) *(Continued)*

Malignancy	Incidence of HCM	Incidence of Bone Metastases	Suggested Etiology of Hypercalcemia
Squamous cell carcinoma of the lung	12.5%–35%	30%–40%	Increased bone resorption mediated by: • PTHrP—secreted by tumor cells • TGF-α • IL-1 • TNF Increased renal calcium reabsorption
Squamous cell carcinoma of the head and neck	2.9%–25%	Uncommon	Increased bone resorption mediated by: • PTHrP—secreted by tumor cells • TGF-α • IL-1 Increased renal calcium reabsorption
Renal cell carcinoma	3%–17%	20%–25%	Increased bone resorption mediated by: • PTHrP—secreted by tumor cells • TGF-α • Prostaglandins Increased renal calcium reabsorption
Lymphomas: Hodgkin	0.6%–5.4%	Rare	Lymphoma metabolizes 1,25-dihydroxyvitamin D (calcitriol), causing increased gut absorption of calcium. Impaired renal calcium clearance
Non-Hodgkin, high grade	14%–33%		
T-cell lymphoma (HTLV-type 1)	50%		HTLV-1—associated with viral induction of *PTHrP* gene and overexpression of RANKL
Other malignancies	7%		Ovary, liver, pancreas, esophagus, cervix
Unknown primary	7%		

GFR—glomerular filtration rate; HTLV—human T-cell lymphotropic virus; IGF—insulin growth factor; IL—interleukin; OPG—osteoprotegerin; PDGF—platelet-derived growth factor; PTHrP—parathyroid hormone-related protein; RANKL—receptor activator of nuclear factor κB ligand; TGF—transforming growth factor; TNF—tumor necrosis factor

Note. Based on information from Block, 2001; Coleman, 2001; Coleman & Rubens, 2004; Grill & Martin, 2000; Guise & Mundy, 1998; Heys et al., 1998; Hofbauer & Schoppet, 2004; Ikeda et al., 1994; Kaplan, 1994; Kvols, 2003; Lipton, 2004; Mundy, 2002; Munshi & Anderson, 2005; Tummula, 1997; Wimalawansa, 1995; Yeung & Gagel, 2003.

2004). Bone is an enormous reservoir of calcium and stores 99% of total body calcium. The remaining 1% of body calcium circulates in the serum, divided into two major fractions: Approximately half is in the form of free calcium ions, and the other half is bound to proteins, especially albumin, the most abundant plasma protein. A small fraction (3%) of serum calcium is neither ionized nor bound to protein but forms complexes with the anions bicarbonate, phosphate, and citrate. Only the free ionized form of calcium is physiologically active and plays a key role in blood coagulation, muscle contraction, and nerve conduction. The protein-bound form of serum calcium is not biologically active and has no clinical significance (Bajournas, 1990; Kaplan, 1994).

Accurate Determination of Serum Calcium Concentration

The normal range of total serum calcium is frequently reported as 8.5–10 mg/dl (Fischbach, 1992; Smith, 2000). In testing for serum calcium, most laboratories measure the concentration of total calcium, which does not distinguish the proportions of free ionized calcium and protein-bound calcium. Although newer, more precise instruments can measure ionized calcium, this testing is more expensive and is not routinely done (Smith). The proportion of free ionized calcium to protein-bound calcium, therefore, must be estimated, or "corrected." To accurately determine the ionized serum calcium concentration, it is essential to recognize the relationship between serum albumin and serum calcium. Because half of the calcium in the blood is bound to serum albumin, it is necessary to determine albumin levels concurrently with serum calcium (Fischbach; Moore, 1998). Serum albumin levels range between 3.5–5.5 g/dl, but in people with cancer, albumin commonly declines, either as a result of cachexia or poor dietary protein intake secondary to the disease process or treatment side effects (Bajournas, 1990; Moore). Any decrease in serum albumin results in an increase in the percentage of active, free ionized calcium, in contrast to the fraction of protein-bound (inactive) calcium, which declines.

When hypoalbuminemia is present, the concentration of serum calcium can be estimated by mathematically adjusting the value reported by the laboratory. Figure 3-1 illustrates a common formula used to correct for decreases in serum albumin. As a general rule, for every 1 g/dl reduction in serum albumin from normal, the total serum calcium is underreported by approximately 0.8 mg/dl (Kaplan, 1994; Kaye, 1995; Wilkes, Ingwersen, & Barton-Burke, 2001). Hypercalcemia exists when the corrected serum calcium is > 10.5 mg/dl (Richerson, 2004; Smith, 2000). Acid-base status also may affect serum calcium levels. When metabolic acidosis is present, less calcium is bound to albumin, increasing the fraction of active ionized serum calcium. With alkalosis, more calcium becomes protein-bound, decreasing the ionized fraction (Kvols, 2003; NCI, 2004).

Figure 3-1. Algorithm for Estimating Corrected Ionized Serum Calcium (Adjusted for Decreases in Serum Albumin)

Formula:
Corrected serum calcium (mg/dl) = measured serum calcium +
[4 (low normal value for albumin) – serum albumin (g/dl)] x 0.8

Example: Laboratory values: albumin = 2.5 g/dl; calcium = 10.5 mg/dl

1. Determine decrease in albumin from normal:
    4 g/dl (low normal)
    – 2.5 g/dl
     1.5 g/dl

2. Estimate underreported serum calcium:

    (For every 1 g/dl reduction in serum albumin, the reported serum calcium is estimated to be too low by 0.8 mg/dl.)

    0.8 mg/dl : 1 g/dl = X mg/dl : 1.5 g/dl

    X = 0.8 x 1.5
    X = 1.2 mg/dl calcium

3. Correct serum calcium concentration: 10.5 mg/dl + 1.2 mg/dl = 11.7 mg/dl

4. Corrected serum calcium = 11.7 mg/dl

5. Hypercalcemia is present.

Regulation of Normal Calcium Homeostasis

In normal calcium homeostasis, the rate of bone formation is approximately equal to the rate of bone resorption, and calcium absorption from the gut is equal to the urinary excretion of calcium (Guyton, 1991). Serum calcium is maintained within its narrow range through a state of dynamic equilibrium between the major forms of body calcium: stored (in bone), and ionized and albumin-bound (in serum). This process is regulated by a sensitive negative feedback loop (see Figure 3-2) that is controlled by the concentration of serum ionized calcium and the actions of three hormones: parathyroid hormone (PTH); calcitriol, the active form of vitamin D (1,25-dihydroxyvitamin D); and calcitonin (Kaplan, 1994).

Role of Parathyroid Hormone

The parathyroid glands release PTH in response to low serum concentration of ionized calcium. PTH acts to increase serum calcium levels to a nor-

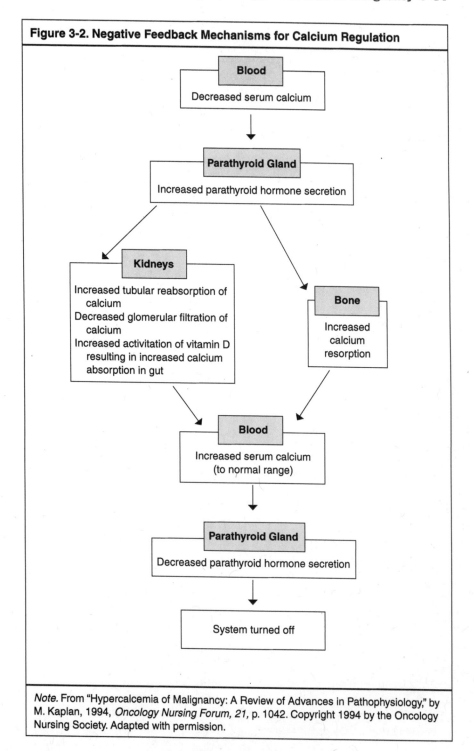

Figure 3-2. Negative Feedback Mechanisms for Calcium Regulation

Blood

Decreased serum calcium

Parathyroid Gland

Increased parathyroid hormone secretion

Kidneys

Increased tubular reabsorption of calcium
Decreased glomerular filtration of calcium
Increased activitation of vitamin D resulting in increased calcium absorption in gut

Bone

Increased calcium resorption

Blood

Increased serum calcium (to normal range)

Parathyroid Gland

Decreased parathyroid hormone secretion

System turned off

Note. From "Hypercalcemia of Malignancy: A Review of Advances in Pathophysiology," by M. Kaplan, 1994, *Oncology Nursing Forum, 21,* p. 1042. Copyright 1994 by the Oncology Nursing Society. Adapted with permission.

mal range through three mechanisms: (a) direct action on bone, (b) direct action on the kidneys, and (c) indirect action on the gastrointestinal tract (Mundy, 1990). In bone, PTH stimulates the activity of osteoclasts, which are multinucleated bone cells that break down (resorb) bone, releasing calcium ions into the circulation. In the kidneys, PTH acts to increase renal excretion of phosphorus, which, in turn, stimulates increased renal reabsorption of calcium. PTH regulates both calcium and phosphorus in inverse proportion to one another; mechanisms that decrease one will increase the other. For this reason, serum phosphate and calcium levels always should be evaluated together (Fischbach, 1992). PTH also stimulates the kidneys to activate vitamin D, which enhances the absorption of ingested calcium from the gastrointestinal tract (Wimalawansa, 1995). When the actions of PTH have elevated serum calcium levels to a normal range, negative feedback mechanisms signal the parathyroid glands to suppress secretion of PTH.

Role of Vitamin D

Vitamin D is a fat-soluble steroid that forms in the skin after exposure to ultraviolet radiation from natural sunlight. It also is absorbed from the fortification of foods, particularly dairy products and some cereals. Several steps of activation must occur before vitamin D can act on target tissues. The first step takes place in the liver with conversion to 25-hydroxyvitamin D (cholecalciferol). Through the stimulus of decreased serum calcium and subsequent PTH secretion, final activation of vitamin D occurs in the kidney, where it is metabolized to its most active form, 1,25-dihydroxyvitamin D (calcitriol) (Wilkes et al., 2001). Calcitriol acts to increase the intestinal absorption of calcium. Researchers have disproved increased dietary intake as a cause of HCM. Typically, vitamin D metabolism and intestinal absorption of calcium are both suppressed in HCM, inhibited by negative feedback mechanisms related to elevated serum calcium (Wimalawansa, 1995). The exceptions are certain lymphomas and multiple myeloma, in which increased activation of calcitriol mediates hypercalcemia. In this situation, patients should avoid dietary intake of calcium (Heys et al., 1998; Seymour & Gagel, 1993).

Role of Calcitonin

Calcitonin, the third hormone involved in serum calcium regulation, is the physiologic antagonist of PTH and has opposing effects. The thyroid gland releases calcitonin in response to increased serum calcium concentration, and this acts to inhibit osteoclastic activity, resulting in decreased calcium resorption from bone. It causes a rapid but short-lived response (Moore, 1998). Calcitonin does not play an important role in the continuing maintenance of calcium homeostasis but, following a calcium-rich meal, exerts a transient effect in reducing bone turnover (Gutierrez et al., 1990).

Role of the Kidneys in Calcium Homeostasis and Hypercalcemia of Malignancy

The kidneys play a major role in calcium homeostasis. The renal glomeruli filter approximately 10 g of calcium from the serum daily, and the renal tubules reabsorb 98% of the filtered calcium and return it to the circulation. Renal calcium reabsorption is linked to sodium and water reabsorption. It takes place primarily in the proximal tubule and ascending loop of Henle, where 90% of the filtered calcium is reabsorbed, independent of hormonal control (Mundy, 1990). The remaining calcium is reabsorbed from the distal tubules and collecting ducts, where fine-tuning of calcium homeostasis occurs in concert with negative feedback mechanisms involving PTH. When ionized serum calcium is low, tubular reabsorption of calcium is very great, so almost no calcium is lost in the urine. On the other hand, even a tiny increase in serum calcium concentration causes greatly increased urinary calcium excretion (Morton & Lipton, 2004).

The normally functioning kidney has great adaptive capacity. Bone resorption can increase by approximately 150% over bone formation before overwhelming the kidneys' capacity to excrete the increased calcium load. In the presence of pathologic destruction of bone, the kidneys can increase calcium excretion as much as fivefold, up to approximately 600 mg of calcium per day (Gutierrez et al., 1990; Morton & Lipton, 2004).

Although renal impairment is rarely the primary cause of hypercalcemia, the kidneys can contribute to the development of hypercalcemia in two important ways: increasing tubular reabsorption of calcium and decreasing glomerular filtration of calcium (Wimalawansa, 1995). In people with malignant disease, depletion of fluids and sodium can occur subsequent to anorexia, nausea, vomiting, mucositis, dysphagia, and fever, all common side effects of the disease, cytotoxic therapy, or existing hypercalcemia. This loss of fluid and sodium stimulates the kidneys to increase tubular reabsorption of sodium, closely followed by calcium (Coward, 1986; Kaplan, 1994). Fluid volume depletion also reduces the glomerular filtration rate, resulting in diminished filtration of calcium from the blood into the urine. The effects of increased tubular reabsorption of calcium and decreased calcium filtration in the kidneys contribute to developing hypercalcemia. The presence of existing hypercalcemia also exacerbates fluid volume depletion (Kaplan). Figure 3-3 illustrates the role of the kidneys in HCM.

Excessive serum calcium interferes with the ability of the kidneys to concentrate urine, which is regulated by antidiuretic hormone (ADH). In the absence of ADH, the distal tubules and collecting ducts become impermeable to water. Water remains in the tubular lumen and is excreted as large volumes of dilute urine (polyuria), stimulating excessive thirst (polydipsia)—both hallmark signs of hypercalcemia (Fojo, 2005). Even with the stimulus of thirst, hypercalcemic patients may not be able to drink enough to replace lost fluid because of other symptoms accompanying hypercalcemia, such as nausea,

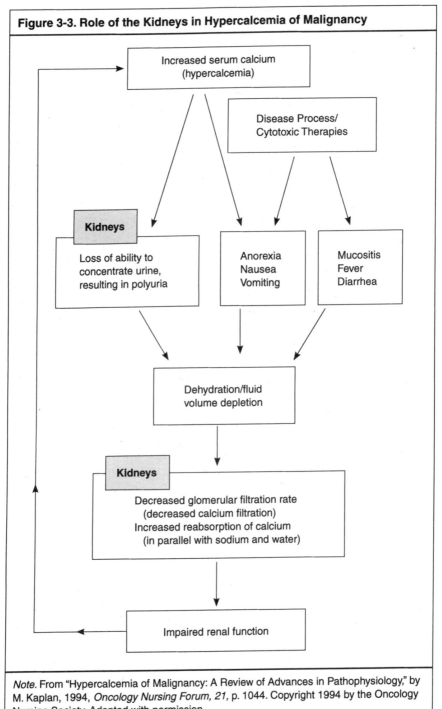

Figure 3-3. Role of the Kidneys in Hypercalcemia of Malignancy

Note. From "Hypercalcemia of Malignancy: A Review of Advances in Pathophysiology," by M. Kaplan, 1994, *Oncology Nursing Forum, 21,* p. 1044. Copyright 1994 by the Oncology Nursing Society. Adapted with permission.

vomiting, confusion, and stupor (Coward, 1986). The ensuing dehydration triggers the kidneys to increase the reabsorption of sodium and water in the proximal tubules, which is closely followed by calcium. These mechanisms further exacerbate the hypercalcemia. Hypovolemia results in diminished glomerular filtration, which can lead to progressive renal insufficiency and renal failure (Fojo; Kovacs et al., 1995). In summary, any condition that con-tributes to or exacerbates dehydration and fluid volume depletion triggers a kidney response that potentiates existing hypercalcemia. This sets into motion a vicious circle of hypercalcemia, dehydration, decreasing renal function, and worsening hypercalcemia.

Normal Bone Remodeling and Effects of Metastatic Disease

Bone is a specialized collagen connective tissue composed of an inner core of spongy trabecular bone covered by an outer matrix of hard min-eralized cortical bone. Normal mineralization of bone requires adequate amounts of vitamin D, calcium, and phosphate. In adults, cortical bone accounts for 85% of the total skeleton and is rich in growth factors that are released from the bone matrix in the process of normal bone remodeling. The remaining 15% of the skeleton is trabecular bone, which gives bone its structural strength. The multicellular marrow within bone is the site of hematopoietic stem cells, stromal cells, and immune cells. Hematopoietic stem cells have the potential to differentiate into blood-forming elements, and into a type of bone cell called an *osteoclast,* a giant, multinucleated cell derived from the fusion of monocyte-macrophage precursors. Osteoclasts mediate bone breakdown, or resorption. Stromal cells in the marrow sup-port the differentiation of bone-forming cells called *osteoblasts,* which are derived from mesenchymal fibroblast-like cells (Coleman & Rubens, 2004; Guise & Mundy, 1998).

Bone is unique among target tissues affected by cancer because it is a dynamic tissue, constantly being remodeled in a cycle of bone disposal and renewal. In healthy individuals, the cycle of bone remodeling follows an orderly sequence, carefully regulated by a mechanism called *coupling,* which involves complex interactions among systemic hormones, local bone-derived growth factors, and cytokines. When metastatic cancer cells arrive in bone, the bone microenvironment, which is rich in growth fac-tors and cytokines, provides a fertile soil for their growth. But even in this fertile soil, the amount of bone destruction seen in metastatic bone disease usually is much greater than would be expected based on the number of malignant cells present (Coleman, 2001). The excessive bone destruction results from the expression of local humoral factors in response to the presence of malignant cells in bone. These local factors further enrich the bone microenvironment, thus enhancing survival of the cancer cells and activating osteoclast-mediated bone resorption (Coleman & Rubens, 2004; Davis, 2004). Metastatic bone involvement characterized by bone loss from osteoclastic overactivity creates *osteolytic lesions*; overgrowths of bone around tumor deposits are called *osteoblastic lesions*. Breast cancer is associated primarily with osteolytic lesions, and prostate cancer with osteoblastic lesions, although mixed osteolytic and osteoblastic lesions may occur in both diseases (Lipton, 2004).

RANKL, RANK, and Osteoprotegerin: Mechanisms Underlying Bone Remodeling

In recent years, researchers have more fully characterized interactions between osteoblasts and osteoclasts. It is now understood that the osteoblasts essentially control the maturation and activity of bone-resorbing osteoclasts in normal bone remodeling (Coleman & Rubens, 2004; Lerner, 2004; Yeung & Gagel, 2003). In the pathologic process associated with HCM, PTH-related protein (PTHrP), a systemic humoral factor released from tumor cells, mimics the physiologic actions of PTH. PTHrP is able to bind with and activate normal PTH receptors on osteoblasts and bone marrow stromal cells. Activation of the PTH receptor stimulates expression of a cell surface protein on the osteoblast called the *receptor activator of nuclear factor κB (RANK) ligand*, or RANK-ligand (RANKL). RANKL is a member of the tumor necrosis factor superfamily and is a powerful inducer of osteoclast formation (Davis, 2004). RANKL stimulates osteoclast activity by binding to its related receptor, RANK, located on undifferentiated, precursor osteoclastic cells. When RANKL activates the RANK receptors, the preosteoclasts fuse and differentiate into mature multinucleated osteoclasts that develop a ruffled border and resorb bone (Teitelbaum, 2000; Yeung & Gagel). Figure 3-4 depicts the interactions underlying normal bone remodeling.

In the normal regulation of bone remodeling, a soluble, free-floating "decoy" receptor called *osteoprotegerin* (OPG) (because it protects against bone loss) acts to turn off osteoclastic differentiation and halt excessive bone resorption. OPG, also produced and secreted by the osteoblast, counteracts the effect of RANKL by binding with it, thus blocking further osteoclastic maturation. The balance between RANKL and OPG, which is regulated by systemic hormones and local bone cytokines, determines osteoclastic functions. In bone that has been invaded by cancer cells, the normal bone microenvironment is deregulated. An imbalance in the RANKL/OPG ratio develops, in which RANKL predominates, causing increased bone destruction (Davis, 2004; Hofbauer & Schoppet, 2004; Lerner, 2004). Myeloma cells have the ability to destroy bone because they can secrete RANKL directly. In breast cancer, RANKL may be secreted by the malignant cells or stimulated by the actions of PTHrP (Morton & Lipton, 2004; Munshi & Anderson, 2005; Rodan & Martin, 2000).

Figure 3-4. Normal Bone Remodeling: A Balanced Process

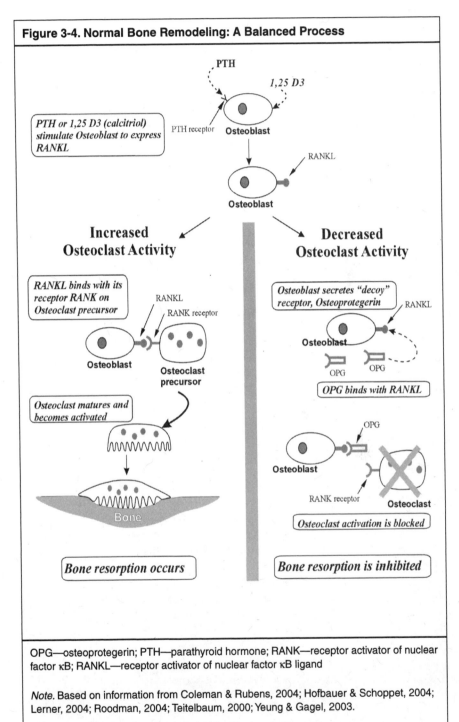

OPG—osteoprotegerin; PTH—parathyroid hormone; RANK—receptor activator of nuclear factor κB; RANKL—receptor activator of nuclear factor κB ligand

Note. Based on information from Coleman & Rubens, 2004; Hofbauer & Schoppet, 2004; Lerner, 2004; Roodman, 2004; Teitelbaum, 2000; Yeung & Gagel, 2003.

Note. Figure courtesy of J. Lubowsky, PhD, PE. Used with permission.

Pathophysiology

Understanding of the complexity of the pathophysiologic mechanisms involved in HCM development continues to evolve. Prior to the late 1980s, this common metabolic complication was thought to develop simply as a consequence of tumor invasion into bone, either through local direct extension or through distant metastasis. Although plausible, certain observations did not fit this conception; 15% of hypercalcemic patients with cancer exhibit little or no evidence of malignant bone destruction, and the occurrence of hypercalcemia does not necessarily correlate with the amount of bone destruction (Kaplan, 1994). More than 100 years ago, Dr. Stephen Paget (associated with Paget disease of bone) noted that "a general degradation of bones sometimes occurs in carcinoma of the breast, yet without the distinct deposition of cancer in them" (Guise & Mundy, 1998, p. 18). In the setting of bronchogenic tumors, both squamous cell and small cell carcinomas of the lung frequently metastasize to bone, but only squamous cell lung cancer is associated with a high incidence of hypercalcemia. Additionally, HCM rarely is seen with prostate cancer, even in the presence of extensive bony metastasis (Block, 2001; Grill & Martin, 2000). Research developments in recent years have explained these inconsistencies, namely through the identification of a variety of cytokines, growth factors, and other humoral and local factors that are expressed or induced by the presence of malignant cells. These tumor-derived biologic mediators, with otherwise normal physiologic roles in the body, act to disrupt normal calcium homeostasis and stimulate increased osteoclastic activity. The characterization of these factors has helped to explain the occurrence of hypercalcemia in diverse malignant settings such as solid tumors with extensive bone metastases, solid tumors without evidence of bone involvement, and hematologic malignancies.

The traditional view has been that HCM is three separate syndromes: humoral hypercalcemia of malignancy (HHM), hypercalcemia related to widespread osteolytic bone metastases, and hypercalcemia of hematologic malignancy (Block, 2001; Grill & Martin, 2000). More recently, however, modern techniques of molecular biology have produced a wealth of knowledge that provides insight into the mechanisms contributing to hypercalcemia. It now is clear that (a) the primary abnormality in HCM is an excessive increase in osteoclastic activity rather than the presence or absence of bone metastases, and (b) the mediators for both HHM and hypercalcemia related to widespread osteolytic bone metastases are mostly the same (Block; Grill & Martin; Mundy & Guise, 1998). Figure 3-5 describes the mediators associated with the development of HCM.

Humoral Hypercalcemia of Malignancy

HHM most frequently occurs with carcinomas of the breast, lung, kidney, and head and neck, which account for approximately 80% of the total incidence of hypercalcemia (Fojo, 2005). Knowledge of the pathophysiologic mechanisms underlying HHM development has greatly expanded since 1987, when PTHrP was identified. Since then, many studies have established the essential role of PTHrP in most types of malignancy-associated hypercalcemia (Davidson, 2001; Grill & Martin, 2000; Mundy & Guise, 1998; Wimalawansa, 1995). PTHrP mimics the physiologic activity of PTH, acting on bone and kidney via authentic PTH receptors, but without the controls of homeostatic negative feedback mechanisms. The unregulated hormonal actions of PTHrP stimulate increased calcium reabsorption and decreased phosphate uptake in the renal tubules, resulting in hypercalcemia and hypophosphatemia (Body, 2004; Rodan & Martin, 2000).

Sensitive radioimmunoassay studies have detected PTHrP expression in a variety of solid tumors, most commonly of squamous cell origin but also in renal cell carcinoma, melanoma, skin tumors, neuroendocrine tumors, and medullary thyroid cancer. Circulating levels of PTHrP are present in 100% of patients who have solid tumors and HCM but no bone metastases, and in two-thirds of hypercalcemic patients with bone involvement (Body, 2004; Grill & Martin, 2000). Most patients with adult T-cell leukemia/lymphoma complicated by hypercalcemia have high circulating PTHrP levels. PTHrP has been detected to a lesser extent in hypercalcemic patients with non-Hodgkin lymphoma, especially the B-cell type, and in patients with multiple myeloma (Ikeda et al., 1994).

Hypercalcemia and Skeletal Metastases

Hypercalcemia develops in 20%–30% of patients who have widespread osteolytic metastases, which occur most frequently in patients with advanced breast cancer (Heys et al., 1998; Mundy & Guise, 1998). Animal models have demonstrated that breast cancer cells metastatic to bone produce PTHrP, which acts to increase osteoclastic activity and release transforming growth factor-beta (TGF-ß) and insulin-like growth factors (IGF I and II) from normal bone (Guise & Mundy, 1998; Rodan & Martin, 2000). TGF-ß and IGF, in turn, stimulate proliferation of the metastatic breast cancer cells, creating a positive feedback loop. Insight into this process has led to the use of bisphosphonates (drugs that inhibit osteoclastic bone resorption) as a strategy to prevent breast cancer metastasis to bone (Yeung & Gagel, 2003). Osteolytic bone destruction also is common in advanced lung cancer and multiple myeloma; both are associated with increased incidence of hypercalcemia (Fojo, 2005).

Metastatic osteoblastic bone disease, characterized by increased bone formation, is much less common. Osteoblastic metastases are seen most frequently in advanced prostate cancer, a cancer in which hypercalcemia occurs in less than 2% of cases, and then usually with prostate tumors of unusual histology (Mundy & Guise, 1998; Yeung & Gagel, 2003).

In addition to PTHrP, a variety of cytokines, growth factors, and other humoral mediators are postulated to cause bone destruction through direct and indirect actions. This group includes the transforming growth factors, tumor necrosis factors, IGFs, prostaglandin E, several interleukins, and hematopoietic colony-stimulating factors (Coleman & Rubens, 2004; Lipton, 2004; Mundy, 2002; Rodan & Martin, 2000; Roodman, 2004; Teitelbaum, 2000; Yeung & Gagel, 2003) (see Figure 3-5).

Figure 3-5. Characteristics of Factors Associated With Development of Hypercalcemia of Malignancy

Parathyroid hormone (PTH)-related protein (PTHrP)
- Released systemically by many solid tumors, especially squamous cell carcinomas
- Secreted locally by cancer cells, particularly breast and myeloma
- Acts by binding to and activating PTH receptors in tissue
- Powerful mediator of osteoclastic bone resorption; enhances renal tubular calcium reabsorption and inhibits phosphate reabsorption
- Stimulates production of RANKL by osteoblasts and bone marrow stromal cells

Local osteoclast-activating factors
- RANKL, RANK, and OPG (see Figure 3-4)
  - Key regulators of osteoclast activity
  - Members of the TNF and TNF-receptor superfamilies
  - RANKL is expressed by osteoblasts, T lymphocytes, breast cancer cells, and multiple myeloma cells.
  - RANK receptor is expressed by osteoclasts.
  - RANKL binds to RANK to stimulate osteoclast activity and bone resorption.
  - OPG is expressed by osteoblasts to turn off osteoclast activity.
  - OPG acts as a decoy receptor and binds to RANKL, inhibiting further bone resorption.
- TNF-α
  - Cytokine produced by activated macrophages and by tumor cells
  - Potent bone-resorbing activity in vitro and in vivo
  - Responsible for cachexia associated with malignancy
- Lymphotoxin (TNF-β)
  - Cytokine produced by activated T lymphocytes and myeloma cells
  - Potent bone-resorbing activity in vitro and in vivo
  - Major mediator of bone resorption in myeloma
- Interleukin (IL)-1
  - Cytokine secreted by monocytes, macrophages, and tumor cells
  - Potent bone-resorbing activity in vitro and in vivo
  - Stimulates expression of M-CSF by marrow stromal cells
  - Stimulates production of RANKL by osteoblasts and bone stromal cells
- IL-6
  - Cytokine secreted by tumor cells
  - Powerful mediator of osteoclastic bone resorption
  - Stimulates production of RANKL by osteoblasts and bone stromal cells

Transforming growth factors (TGFs)
- TGF-α
  - Potent agent of osteoclastogenesis
  - Produced by many solid tumors
  - Potent bone resorber in vitro
  - TNF/IL-1 work synergistically with TGF-α/PTHrP in some malignancies.

(Continued on next page)

Figure 3-5. Characteristics of Factors Associated With Development of Hypercalcemia of Malignancy *(Continued)*

- TGF-β
  - High concentration in bone, platelets, and placenta
  - Osteoblast growth factor—indirectly stimulates bone resorption
  - Mediator of osteoblastic metastases
  - Expressed at high levels by prostate cancer cells
  - Released from bone in response to PTHrP secretion by breast cancer cells metastatic to bone; accelerates growth of those breast cancer cells

Platelet-derived growth factor
- Abundant in platelets and bone
- Osteoblast growth factor—indirectly stimulates bone resorption
- May potentiate effects of TGF-α and TGF-β

Insulin-like growth factors (IGFs) I and II
- Abundant in bone
- Released into bone microenvironment by osteoclastic bone resorption
- Act with TGF-β to stimulate growth of breast cells metastatic to bone

Hematopoietic colony-stimulating factors (CSFs)
- Granulocyte macrophage–CSF
  - Supports all steps of myelopoiesis
  - Produced by fibroblasts and osteoblasts following IL-1 stimulation
  - Released by melanoma cells in vitro
  - Activates osteoclastic bone resorption
- M-CSF
  - Imperative for macrophage maturation
  - Secreted by osteoblasts and bone marrow stromal cells in response to IL-1, TNF-α, and prostaglandin E stimulation
  - Stimulates proliferation of osteoclast precursors
  - Stimulates macrophages to become osteoclasts

Prostaglandins—E series
- Secreted by tumor cells, especially breast cancer
- Bone-resorbing activity in vitro
- Subsidiary role in bone resorption associated with humoral hypercalcemia of malignancy

1,25-dihydroxyvitamin D (calcitriol)
- Mediates hypercalcemia of malignancy in lymphoma malignancies
- Lymphoma tumor cells metabolize vitamin D—increase gut absorption of calcium.
- Induces expression of RANKL by bone stromal cells and osteoblasts and unbalances the RANKL-OPG signaling pathway
- Inhibited by PTHrP secreted by solid tumors

M-CSF—macrophage colony-stimulating factor; OPG—osteoprotegerin; RANK—receptor activator of nuclear factor κB; RANKL—receptor activator of nuclear factor κB ligand; TNF—tumor necrosis factor

Note. Based on information from Coleman & Rubens, 2004; Davis, 2004; Guise & Mundy, 1998; Kaplan, 1994; Lipton, 2004; Mundy, 2002; Rodan & Martin, 2000; Roodman, 2004; Seymour & Gagel, 1993; Sezer et al., 2003; Teitelbaum, 2000; Wimalawansa, 1995; Yeung & Gagel, 2003.

Hypercalcemia and Hematologic Malignancy

Multiple Myeloma

Osteolytic bone destruction, renal failure, and hypercalcemia are clinical hallmarks of multiple myeloma (Kyle & Rajkumar, 2004). Approximately one-third of patients diagnosed with this disease will develop HCM (Grill & Martin, 2000). The bone lesions characteristic of myeloma are purely lytic; they have no osteoblastic component. The bone destruction arises from an unbalanced process of increased osteoclastic and suppressed osteoblastic activity, mediated by RANKL overexpression (Kyle & Rajkumar; Roodman, 2004). Myeloma cells are able to secrete RANKL and also can induce RANKL expression in bone marrow stromal cells, which leads to local osteoclastic proliferation. At the same time, OPG, the receptor that blocks osteoclast overactivity, is inhibited and degraded. This imbalance between RANKL and OPG, mediated by the myeloma cells, favors formation and activation of osteoclasts (Hofbauer & Schoppet, 2004; Munshi & Anderson, 2005; Sezer, Heider, Zavrski, Kuhne, & Hofbauer, 2003). Increased understanding of myeloma-associated bone disease has led to the use of bisphosphonates as prophylactic therapy (Kyle & Rajkumar).

Adult T-Cell Leukemia and Lymphoma

Hypercalcemia develops in more than 50% of patients with adult T-cell leukemia/lymphoma, a malignancy associated with human T-cell leukemia virus type 1 (HTLV-1) infection (Ikeda et al., 1994; Tummula, 1997). The underlying mechanism involves activation of the *PTHrP* gene, possibly induced by the HTLV-1 virus. PTHrP stimulates overexpression of RANKL in the malignant T cells, resulting in excessive osteoclast formation and activity (Block, 2001; Morton & Lipton, 2004).

Hodgkin Disease and Non-Hodgkin Lymphoma

Calcitriol mediates hypercalcemia in Hodgkin disease and non-Hodgkin lymphoma (NHL). The lymphoma tissue itself, without hormonal stimulation by either PTH or PTHrP, metabolizes 25-hydroxyvitamin D (cholecalciferol) to its active form, 1,25-dihydroxyvitamin D (calcitriol), which acts to increase intestinal calcium absorption and enhance osteoclastic activity. Another contributing factor may relate to alterations in renal function that impair renal clearance of calcium (Block, 2001; Grill & Martin, 2000; Guise & Mundy, 1998). Hypercalcemia associated with Hodgkin disease has an incidence of 1.6%–5.4%, mostly in older patients with stage III or IV bulky disease below the diaphragm. HCM is very uncommon in low-grade NHL, but incidence can reach 30% in intermediate and aggressive high-grade NHL, in both B- and T-cell phenotypes associated with bulky disease (Block; Tummula, 1997). The characteristic clinical features of lymphoma-associated hypercalcemia include suppressed serum PTH, normal or slightly increased phosphorus levels (caused by suppressed PTH), hypercalciuria, and an absence of bone metastases. Approximately 50% of patients have elevated serum calcitriol levels (Yeung & Gagel, 2003).

Nonmalignant Causes of Hypercalcemia

In determining the etiology of hypercalcemia, healthcare providers should consider the possibility of causes other than malignancy. Primary hyperparathyroidism and benign causes of hypercalcemia are not unusual in patients with cancer. The most common causes of hypercalcemia in the general population are primary hyperparathyroidism (54%), malignancy (35%), and a variety of other conditions (12%), including vitamin D toxicity, sarcoidosis, and hyperthyroidism (Kovacs et al., 1995; Wimalawansa, 1995). The elevated serum calcium levels seen in most cases of primary hyperparathyroidism are related to increased intestinal absorption of calcium (mediated by PTH-induced calcitriol synthesis) rather than bone breakdown (Hemphill, 2005). Hypercalcemia associated with hyperparathyroidism tends to be mild and prolonged and often is undiagnosed until routine blood tests are performed. In general, serum calcium levels that are mildly elevated over a long period are caused by nonmalignant conditions, but rapidly rising calcium levels should increase the suspicion for malignancy (Agraharkar & Dellinger, 2004; Keenan & Wickham, 2005). In addition, with primary hyperparathyroidism the normal balance still exists between bone breakdown and bone deposition, in contrast to malignancy-induced hypercalcemia, in which an uncoupling occurs between bone resorption and formation (Fojo, 2005; Hemphill). Figure 3-6 lists nonmalignant conditions contributing to hypercalcemia.

Clinical Manifestations

In general, the clinical manifestations seen in hypercalcemia occur because of the depressant effects that elevated serum calcium levels exert on the excitability of nerve tissue and on the contractility of cardiac, skeletal, and smooth muscle (Kaplan, 1994). The organ systems affected by hypercalcemia include the central nervous system (CNS), cardiovascular system, and the gastrointestinal, musculoskeletal, and renal systems (see Figure 3-7), but the effects are especially profound in the CNS and the kidneys (Agraharkar & Dellinger, 2004).

Neurologic Effects

CNS changes reflect the direct depressant effect of hypercalcemia on the transmission of nerve impulses. Neurologic symptoms begin with vague muscle

Figure 3-6. Nonmalignant Causes of Hypercalcemia

Related to increased parathyroid hormone (PTH) levels
- Primary hyperparathyroidism
- Hyperthyroidism—negative feedback regulation of serum calcium is lost.
- Lithium-related release of PTH
- Familial causes of parathyroid adenomas and elevated PTH levels:
  - Inherited autosomally dominant syndromes:
    * Inactivation of multiple endocrine neoplasia *(MEN)* tumor suppressor genes; implicated in 12%–20% of parathyroid adenomas
    * Abnormal gene regulating the cell cycle:
      - Activation of *PRAD1* proto-oncogene leads to overexpression of *cyclin D1,* a key regulator of the G1 growth phase of the cell cycle; implicated in 20%–40% of parathyroid adenomas.

Related to increased bone breakdown
- Hyperthyroidism
- Immobilization (especially with Paget disease of bone)

Related to renal function
- Chronic renal failure
- Thiazide diuretics—increased renal calcium reabsorption
- Milk-alkali syndrome—excessive consumption of milk (high in calcium and added vitamin D) and soluble alkali-like antacids (for peptic ulcer disease) or chewable calcium carbonate (to prevent osteoporosis) leads to mild metabolic alkalosis and increased renal reabsorption of calcium.
- Hypophosphatemia—inverse relationship between serum phosphate and calcium; decreased phosphorus levels lead to excess calcium.

Related to increased intestinal calcium absorption
- Excessive oral intake of calcium
- Excessive oral intake of vitamin D
- Milk-alkali syndrome
- Granulomatous disease—especially sarcoidosis, tuberculosis, histoplasmosis, coccidioidomycosis
  - Associated macrophages produce 1,25-dihydroxyvitamin D (calcitriol)

Related to mutations in calcium-sensing receptor gene
- Familial hypocalciuric hypercalcemia—dominantly inherited:
  - Increased set point for extracellular calcium results in mild hypercalcemia and low urinary calcium excretion—nonprogressive, asymptomatic.

Other rare causes
- Adrenal insufficiency (Addison disease)
- Estrogen/antiestrogen therapy
- Pheochromocytoma (may be part of *MEN 2* syndrome)
- Vitamin A intoxication
- Theophylline toxicity
- Parenteral nutrition

Note. Based on information from Agraharkar & Dellinger, 2004; Bajournas, 1990; Kovacs et al., 1995; Kvols, 2003; Lairmore & Moley, 2005; Smith, 2000; Tummula, 1997; Wimalawansa, 1995; Yeung & Gagel, 2003.

Figure 3-7. Signs and Symptoms of Hypercalcemia of Malignancy*

Renal
Early: Polyuria, polydipsia, nocturia, dehydration, decreased glomerular filtration,
  hypercalciuria, kidney stones, renal insufficiency
Late: Renal failure

Musculoskeletal
Early: Muscle weakness, fatigue, hypotonia, bone pain
Late: Ataxia, pathologic fractures

Gastrointestinal
Early: Anorexia, nausea, vomiting, constipation, vague abdominal pain, weight loss,
  peptic ulcers, acute pancreatitis
Late: Atonic ileus, obstipation

Neurologic
Early: Drowsiness, lethargy, weakness, decreased deep tendon reflexes, apathy, restlessness, irritability, depression, confusion, personality changes, cognitive dysfunction,
  disorientation, delirium, psychotic behavior, visual disturbances
Late: Seizures, stupor, coma

Cardiovascular
Early: Electrocardiographic changes indicating slowed conduction, including prolonged
  PR interval, widened QRS complex, shortened QT interval, shortened or absent ST
  segments; broadened T wave, digitalis sensitivity, sinus bradycardia, arrhythmias
Late: Heart block, cardiac arrest

---

* Signs and symptoms of hypercalcemia vary considerably from person to person regardless of serum calcium levels.

Note. Based on information from Kaplan, 1994; Meriney & Reeder, 1998; Moore, 1998;
National Cancer Institute, 2004; Richerson, 2004; Wimalawansa, 1995.

---

weakness, lethargy, apathy, and hyporeflexia. As the calcium level continues
to rise, the symptoms progress to profound alterations in mental status, psychotic behavior, seizures, coma, and ultimately death (Barnett, 1999; Meriney
& Reeder, 1998; NCI, 2004).

Renal Effects

Hypercalcemia is toxic to the renal tubules. It impairs the ability of the kidneys to concentrate urine, causing some of the hallmark clinical manifestations
of HCM—polydipsia, polyuria, and nocturia (Kaplan, 1994). Calcium deposition within the renal tubules inhibits the urine-concentrating action of ADH,
creating nephrogenic diabetes insipidus and diuresis of large volumes of dilute
urine (Block, 2001). Kidney stones may develop secondary to hypercalciuria.
Prolonged hypercalcemia may cause calcium to be deposited in any soft tissue
in the body, especially when associated with hyperphosphatemia related to

renal failure (Agraharkar & Dellinger, 2004). The degree of renal impairment frequently determines the course of hypercalcemia; increasingly severe renal dysfunction often portends a fatal outcome (Wimalawansa, 1995).

Cardiac Effects

High serum calcium levels depress the electrical conduction system of the heart and increase cardiac muscle contractility and irritability. Electrocardiographic (EKG) changes, such as prolonged PR and QRS intervals, reflect slowed conduction through the heart. Cardiac arrhythmias may result from decreases in serum potassium and magnesium. Clinical effects related to arrhythmias range from feeling light-headed, to fainting, to sudden death if serum calcium rises acutely (Glick & Glover, 1995). Elevations in serum calcium also can potentiate the effects of digitalis and cause digitalis toxicity. Hypertension may be present, caused by the vasoconstrictive effect of calcium on arterial smooth muscle, but more often is associated with hypercalcemia from nonmalignant causes (Barnett, 1999; Moore, 1998).

Gastrointestinal Effects

Most of the gastrointestinal manifestations associated with hypercalcemia arise because of the depressive effects of elevated serum calcium on the autonomic nervous system and the resulting hypotonicity of smooth muscle in the gastrointestinal tract. Anorexia, nausea, vomiting, and constipation are common, caused by delayed gastric emptying and slowed gastrointestinal motility. Prolonged hypercalcemia stimulates increased gastrin release, which may cause peptic ulcer disease. Acute pancreatitis also may develop secondary to phospholipase activation by calcium (Moore, 1998; NCI, 2004).

Musculoskeletal Effects

Elevation of serum calcium levels decreases neuromuscular excitability, causing hypotonicity of smooth and striated muscle. Neuromuscular manifestations usually are more marked in older patients. Bone pain may be present with or without metastatic bone involvement because calcium has neurosensitizing actions that diminish the pain threshold (Barnett, 1999). Pathologic fractures and skeletal deformities may develop with progressive disease (NCI, 2004).

Patient Assessment

Grading Hypercalcemia in Malignant Disease

Nurses must be able to recognize which patients are at increased risk for developing hypercalcemia. The signs and symptoms of increasing serum calcium often are so general and nonspecific that it may be difficult to distinguish them from side effects arising from the underlying malignancy or from the treatment process. Typical nonspecific symptoms include fatigue, anorexia, nausea, vomiting, thirst, muscle weakness, polyuria, and constipation (Barnett, 1999; Kovacs et al., 1995; Wimalawansa, 1995). Although considerable individual variation exists, the severity of symptoms is most closely associated with the rapidity of onset of the hypercalcemia, the degree of serum calcium elevation, and the age and performance status of the patient (Kaplan, 1994). Hypercalcemia grading categories are mild, moderate, and severe based on corrected serum calcium levels, but there is often a lack of correlation between symptom severity and serum calcium levels. Older adult or debilitated patients may become symptomatic with only a slight rise in ionized calcium, especially if it is rapid. In contrast, patients with longstanding hypercalcemia are able to tolerate high serum calcium levels with few symptoms (NCI, 2004).

Asymptomatic patients with a corrected serum calcium concentration < 12 mg/dl are considered to have mild hypercalcemia and may not require intervention beyond close monitoring, oral hydration, and ambulation (Davidson, 2001; Meriney & Reeder, 1998; Tummula, 1997). A corrected calcium concentration of 12–13.5 mg/dl indicates moderate hypercalcemia; severe hypercalcemia exists at levels > 13.5 mg/dl. Patients with corrected serum calcium concentrations > 14 mg/dl are invariably symptomatic and require urgent intervention (Bajournas, 1990; Kaye, 1995; Morton & Ritch, 2002). Patient prognosis depends on how quickly the hypercalcemia can be recognized and treated. Early intervention can help to prevent secondary organ damage, which would add greatly to patients' morbidity and mortality (Wimalawansa, 1995). As a general rule, clinicians should treat patients with symptoms clearly related to HCM as though they have severe cases, regardless of the measured increase in serum calcium (Block, 2001). Without proper intervention, almost 50% of hypercalcemic patients will die as a consequence of either renal failure, coma, or cardiac arrest (Moore, 1998; Wimalawansa).

Diagnostic Evaluation

In patients with known malignant disease, determining the serum calcium level is the most important laboratory test in the diagnostic workup for hypercalcemia (Morton & Ritch, 2002; Wimalawansa, 1995). The level of ionized calcium is the best measurement to obtain, but that test is often expensive and not readily available. Instead, clinicians measure the serum calcium concentration along with the albumin level, using a correction algorithm to arrive at the estimated corrected value for ionized serum calcium, as discussed earlier (see Figure 3-1). Urinary calcium also may be measured because increases in urine may be detected before serum calcium rises (Myers, 2001).

Other blood chemistry laboratory values that are mandatory to review in the initial HCM workup are blood urea nitrogen (BUN) and creatinine to provide information about renal function. Serum electrolyte levels should be checked with attention to phosphorus, magnesium, and potassium (Morton & Ritch, 2002). Phosphorus and calcium have an inverse relationship regulated by PTH and should be evaluated together (Fischbach, 1992). Serum phosphorus levels may be decreased or normal but also can be elevated depending on the extent of bone metastasis (Smith, 2000). Magnesium levels are important; they may be decreased, aggravating the neuromuscular effects of hypercalcemia (Barnett, 1999). Serum alkaline phosphatase levels also may be elevated in patients with breast cancer metastatic to bone (Barnett; Myers, 2001), reflecting increased osteoblast activity (Mundy, 2002). Hypokalemia may be revealed and may relate to inadequate dietary intake of potassium (Morton & Ritch). An EKG may show a shortened QT interval; orthostatic hypotension and signs of dehydration may indicate compromised renal function (Block, 2001). Determinations of serum calcitriol (1,25-dihydroxyvitamin D) concentrations may be useful in patients with lymphoma.

Appropriate radiographic imaging tests may demonstrate the presence of either lung cancer, bone metastases, myeloma, or breast cancer (NCI, 2004). In patients with nonspecific symptoms, an immunoassay of serum intact parathyroid hormone (iPTH) can rule out nonmalignant causes of hypercalcemia. In general, iPTH levels are elevated in patients with primary hyperparathyroidism and suppressed in patients with cancer (Kaye, 1995; Yeung & Gagel, 2003). See Table 3-2 for laboratory variables used to distinguish between primary hyperparathyroidism and HCM.

Treatment Modalities

General Measures

The overall goals of antihypercalcemic treatment are to improve renal function, mental status, and quality of life and to provide effective antitumor therapy, shorten length of hospitalization, and prolong life. To achieve these goals, treatment of cancer-induced hypercalcemia is individualized for each patient based on several factors: elevation of serum calcium, severity of symptoms, status of disease, and prognosis for survival (Kaplan, 1994). Asymptomatic patients with mild hypercalcemia (< 12 mg/dl corrected serum calcium) who are receiving antineoplastic therapy may only require careful observation plus a variety of preventive measures.

Preventive measures include increasing oral fluid intake to 3 L per day to expand the intravascular fluid volume, controlling nausea and vomiting to prevent dehydration, and maintaining weight-bearing activities to decrease bone resorption. In addition, patients should avoid medications that might potentiate hypercalcemia, such as thiazide diuretics that decrease renal excretion of calcium and nonsteroidal anti-inflammatory drugs that inhibit renal blood flow, as well as supplements for vitamins A and D. Minimize the use of

Table 3-2. Laboratory Variables in the Differential Diagnosis of Hypercalcemia

Serum—Adult Reference Range*	Primary Hyperparathyroidism	Hypercalcemia of Malignancy
Calcium: 8.5–10.5 mg/dl	H	H
Phosphate: 3–4.5 mg/dl	L	L/N/H
Chloride: 98–106 mEq/L	H	L
Bicarbonate: 23–30 mmol/L	L	H
Sodium: 135–147 mEq/L	N	L
Potassium: 3.5–5 mEq/L	N	L
Alkaline phosphatase: 25–92 U/L	H	H/may be normal in myeloma
Magnesium: 1.3–2.1 mEq/L		L/N
Creatinine: 0.6–1.2 mg/dl		H
Blood urea nitrogen: 8–18 mg/dl		H
iPTH	H	L/N
iPTHrP	Undetectable	H
pH	Metabolic acidosis	Metabolic alkalosis
Urine		
cAMP	H	H
Phosphate: 0.82–0.95 mg/day	H	H/N
Calcium: 300 mg/day	H	Higher than with PHP
Gut		
1,25-dihydroxyvitamin D (calcitriol): 8–72 ng/ml	H	L/except in calcitriol-mediated HCM
Bone		
Resorption	Increased	Increased
Formation	Increased	Decreased

* Data from Fischbach, 1992; Meriney & Reeder, 1998.
cAMP—cyclic adenosine monophosphate; H—high; HCM—hypercalcemia of malignancy; iPTH—immunoreactive parathyroid hormone; iPTHrP—immunoreactive parathyroid hormone-related protein; L—low; N—normal; PHP—primary hyperparathyroidism

Note. Based on information from Bajournas, 1990; Block, 2001; Fischbach, 1992; Grill & Martin, 2000; Kvols, 2003; Meriney & Reeder, 1998; Smith, 2000; Solimando, 2001; Wimalawansa, 1995.

sedating medications, which may affect patients' level of consciousness, and encourage adequate salt intake to help to promote expansion of fluid volume. In general, restricting dietary calcium is unnecessary because gastrointestinal absorption of calcium is very low. The exception is certain lymphomas in which calcitriol mediates the hypercalcemia (Barnett, 1999; Morton & Ritch, 2002; NCI, 2004). When antihypercalcemic treatment becomes necessary, it focuses on (a) expanding fluid volume and correcting dehydration, (b) increasing renal excretion of calcium, (c) reducing calcium resorption from bone, and (d) controlling the underlying precipitating malignancy (Kaplan, 1994; Tummula, 1997). See Table 3-3 for an overview of antihypercalcemic therapy and associated nursing management.

Antineoplastic Therapy

Cancer-induced hypercalcemia is a reflection of tumor activity. The most effective long-term treatment of HCM is antineoplastic therapy targeted to the underlying malignancy, thus abolishing the mechanisms precipitating the hypercalcemia. Ablative surgery and/or appropriate cytotoxic therapies are initiated in patients for whom effective treatment exists, in combination with measures to enhance patients' renal function (Morton & Ritch, 2002).

Water and Electrolyte Repletion and Sodium Diuresis

The cornerstone of antihypercalcemic treatment is to reverse the dehydration, the depletion of intravascular volume, and the decreased glomerular filtration that result from the combined effects of polyuria, vomiting, anorexia, and nephrogenic diabetes insipidus (Fojo, 2005). Although oral hydration with 3–4 L of fluid per day may be sufficient for patients with asymptomatic or mild hypercalcemia, symptomatic patients require vigorous rehydration with IV normal saline. Infusion rates of 100–300 ml/hour can lower the serum calcium by 10%–40% over a 6–12-hour period (Yeung & Gagel, 2003). The rate of the saline infusion is dependent on the severity of the hypercalcemia, the degree of dehydration, and patients' cardiovascular status. During rehydration, nurses need to assess patients for fluid overload and renal function, with monitoring of intake and output and electrolytes. Closely monitor the laboratory values of BUN, creatinine, sodium, potassium, calcium, and magnesium at this time, and institute electrolyte replacement as necessary (Richerson, 2004).

The effect of the saline diuresis is increased calcium loss in the urine because sodium and calcium are excreted in parallel by the renal tubules. The sodium diuresis also increases the excretion of potassium and magnesium from the kidneys, and patients may require supplementation of these electrolytes to prevent cardiac arrhythmias, especially if they are taking digitalis (Glick & Glover, 1995; Morton & Ritch, 2002). Although rehydration is effective at increasing urinary output and renal calcium excretion, achieving normocalcemia through saline diuresis alone is unlikely (Hussein & Cullen, 2002; Morton & Ritch; Wimalawansa, 1995). After restoration of normal fluid volume, saline administration is maintained at 2.5–4 L per

Table 3-3. Overview of Interventions for Hypercalcemia of Malignancy (HCM)

Treatment Modality	Mechanism of Action	Dosage	Management/Side Effects
Tumor-specific treatment			
Treat underlying malignancy: Surgery, chemotherapy, hormonal therapy, immunotherapy, radiation therapy	Goals of antineoplastic therapy are to ablate disease and abolish precipitating factors.	—	Chemotherapy and hormonal therapies may be effective in producing normocalcemia in patients with multiple myeloma or breast cancer. Tamoxifen for bone metastases in breast cancer may cause transient increased serum calcium ("flare" reaction).
General measures			
Identify patients at risk.	Certain cancers are associated with increased risk for HCM (see Table 3-1).	—	Emphasize need for adequate oral hydration. Perform serial checks of serum calcium, phosphorus, and albumin levels.
Water and electrolyte repletion: Oral fluids Saline hydration	Expands fluid volume; reverses dehydration; improves renal function	Oral hydration 3–4 L/day Initial IV: 0.9% NaCl 100–300 ml/hr Maintenance IV: 2.5–4 L/day	Encourage oral fluids. Monitor intake and output for fluid overload. Monitor electrolytes for sodium, potassium, and magnesium depletion.
Sodium diuresis	Calcium is excreted in the urine alongside sodium.		Patients may need replacement of potassium and magnesium to prevent cardiac arrhythmias, especially with digitalis.
Loop diuretics (furosemide)	Blocks calcium and sodium reabsorption in loop of Henle	Given after rehydration IV: 20–40 mg q 12 hours Aggressive treatment: IV: 80–100 mg q 2–4 hours	Administer after volume expansion is achieved. Monitor intake and output and electrolytes. Requires intensive care setting to monitor central venous pressure and electrolytes Can cause hypovolemia and life-threatening decreases in potassium, phosphorus, and magnesium

(Continued on next page)

Table 3-3. Overview of Interventions for Hypercalcemia of Malignancy (HCM) (Continued)

Treatment Modality	Mechanism of Action	Dosage	Management/Side Effects
Mobilization	Weight-bearing activities decrease bone resorption.	—	Ambulate tid if possible. Initiate active resistive exercises with pain management for patients on bed rest. Evaluate for pathologic fracture if bone pain is present.
Drugs to avoid Thiazide diuretics	Increase renal calcium absorption	—	Withhold drugs that may potentiate hypercalcemia.
Nonsteroidal anti-inflammatory drugs (NSAIDs), H_2-receptor agonists	Inhibit renal blood flow		
Vitamins A and D	Increase bone resorption		
Dietary recommendations Maintain salt intake.	Sodium promotes fluid volume expansion.	—	Encourage adequate salt intake.
Dietary calcium restriction usually is not necessary.	Calcium is poorly absorbed from the gut.		Exception is hematologic malignancies with increased vitamin D synthesis.
Dialysis	Rapidly lowers serum calcium concentration but is short-acting	—	Used for select patients with preexisting renal failure who cannot tolerate saline diuresis

(Continued on next page)

Table 3-3. Overview of Interventions for Hypercalcemia of Malignancy (HCM) (Continued).

Treatment Modality	Mechanism of Action	Dosage	Management/Side Effects
Agents to inhibit bone resorption			
Bisphosphonates	All drugs in this class inhibit osteoclastic activity.	—	All bisphosphonates are potentially nephrotoxic. Administer saline hydration to maintain urine output at 2 L/day throughout treatment for all bisphosphonates.
Etidronate (Didronel®)	First generation No longer used in managing HCM	IV: 7.5 mg/kg/day over 2–4 hours for 3–7 days	Slight increase in blood urea nitrogen, creatinine; altered taste; transient fever, nausea, and hyperphosphatemia
Clodronate (Bonefos®) Available in Europe and Canada. No longer marketed in the United States.	Second generation	IV: 300–500 mg/day over 4 hours for 3–7 days; or 1,500 mg over 4–30 hours po: 1,600–2,400 mg/day In palliative setting, can be given as SC infusion	Mild local reaction Increased creatinine Decreased phosphorus
Pamidronate (Aredia®)	Second generation Approved for treating HCM Also indicated for osteolytic bone lesions in multiple myeloma and breast cancer in conjunction with standard antineoplastic therapy	HCM: IV: Single dose of 60–90 mg over 2–24 hours Dose may be repeated after a minimum of 7 days.	Monitor serum creatinine prior to each dose to assess renal function and the need for dose adjustment. Fever Local infusion site reaction Nausea Mild decrease in phosphorus, potassium, and magnesium ONJ associated with invasive dental procedures

(Continued on next page)

Table 3-3. Overview of Interventions for Hypercalcemia of Malignancy (HCM) *(Continued)*

Treatment Modality	Mechanism of Action	Dosage	Management/Side Effects
Zoledronate (zoledronic acid, Zometa®)	Third generation Most potent bisphosphonate now available Approved for treatment of HCM Also indicated for multiple myeloma and bone metastases from solid tumors in conjunction with standard antineoplastic therapy	HCM: IV: Single dose of 4 mg over no less than 15 minutes Dose may be repeated after a minimum of 7 days.	Monitor serum creatinine prior to each dose to assess renal function and the need for dose adjustment. Fever; flu-like syndrome; nausea and vomiting, infusion site reaction; mild decreased potassium, phosphorus, and magnesium ONJ associated with invasive dental procedures
Ibandronate (Bondronat®)	Third generation Licensed in Europe for HCM treatment Also indicated for bone metastases and prevention of skeletal events with breast cancer (e.g., pathologic fractures)	HCM: IV: Single dose of 2–4 mg over 2 hours Oral tablet available	Favorable renal safety profile; mandatory monitoring of renal function not required. Dose adjustments only required in patients with severe renal impairment. Drug-induced fever
Calcitonin—salmon (Calcimar®)	Thyroid hormone Rapid action; direct inhibition of osteoclast receptors; increased renal calcium excretion Small analgesic effect	SC or IM: 4–8 IU/kg q 6–12 hours for 2 days	Safe in dehydrated patients and those with preexisting renal failure Brief effect; resistance develops. Useful as rapid-acting adjunct in severe HCM; minimal toxicity, nausea, and hypersensitivity

(Continued on next page)

Table 3-3. Overview of Interventions for Hypercalcemia of Malignancy (HCM) (Continued)

Treatment Modality	Mechanism of Action	Dosage	Management/Side Effects
Plicamycin (mithramycin) No longer marketed in the United States	Direct toxic effect on osteoclasts; blocks RNA synthesis	IV: 25 mcg/kg over 4–6 hours (ideally through central line)	Avoid extravasation; drug is an irritant. Side effects: Nausea, vomiting, thrombocytopenia; coagulopathy; renal, hepatic, and neurotoxicities Used where HCM is resistant to safer drugs
Gallium nitrate (Ganite®)	Inhibits osteoclastic activity	Given after adequate rehydration IV: 200 mg/m²/day continuous for 5 days	Renal toxicity Administer saline hydration to maintain urine output at 2 L/day throughout treatment. Not marketed in the United States since 1995
NSAID Indomethacin (Indocin®)	Inhibits prostaglandins, which stimulates bone resorption	po: 75–100 mg/day in divided doses	Gastric upset is common. Give with food or antacids. Rarely is effective in clinical practice. May be useful in patients unable to tolerate other agents, especially where NSAIDs are part of pain palliation
Other hypocalcemic agents **Corticosteroids** Prednisone	Therapy of choice for steroid-sensitive, calcitriol-mediated malignancies: multiple myeloma and lymphomas	po: 40–100 mg/day IV: 200–400 mg/day for 3–5 days	Long-term use of steroids can cause hyperglycemia, hypokalemia, immunosuppression, Cushingoid symptoms, gastritis, osteoporosis, and muscle wasting.
Hydrocortisone	Inhibits vitamin D metabolism		No role in solid tumors

(Continued on next page)

Table 3-3. Overview of Interventions for Hypercalcemia of Malignancy (HCM) (Continued)

Treatment Modality	Mechanism of Action	Dosage	Management/Side Effects
Phosphates Neutra-Phos®	Used to correct hypophosphatemia, which stimulates increased calcium resorption from bone	po: 250–375 mg four times a day	Oral use: Diarrhea increases with dose; soft tissue calcifications IV phosphates have no role because of risks for extraskeletal calcium precipitation and renal insufficiency.

IM—intramuscular; IV—intravenous; ONJ—osteonecrosis of the jaw; po—by mouth; SC—subcutaneous

Note. Based on information from Body, 2004; Davidson, 2001; Fojo, 2005; Hussein & Cullen, 2002; Morton & Lipton, 2004; Novartis Pharmaceuticals Corp., 2005a, 2005b; Smith, 2000; Tummula, 1997; von Moos, 2005; Wilkes et al., 2001.

day with careful monitoring of fluid and electrolyte status (Kaye, 1995; Tummula, 1997). Patients also should increase their oral fluid intake.

Loop Diuretics (Furosemide)

Once hypercalcemic patients have rehydrated sufficiently to maintain a urine output of 3–4 L per day, a loop diuretic, such as furosemide, may be added to augment the effects of saline rehydration. Loop diuretics block calcium and sodium reabsorption in the ascending loop of Henle, further increasing calcium excretion. Moderate doses of furosemide (20–40 mg every 12 hours) may be useful in preventing or managing fluid overload in adequately hydrated patients (Hussein & Cullen, 2002). Clinicians should reserve aggressive treatment with high doses of furosemide or other powerful loop diuretics only for acute situations or fluid overload. High doses are dangerous in the presence of compromised renal function and can exacerbate hypercalcemia by causing hypovolemia (Morton & Lipton, 2004; Wimalawansa, 1995). In an intensive care setting, where nurses can closely monitor central venous pressures and urinary electrolyte losses, administering furosemide in large doses (80–100 mg every two hours) can be effective in decreasing serum calcium (Grill & Martin, 2000; Wimalawansa). Obtaining serial urine volumes and electrolyte measurements is critical with this aggressive treatment to identify potential hypovolemia and electrolyte losses that can lead to hypokalemia, hypophosphatemia, and hypomagnesemia, which can be life-threatening (Hussein & Cullen; NCI, 2004). The availability of safer, more potent antiresorptive agents, such as bisphosphonates, has made the use of loop diuretics debatable in HCM management (Grill & Martin; Morton & Lipton; Tummula, 1997). Thiazide diuretics are contraindicated because they increase renal tubular absorption of calcium and may exacerbate hypercalcemia (Hussein & Cullen; Richerson, 2004; Smith, 2000).

Antiresorptive Therapy

Bisphosphonates

Bisphosphonate therapy, along with volume repletion, is the current standard of care for the treatment and prevention of malignancy-associated hypercalcemia (Fojo, 2005; Gucalp, 2004). The bisphosphonates have supplanted all other drugs in the management of HCM, except with steroid-sensitive malignancies, such as myeloma and lymphoma (Body, 2004). Bisphosphonates are simple chemical compounds that have a composition similar to pyrophosphate in bone. They possess an inherent ability to inhibit bone resorption by altering osteoclast activity, and they provide an antitumor effect as well. Bisphosphonates are poorly absorbed from the gastrointestinal tract after oral administration and are cleared from the body via renal excretion (Berenson, 2001; Fojo). Nephrotoxicity is the most significant side effect of bisphosphonates and may be related to calcium-phosphonate crystallization in the blood and the rapidity of the infusion (Block, 2001). Assessment of renal function by measuring serum creatinine is required prior to initiation of bisphosphonate therapy and prior to each dose. All patients receiving bisphosphonates should receive sufficient hydration to maintain a daily urine output of 2 L throughout treatment (Wilkes et al., 2001). As a group, bisphosphonates are well tolerated but frequently are associated with a low-grade fever and transient local infusion reactions that diminish with subsequent treatments (Berenson, 2005).

Osteonecrosis of the jaw (ONJ) recently has been recognized as a potential risk of bisphosphonate therapy. Although little is known of the pathogenesis of ONJ, it has been reported in patients who were receiving chemotherapy and corticosteroids in addition to bisphosphonates and had undergone invasive dental procedures. It now is recommended that dental procedures requiring bone healing should be completed before beginning IV bisphosphonate therapy and that patients maintain good dental and oral hygiene throughout treatment. There is no evidence that interrupting bisphosphonate therapy to perform invasive dental procedures will lower the risk of ONJ; conservative dental management is advised for these patients (Ruggiero et al., 2006). Several generations of bisphosphonates have been used over the years in HCM treatment.

Etidronate was the first bisphosphonate to receive U.S. Food and Drug Administration (FDA) approval for the treatment of HCM. It is administered as an IV infusion over two to four hours at a maximum dose of 7.5 mg/kg/day, which is repeated over three to seven days (Tummula, 1997). Studies demonstrated that etidronate decreased serum calcium concentration by more than 1 mg/dl per dose and achieved normocalcemia in 40%–92% of cases over several days. Typical side effects of etidronate include slightly increased serum creatinine and BUN, transient fever, rash, metallic taste, and transient elevation of serum phosphorus (Davidson, 2001). Because of its inconvenient dosing schedule and variable duration of action, healthcare providers no longer use etidronate in the management of hypercalcemia (Morton & Lipton, 2004).

Clodronate is a second-generation bisphosphonate with intermediate potency. A single IV infusion of 1,500 mg administered over 4–30 hours has been found to be as effective as daily 300 mg infusions repeated for five days; clodronate achieved normocalcemia in 50%–80% of cases with the single-dose schedule. An oral formulation also is available (Body, 2004). An advantage to clodronate is that it also can be given as a subcutaneous infusion in the palliative care setting (Kovacs et al., 1995). The principal side effect of clodronate is mild local reaction, but hypophosphatemia also has occurred (Fojo, 2005). Parenteral clodronate is used in Europe and Canada but is no longer marketed in the United States following reports of leukemia in patients receiving the drug (Agraharkar & Dellinger, 2004).

Pamidronate, the first of the more-potent group of nitrogen-containing bisphosphonates (aminobisphosphonates), received FDA approval for HCM treatment in 1991. Studies have demonstrated that it is more effective than clodronate or etidronate, restoring normocalcemia in 90% of patients for a significantly longer period. A 60 mg dose of pamidronate administered as a single-dose IV infusion over 2–24 hours is effective for patients with moderate hypercalcemia. For more severe cases and those with a humoral component, a single dose of 90 mg is infused over 2–24 hours (Fojo, 2005; Novartis Pharmaceuticals Corp. [Novartis], 2005a). Pamidronate decreases serum calcium levels by more than 1 mg/dl per dose and can be repeated weekly if necessary (Davidson, 2001). A minimum of seven days should elapse to allow for full response to the initial dose of pamidronate before retreatment at the same dosing schedule is considered. Nurses should monitor serum creatinine before each dose to assess renal function, and patients should maintain urine output at 2 L per day throughout treatment (Novartis, 2005a). Fever is a frequent side effect, and induration and pain at the injection site are common with the 90 mg dose. Transient decreases in serum levels of potassium, phosphate, and magnesium may occur but are rarely of clinical significance (Davidson; Richerson, 2004; Wilkes et al., 2001). ONJ, associated with invasive dental procedures, has been reported in patients with cancer who have received pamidronate as a component of their therapy. A dental examination, oral preventive care, and completion of invasive dental procedures are recommended prior to initiating pamidronate treatment (FDA Center for Drug Evaluation and Research, 2005; Novartis, 2005a; Ruggiero et al., 2006).

Zoledronate is a third-generation, nitrogen-containing bisphosphonate that received FDA approval for HCM treatment in 2001. It currently is the most potent bisphosphonate available. Comparison studies have shown that zoledronate is significantly more effective than pamidronate in terms of higher response rate, faster onset, and longer duration of action (Major et al., 2001). Zoledronate is associated with renal toxicity; healthcare providers should consider instituting therapy in patients with HCM complicated by severe renal impairment only after evaluating the risks and benefits of treatment. The recommended dose of zoledronate is 4 mg delivered as a single-dose IV infusion over no less than 15 minutes. Retreatment at the same dose may be considered after a minimum period of seven days to allow for full response to the initial dose. Prior to retreatment with zoledronate, nurses should assess renal function by carefully monitoring serum creatinine; dose reduction or withholding of treatment is based on the extent of renal dysfunction as indicated by increases in serum creatinine. Patients should maintain hydration to sustain a urine output of 2 L per day throughout treatment (Novartis, 2005b). Common side effects of zoledronate include fever, flu-like syndrome, nausea and vomiting, and infusion site reaction. Mild decreases in potassium, phosphorus, and magnesium levels may occur as well (Davidson, 2001; Wilkes et al., 2001). In addition, ONJ has been reported in patients with cancer who have received bisphosphonates as a component of their therapy. As with pamidronate, patients should have pretreatment dental examinations and necessary dental care completed prior to initiating zoledronate therapy (FDA Center for Drug Evaluation and Research, 2005; Novartis, 2005b). Invasive dental procedures should be avoided while patients are receiving bisphosphonate therapy. In these patients, interrupting therapy to perform dental care that requires bone healing does not preclude the risk of ONJ (Ruggiero et al., 2006).

Ibandronate is a third-generation bisphosphonate that was licensed in Europe in 2003 for treating HCM (Body, 2004; von Moos, 2005). It has been shown to be approximately 50 times more potent than pamidronate in animal models. A dose of 6 mg administered as a two-hour IV infusion normalized serum calcium in 77% of patients (Fojo, 2005; Morton & Lipton, 2004). A phase II study demonstrated that patients with myeloma or breast cancer had a better hypocalcemic response to ibandronate than those with other tumor types (Body, 2004). Studies have shown that ibandronate has a renal safety profile comparable to that of placebo and does not require mandatory monitoring of renal function prior to each infusion. Only patients with severe renal impairment require dose reductions (von Moos). Reported side effects include fever, hypocalcemia, hypophosphatemia, and, less commonly, flu-like symptoms and gastrointestinal disturbance (Hussein & Cullen, 2002).

Bisphosphonate Therapy for Metastatic Bone Disease

In addition to being the current standard of care for HCM, bisphosphonate therapy has an important role in the management of metastatic bone disease and supportive cancer care. Bisphosphonates have demonstrated antitumor effects and significant reduction in the incidence of or delay in the onset of bone lesions in multiple myeloma, breast cancer, prostate cancer, and other solid tumors. Bisphosphonates also can reduce bone pain in at least 50% of patients (Berenson, 2001; Body, 2003; Gucalp, 2004). In conjunction with standard antineoplastic therapy, zoledronate has approval for the treatment of patients with multiple myeloma and for patients with documented bone metastases secondary to all solid tumor types (Berenson, 2005; Novartis, 2005b). Pamidronate is approved for the treatment of osteolytic bone lesions secondary to multiple myeloma and breast cancer in conjunction with standard antineoplastic therapy and has demonstrated long-term effectiveness in those patients (Major et al., 2001; Novartis, 2005a). In Europe, ibandronate is indicated for treating bone metastases and preventing bone complications such as pathologic fractures in patients with breast cancer. It is available as an IV infusion or a daily oral tablet; both formulations have demonstrated similar efficacy (von Moos, 2005).

Calcitonin

Calcitonin is a peptide hormone secreted by the thyroid gland and is one of the oldest drugs used to treat HCM. It produces antihypercalcemic effects by directly inhibiting osteoclastic bone resorption and increasing renal calcium excretion. It has a rapid onset of action and lowers the plasma calcium by approximately 2–3 mg/dl within two to six hours of administration (Davidson, 2001; Fojo, 2005; Tummula, 1997). Calcitonin is especially safe in the acute management of hypercalcemia in patients with renal or cardiac failure who cannot tolerate large sodium loads (Grill & Martin, 2000; Hussein & Cullen, 2002). It is administered by either a subcutaneous or intramuscular route in doses of 4–8 IU/kg body weight every 6–12 hours over two days (Davidson; Morton & Lipton, 2004; Tummula). Common side effects include nausea, rash, flushing, and malaise (Davidson). Calcitonin is not appropriate for long-term management of HCM because most patients quickly become resistant to its action. In the past, concomitant administration of corticosteroids was used to reverse resistance to calcitonin and prolong its action, but with the availability of effective bisphosphonates, healthcare providers rarely use the combination of calcitonin and corticosteroids (Davidson). The present role of calcitonin is as a rapidly acting adjunct in patients with severe HCM given while waiting for more potent inhibitors of bone resorption, such as bisphosphonates, to demonstrate an effect (Fojo; Grill & Martin; Morton & Lipton). In the palliative setting, studies have shown parenteral calcitonin to provide a strong analgesic effect in reducing the pain associated with bone metastases and pathologic fractures (Kovacs et al., 1995).

Plicamycin

Before bisphosphonates became available, healthcare providers frequently used plicamycin, a cytotoxic antibiotic, to treat cancer-induced hypercalcemia. Plicamycin produces a direct toxic effect on osteoclasts by blocking RNA synthesis and is more potent than calcitonin. The usual dose is 25 mcg/kg/day administered by slow infusion over four to six hours, ideally via a central IV line because plicamycin is an irritant drug (Davidson, 2001). Plicamycin reduces serum calcium levels within 12 hours of treatment, reaching a peak effect at 48 hours (Fojo, 2005). Plicamycin is used with caution because it has significant side effects that are cumulative with repeated doses, such as thrombocytopenia, nausea and vomiting, hypotension, and renal, hepatic, and neurotoxicities (Barnett, 1999; Grill & Martin, 2000; Tummula, 1997). Although safer and more effective bisphosphonates have replaced plicamycin as first-line antiresorptive therapy, the drug is effective at restoring normocalcemia in approximately 80% of patients, and many consider its toxic effects to be overstated (Morton & Lipton, 2004). Plicamycin has been used to treat patients whose HCM is resistant to safer drugs; however, it is currently not marketed in the United States.

Gallium Nitrate

Gallium nitrate originally was developed as a chemotherapeutic agent and incidentally produced hypocalcemic effects in people being treated for lymphoma (Morton & Lipton, 2004; Tummula, 1997). Researchers do not fully understand its mechanism of action, but it appears to involve multiple effects on the skeleton without being cytotoxic to bone (Leyland-Jones, 2004). Randomized studies have shown gallium nitrate to be significantly superior to calcitonin, etidronate, and pamidronate; it restores normocalcemia in 75%–85% of patients (Hussein & Cullen, 2002; Leyland-Jones). Gallium nitrate is administered by continuous IV infusion over five days in a daily dose of 200 mg/m^2 (Myers, 2001). Nephrotoxicity is a major side effect, occurring in approximately 10% of patients (Fojo, 2005), and the drug should be administered only after adequate saline rehydration to maintain urinary output at 2 L per day during treatment. Avoid concurrent use of nephrotoxic drugs (Wilkes et al., 2001). Other potential side effects include nausea, vomiting, and hypophosphatemia (Tummula). Although drawbacks to its use include the five-day administration schedule and its potential for nephrotoxicity, gallium nitrate can be effective in patients who are refractory to bisphosphonates, particularly those with recurrent HCM (Fojo; Gucalp, 2004).

Prostaglandin Synthesis Inhibitors

Prostaglandin E$_2$ is known to stimulate bone resorption in breast cancer. Although animal models have demonstrated some benefit with prostaglandin synthesis inhibitors, such as indomethacin and aspirin, in clinical practice, they are rarely effective in lowering serum calcium and have not shown a benefit in metastatic bone disease associated with breast cancer. Prostaglandin synthesis inhibitors sometimes are useful for patients who are unable to tolerate other agents, particularly in cases where nonsteroidal drugs are part of palliative pain management (Morton & Lipton, 2004).

Other Antihypercalcemic Therapies

Corticosteroids

Corticosteroids frequently are employed in managing HCM, despite strong evidence that their usefulness is limited (Block, 2001; Morton & Lipton, 2004). They have no role in solid tumors; their predominant use is with steroid-sensitive hematologic malignancies associated with calcitriol-mediated hypercalcemia, such as lymphoma, leukemia, and multiple myeloma (Block; Davidson, 2001; Tummula, 1997). Corticosteroids, such as prednisone, act to inhibit vitamin D metabolism, blocking calcitriol-induced gastrointestinal calcium absorption and increasing urinary calcium excretion. They also comprise part of the antineoplastic regimens used for lymphoid malignancies and multiple myeloma (Morton & Lipton). Following initiation of corticosteroid therapy, the maximal antihypercalcemic effect does not occur for days to weeks. The minimum effective dose is uncertain, but generally the given dose is 40–100 mg prednisone per day (Morton & Lipton; Tummula). Long-term use of steroids can produce undesirable side effects, including immunosuppression, hyperglycemia, hypokalemia, gastrointestinal hemorrhage, bone destruction, and muscle wasting (Davidson).

Phosphates

Oral phosphates are effective in treating mild to moderate hypercalcemia, particularly when hypophosphatemia is present. Hypophosphatemia stimulates increased osteoclastic activity, leading to calcium resorption from bone. Oral phosphate usually is taken in doses of 250–375 mg four times a day to minimize the potential for hyperphosphatemia (Hussein & Cullen, 2002) but is contraindicated with renal failure or when serum phosphorus is > 3.8 mg/dl (Myers, 2001; Smith, 2000). Diarrhea is a dose-limiting side effect of oral phosphate administration but initially may counteract the constipation that patients experience secondary to hypercalcemia (Hussein & Cullen). Patients should avoid magnesium- and aluminum-containing antacids during therapy because they bind to phosphate (Agraharkar & Dellinger, 2004; Smith). IV phosphate is very effective at rapidly decreasing serum calcium levels but also is very dangerous because of the risk of hypotension, renal failure, severe hypocalcemia, and precipitation of calcium-phosphate complexes in tissues throughout the body. The use of IV phosphate, therefore, is restricted to extreme, life-threatening HCM not responding to any other form of therapy (Tummula, 1997).

Dialysis

Peritoneal or hemodialysis can be a rapid and effective initial method for removing serum calcium from patients with renal failure who cannot undergo saline diuresis. Dialysis can remove 200–2,000 mg of calcium in 24–48 hours but is effective for only brief periods. Patients lose large quantities of phosphate, as well as calcium, during dialysis; therefore, nurses should monitor serum phosphate levels after each session and initiate replacement in the dialysate or diet as necessary (Hussein & Cullen, 2002). Dialysis usually is a consideration for only those patients whose malignancies are expected to respond favorably to antineoplastic treatment. Occasionally, patients with severe acute HCM may require dialysis on an emergent basis to lower serum calcium levels in order to prevent cardiac arrhythmias or severe neurologic complications (Wimalawansa, 1995).

Mobilization

Whenever possible, encourage weight-bearing ambulation to prevent increased bone resorption of calcium resulting from immobility. For patients on bed rest, active resistive exercises coupled with a pain management program may be helpful in controlling the loss of calcium from bone (Richerson, 2004).

Dietary Restriction

Dietary restriction of calcium usually is not necessary in treating HCM because negative feedback mechanisms reduce calcium absorption from the gut in most hypercalcemic patients. The exception is patients who are experiencing calcitriol-mediated hypercalcemia, in which case patients should avoid dietary calcium.

Future Directions

Although bisphosphonates have supplanted all other therapeutic agents and can normalize calcium in more than 90% of patients with HCM, they are not as effective when hypercalcemia recurs (Body, 2000). New therapies that show promise in treating HCM by inhibiting tumor-induced bone resorption are in early stages of development and focus on interrupting the RANKL/RANK signaling pathway and neutralizing the effects of PTHrP (Hofbauer & Schoppet, 2004; Rodan & Martin, 2000; Yeung & Gagel, 2003). One approach under investigation is the use of soluble recombinant OPG. OPG is the natural decoy receptor for RANK and is a powerful inhibitor of bone resorption. It prevents RANKL from binding with its receptor (RANK) and stimulating osteoclastic activity (Body, 2000; Mundy, 2002). (See Figure 3-4 and earlier discussion of bone remodeling for a fuller description.) Preliminary studies of recombinant OPG have shown that it inhibited osteoclast formation and lowered serum calcium concentration (Body, 2000). Research into the use of antibodies against RANKL and the use of a RANK-type decoy molecule that acts in identical fashion to OPG may be promising (Mundy, 2002). Another therapeutic approach involves using humanized PTHrP monoclonal antibodies to counteract the effects of PTHrP in the pathogenesis of HCM (Yeung & Gagel). Further understanding of these key molecules ultimately will lead to new ways to treat hypercalcemia and limit bone destruction by metastatic tumors.

Nursing Management

Nursing management in the care of patients with cancer-induced hypercalcemia is multifaceted and is directed at prevention, early detection, treatment management, and support of patients and family. Table 3-4 presents an overview of nursing management. Whatever the patient setting—acute care, ambulatory care, home care, or palliative care—nurses must be able to identify patients whose malignancies place them at increased risk for hypercalcemia. Those patients require close observation, continual assessment of their physical and mental status, and frequent monitoring of their levels of serum calcium, albumin, and phosphate to distinguish between the effects of their disease and treatment and the early signs and symptoms of developing hypercalcemia. Although cancer-induced hypercalcemia may not be preventable, early recognition and prompt treatment may deter it from becoming a life-threatening oncologic emergency. Additionally, once an individual has experienced HCM, the chance of future recurrence increases.

Patients with mild or asymptomatic HCM and those who have achieved normocalcemia may be followed on an outpatient basis. Patients who are receiving hypocalcemic therapy should have their serum calcium levels and renal function monitored daily until the calcium concentration normalizes (Moore, 1998). Initially, during the volume expansion and diuresis phase of treatment, potassium and magnesium levels may decline steeply as the calcium is corrected and the glomerular filtration rate increases. Patients may require supplementation of potassium and magnesium, as well as phosphorus if serum phosphate levels fall in response to potent antiresorptive therapy (Morton & Ritch, 2002). Once serum calcium levels are normalized, nurses should perform weekly measurements to assess the need for further antihypercalcemic treatment. The need for other laboratory tests depends on the individual's clinical condition and response to therapy (Morton & Ritch).

Supportive care of hypercalcemic patients focuses on multiple issues. Nurses must manage fluid and electrolyte imbalances; evaluate treatment effectiveness and side effects; and monitor patients for changes in mental status, gastrointestinal disturbances, and alterations in renal and cardiac function. They also should establish an appropriate weight-bearing or exercise regimen

Table 3-4. Nursing Management of Hypercalcemia of Malignancy (HCM)

Issue	Management Measures
Early detection of HCM	Identify patients at risk: Obtain history related to type of cancer, presence of bone metastases, and treatment regimens. Check vital signs, serum electrolytes, blood chemistries (particularly calcium, phosphorus, albumin, blood urea nitrogen [BUN], and creatinine levels), urine calcium, and electrocardiogram, if done. Review medications and supplements to identify drugs and vitamins that may contribute to hypercalcemia and should be discontinued (e.g., thiazide diuretics, vitamins A and D). Evaluate for early signs of hypercalcemia (see Figure 3-7). Conduct physical assessment, looking for signs of dehydration: Poor skin turgor; dry mucous membranes; rapid, weak pulse; weight loss; and orthostatic hypotension. Assess muscle strength and neurologic/mental status; record baseline.
Prevention Measures High-risk patients	
• Hydration	Explain need for maintaining oral fluid intake of 3 L per day.
• Mobilization	Emphasize the importance of weight-bearing activity. Establish an activity and exercise regimen based on the patient's physical ability and the physician's orders. Patients unable to ambulate can be helped to stand at the bedside four to six times a day. Encourage patients at home to ambulate as much as possible. Provide assistive devices as necessary: cane, walker, handrails, etc. Patients on bed rest: Provide active resistive exercises every hour while awake; couple with a pain management program if necessary. Pain management: Achieve a narcotic-sedation level that promotes increased physical activity rather than oversedation.
Supportive nursing care	Supportive care for patients with HCM focuses on 　Evaluating treatment effectiveness and side effects 　Managing fluid and electrolyte imbalances 　Assessing mental status changes, gastrointestinal disturbances, and alterations in renal and cardiac function 　Instituting safety measures, pain management, and comfort measures 　Providing emotional support to patients and caregivers.
Antihypercalcemic therapy	Administer fluids and hypocalcemic agents as ordered, and observe for side effects (see Table 3-3). Monitor daily serum calcium levels to evaluate treatment response. Observe for clinical manifestations related to HCM (see Figure 3-7). Assess for bone pain and pathologic fractures; administer analgesics as ordered.

(Continued on next page)

Table 3-4. Nursing Management of Hypercalcemia of Malignancy (HCM) (Continued)

Issue	Management Measures

Fluid and electrolyte balance	Mild HCM: Encourage oral fluid intake of 2–4 L/day if possible.
	Correction of fluid volume depletion
	    Administer saline infusion as ordered.
	    Continue to monitor blood pressure, pulse, and breath sounds.
	    Measure intake/output q 2 hours for first 24 hours, then every 4–8 hours.
	    Check for signs of fluid overload (e.g., rales, shortness of breath, weight gain, peripheral edema, distended neck veins) every 4 hours and as necessary.
	Record daily weights.
	Administer loop diuretics after rehydration, as ordered.
	Thiazide diuretics are contraindicated; they impair renal excretion of calcium.
	Monitor electrolytes daily for decreases in serum sodium, potassium, calcium, phosphorus, and magnesium.
	Correct hypokalemia, hypophosphatemia, and hypomagnesemia, as ordered.

Renal function	Assess for diminishing renal function: increases in BUN and creatinine; oliguria; and anuria.
Cardiac changes	Monitor heart rate and rhythm for bradycardia and arrhythmias. Observe electrocardiogram for delayed cardiac conduction. Reduce digoxin doses as ordered.
Mental status alterations	Monitor for lethargy, restlessness, disorientation, personality changes, and progressive changes in level of consciousness. Institute falls, safety, and seizure precautions as per protocols.
Gastrointestinal disturbances	Administer antiemetics for nausea and vomiting and stool softeners and laxatives for constipation, as ordered.

Patient and caregiver teaching and advocacy	Teaching focuses on several areas of self-care, including
	    Understanding preventive measures (i.e., ensuring adequate fluid and salt intake, maintaining weight-bearing activities) and the importance of early treatment interventions
	    Recognizing/reporting conditions that prevent oral intake or increase fluid loss (e.g., confusion, vomiting, diarrhea, fever)
	    Recognizing/reporting manifestations of HCM (e.g., anorexia, lethargy, nausea, vomiting, constipation, excessive thirst)
	    Understanding the importance of following prescribed medical regimens; avoiding drugs and supplements that potentiate HCM; and maintaining follow-up schedules
	    Managing pain and coping with changes in mental status
	Nurses provide emotional support, help to identify and support coping strategies, communicate acceptance of patients' beliefs, and act as patient advocates in discussions related to discontinuing antihypercalcemic treatment, if applicable.

Note. Based on information from Agraharkar & Dellinger, 2004; Barnett, 1999; Kaplan, 1994; Meriney & Reeder, 1998; Moore, 1998; Morton & Lipton, 2004; Myers, 2001; National Cancer Institute, 2004; Richerson, 2004; Smith, 2000.

for patients; institute safety measures and fall-prevention strategies; manage pain; and provide comfort and emotional support to patients and caregivers (see Table 3-4).

End-of-Life Considerations

Patients and caregivers may have to face profound decisions regarding continuation of antihypercalcemic treatment. If antineoplastic therapies have been adequate and yet hypercalcemia develops, this usually indicates tumor progression. If antineoplastic therapies have not been effective in controlling the precipitating malignancy, hypercalcemia is likely to recur. Both of these situations portend a shortened life span. Death usually results from renal failure or cardiac arrhythmias secondary to hypercalcemia or from disease progression (Yeung & Gagel, 2003). Severe hypercalcemia frequently depresses cerebral function, so the decision not to begin treatment or to discontinue treatment may be appropriate in order to spare the hypercalcemic patient from further suffering and futile treatments, especially if it is expected that the patient will rapidly become comatose and die without pain (Coward, 1986; Yeung & Gagel).

In recent years, the mentality regarding treatment interventions at the end of life has been changing because of the availability of potent, well-tolerated drugs such as bisphosphonates. Antihypercalcemic therapy can ameliorate or reverse the many unpleasant and distressing side effects, such as anorexia, nausea, vomiting, constipation, and confusion, that accompany the hypercalcemic state (Kovacs et al., 1995; Moore, 1998). Bisphosphonates and calcitonin also provide an analgesic effect that reduces bone pain (Kovacs et al.). If patients respond poorly to bisphosphonate therapy, alternative antiresorptive treatments using gallium nitrate can be attempted (Morton & Lipton, 2004). Second-line, noninvasive therapies, such as subcutaneous calcitonin and oral bisphosphonates, also are an option in the palliative care setting, and their use can improve end-of-life quality (Kovacs et al.). Nurses can provide patients with comfort measures to alleviate distressing symptoms while offering their caregivers continuing support, reassurance, and solace as they cope with decisions about continuing treatment and face the progressive deterioration and the end of their loved one's life.

Patient and Caregiver Education

Education of patients and caregivers focuses on providing them with information about strategies designed to prevent, recognize, and manage the manifestations of HCM. Nurses teach them to (a) practice preventive measures, such as maintaining adequate hydration and safe weight-bearing activities, (b) recognize and report any condition, such as diarrhea or vomiting, that can contribute to fluid loss and exacerbate dehydration, and (c) recognize and report the nonspecific manifestations of hypercalcemia, such as anorexia, nausea, constipation, and lethargy. Teaching of safety precautions should include prevention of falls, the need for close observation of confused or restless patients, and the importance of careful movement and transfers of bedbound patients to decrease the risk of pathologic fractures (Myers, 2001). Patients and caregivers must recognize the importance of taking medications as prescribed and avoiding drugs and vitamin supplements that can potentiate hypercalcemia. Nurses also instruct them in methods for managing pain, ideally without oversedating hypercalcemic patients.

Conclusion

HCM results from disruption of normal calcium homeostasis and impaired renal excretion of calcium. Early signs and symptoms of hypercalcemia are general and nonspecific and can be difficult to distinguish from disease- or cytotoxic treatment–related side effects. It is essential for nurses to recognize which malignancies confer increased risk and to have an understanding of the pathologic mechanisms that can precipitate and/or contribute to HCM. Successful clinical management of HCM depends on correcting the abnormalities of bone, kidney, and intestinal calcium absorption associated with HCM. Essential components of antihypercalcemic treatment include instituting preventive measures, controlling the precipitating malignancy, reversing dehydration, and inhibiting bone resorption. Knowledge of the rationales for the various treatment modalities will assist nurses in implementing antihypercalcemic treatments, evaluating treatment effectiveness and side effects, and instituting pain management and safety and comfort measures. Although cancer-induced hypercalcemia may not be preventable, early recognition and appropriate treatment may deter it from becoming a life-threatening oncologic complication.

References

Agraharkar, M., & Dellinger, D.O. (2004, May). *Hypercalcemia*. Retrieved January 22, 2005, from http://www.emedicine.com/med/topic1068.htm

Bajournas, D.R. (1990). Clinical manifestations of cancer-related hypercalcemia. *Seminars in Oncology, 17*(2 Suppl. 5), 16–25.

Barnett, M.L. (1999). Hypercalcemia. *Seminars in Oncology Nursing, 15,* 190–201.

Berenson, J.R. (2001). Advances in the biology and treatment of myeloma bone disease. *American Journal of Health-System Pharmacy, 58*(Suppl. 3), S16–S20.

Berenson, J.R. (2005). Recommendations for zoledronic acid treatment of patients with bone metastases. *Oncologist, 10,* 52–62.

Block, J.B. (2001). Paraneoplastic syndromes. In C.H. Haskell (Ed.), *Cancer treatment* (5th ed., pp. 302–326). Philadelphia: Saunders.

Body, J.J. (2000). Current and future directions in medical therapy: Hypercalcemia. *Cancer, 88*(Suppl. 12), 3054–3058.

Body, J.J. (2003). Effectiveness and cost of bisphosphonate therapy in tumor bone disease. *Cancer, 97*(Suppl. 3), 859–865.

Body, J.J. (2004). Hypercalcemia of malignancy. *Seminars in Nephrology, 24*, 48–54.

Coleman, R.E. (2001). Metastatic bone disease: Clinical features, pathophysiology and treatment strategies. *Cancer Treatment Reviews, 27*, 165–176.

Coleman, R.E., & Rubens, R.D. (2004). Bone metastases. In M.D. Abeloff, J.O. Armitage, J.E. Niederhuber, M.B. Kasten, & W.G. McKenna (Eds.), *Clinical oncology* (3rd ed., pp. 1091–1128). Philadelphia: Elsevier Churchill Livingstone.

Coward, D.D. (1986). Cancer-induced hypercalcemia. *Cancer Nursing, 9*, 125–132.

Davidson, T.G. (2001). Conventional treatment of hypercalcemia of malignancy. *American Journal of Health-System Pharmacy, 58*(Suppl. 3), S8–S15.

Davis, E.O. (2004). Stuck on the TRAIL of osteoclast differentiation. *Blood, 104*, 1914–1915.

Fischbach, F.T. (1992). *A manual of laboratory and diagnostic tests* (4th ed.). Philadelphia: Lippincott.

Fojo, A.T. (2005). Metabolic emergencies. In V.T. DeVita, S. Hellman, & S.A. Rosenberg (Eds.), *Cancer: Principles and practice of oncology* (7th ed., pp. 2292–2300). Philadelphia: Lippincott Williams & Wilkins.

Food and Drug Administration Center for Drug Evaluation and Research. (2005, March 4). *Aredia/Zometa: Questions to the committee.* Retrieved August 12, 2005, from http://www.fda .gov/ohrms/dockets/ac/05/questions/2005-4095Q2_02_Zometa-Aredia-Questions.pdf

Glick, J.H., & Glover, D. (1995). Oncologic emergencies: Hypercalcemia. In G.P. Murphy, W. Lawrence, & E.L. Raymond (Eds.), *American Cancer Society textbook of clinical oncology* (2nd ed., pp. 597–618). Atlanta, GA: American Cancer Society.

Grill, V., & Martin, T.J. (2000). Hypercalcemia of malignancy. *Reviews in Endocrine and Metabolic Disorders, 1*, 253–263.

Gucalp, R. (2004). Hypercalcemia and gallium nitrate. *Journal of Supportive Oncology, 2*, 518–520.

Guise, T.A., & Mundy, G.R. (1998). Cancer and bone. *Endocrine Reviews, 19*, 18–54.

Gutierrez, G.E., Poser, J.W., Katz, M.S., Yates, A.J., Henry, H.L., & Mundy, G.R. (1990). Mechanisms of hypercalcemia of malignancy. *Bailliere's Clinical Endocrinology and Metabolism, 4*, 119–138.

Guyton, A.C. (1991). *Textbook of medical physiology* (8th ed.). Philadelphia: Saunders.

Hemphill, R.H. (2005, January). *Hypercalcemia.* Retrieved August 12, 2005, from http://www .emedicine.com/emerg/topic260.htm

Heys, S.D., Smith, I.A., & Eremin, O. (1998). Hypercalcemia in patients with cancer: Aetiology and treatment. *European Journal of Surgical Oncology, 24*, 139–142.

Hofbauer, L.Z., & Schoppet, M. (2004). Clinical implications of the osteoprotegerin/RANKL/RANK system for bone and vascular diseases. *JAMA, 292*, 490–495.

Hussein, M., & Cullen, K. (2002). Metabolic emergencies. In P.G. Johnston & R.A.J. Spence (Eds.), *Oncologic emergencies* (pp. 51–73). New York: Oxford University Press.

Ikeda, K., Ohno, H., Hane, M., Yokoi, H., Okada, M., Honma, T., et al. (1994). Development of a sensitive two-site immunoradiometric assay for parathyroid hormone-related peptide: Evidence for elevated levels in plasma from patients with adult-T-cell leukemia/lymphoma and B-cell lymphoma. *Journal of Clinical Endocrinology and Metabolism, 79*, 1322–1327.

Kaplan, M. (1994). Hypercalcemia of malignancy: A review of advances in pathophysiology. *Oncology Nursing Forum, 21*, 1039–1046.

Kaye, T.B. (1995). Hypercalcemia: How to pinpoint the cause and customize treatment. *Postgraduate Medicine, 97*(1), 153–160.

Keenan, A.K., & Wickham, R.S. (2005). Hypercalcemia. In C.H. Yarbro, M.H. Frogge, & M. Goodman (Eds.), *Cancer nursing: Principles and practice* (6th ed., pp. 791–807). Sudbury, MA: Jones and Bartlett.

Kovacs, C.S., MacDonald, S.M., Chik, C.L., & Bruera, E. (1995). Hypercalcemia of malignancy in the palliative care patient: A treatment strategy. *Journal of Pain and Symptom Management, 10*, 224–232.

Kvols, L.K. (2003). Neoplasms of the diffuse endocrine system. In D.W. Kufe, R.E. Pollock, R.R. Weichselbaum, R.C. Bast, T. Gansler, J.F. Holland, et al. (Eds.), *Holland-Frei cancer medicine* (6th ed., pp. 1275–1323). Hamilton, Ontario, Canada: BC Decker.

Kyle, R.A., & Rajkumar, S.V. (2004). Drug therapy: Multiple myeloma. *New England Journal of Medicine, 351,* 1860–1873.

Lairmore, T.C., & Moley, J.F. (2005). Cancer of the endocrine system. In V.T. DeVita, S. Hellman, & S.A. Rosenberg (Eds.), *Cancer: Principles and practice of oncology* (7th ed., pp. 1489–1501). Philadelphia: Lippincott Williams & Wilkins.

Lamy, O., Jenzer-Closut, A., & Burckhardt, P. (2001). Hypercalcemia of malignancy: An undiagnosed and undertreated disease. *Journal of Internal Medicine, 250,* 73–79.

Lerner, U.H. (2004). New molecules in the tumor necrosis factor ligand and receptor superfamilies with importance for physiological and pathological bone resorption. *Critical Reviews in Oral Biology and Medicine, 15,* 64–81.

Leyland-Jones, B. (2004). Treating cancer-related hypercalcemia with gallium nitrate. *Journal of Supportive Oncology, 2,* 509–516.

Lipton, A. (2004). Pathophysiology of bone metastases: How this knowledge may lead to therapeutic intervention. *Journal of Supportive Oncology, 2,* 205–220.

Major, P., Lortholary, A., Hon, J., Abdi, E., Mills, G., Menssen, H.D., et al. (2001). Zoledronic acid is superior to pamidronate in the treatment of hypercalcemia of malignancy: A pooled analysis of two randomized, controlled clinical trials. *Journal of Clinical Oncology, 19,* 558–567.

Meriney, D.K., & Reeder, S.J. (1998). Hypercalcemia. In C.C. Chernecky & B.J. Berger (Eds.), *Advanced and critical care oncology nursing: Managing primary complications* (pp. 254–269). Philadelphia: Saunders.

Moore, J.M. (1998). Metabolic emergencies: Hypercalcemia. In B.L. Johnson & J. Gross (Eds.), *Handbook of oncology nursing* (3rd ed., pp. 687–702). Sudbury, MA: Jones and Bartlett.

Morton, A.R., & Lipton, A. (2004). Hypercalcemia. In M.D. Abeloff, J.O. Armitage, J.E. Niederhuber, M.B. Kasten, & W.G. McKenna (Eds.), *Clinical oncology* (3rd ed., pp. 957–972). Philadelphia: Elsevier Churchill Livingstone.

Morton, A.R., & Ritch, P.S. (2002). Hypercalcemia. In A.M. Berger, R.K. Portenoy, & D.E. Weissman (Eds.), *Principles and practice of palliative care and supportive oncology* (2nd ed., pp. 493–507). Philadelphia: Lippincott Williams & Wilkins.

Mundy, G.R. (1990). Pathophysiology of cancer-associated hypercalcemia. *Seminars in Oncology, 17*(2 Suppl. 5), 10–15.

Mundy, G.R. (2002). Metastasis to bone: Causes, consequences and therapeutic options. *Nature Reviews Cancer, 2,* 584–593.

Mundy, G.R., & Guise, T.A. (1998). Role of parathyroid-related peptide in hypercalcemia of malignancy and osteolytic bone disease. *Endocrine-Related Cancer, 5,* 15–26.

Munshi, N.C., & Anderson, K.C. (2005). Plasma cell neoplasms. In V.T. DeVita, S. Hellman, & S.A. Rosenberg (Eds.), *Cancer: Principles and practice of oncology* (7th ed., pp. 2160–2164). Philadelphia: Lippincott Williams & Wilkins.

Myers, J.S. (2001). Oncologic complications. In S.E. Otto (Ed.), *Oncology nursing* (4th ed., pp. 498–581). St. Louis, MO: Mosby.

National Cancer Institute. (2004, November). *Hypercalcemia (PDQ®).* Retrieved January 22, 2005, from http://www.cancer.gov/cancerinfo/pdq/supportivecare/hypercalcemia

Novartis Pharmaceuticals Corp. (2005a, April). Aredia (pamidronate) [Package insert]. East Hanover, NJ: Author.

Novartis Pharmaceuticals Corp. (2005b, April). Zometa (zoledronic acid) [Package insert]. East Hanover, NJ: Author.

Richerson, M.T. (2004). Electrolyte imbalances: Hypercalcemia. In C.H. Yarbro, M.H. Frogge, & M. Goodman (Eds.), *Cancer symptom management* (3rd ed., pp. 440–453). Sudbury, MA: Jones and Bartlett.

Rodan, G.A., & Martin, J. (2000). Therapeutic approaches to bone disease. *Science, 289,* 1508–1514.

Roodman, G.D. (2004). Mechanisms for bone metastasis. *New England Journal of Medicine, 350,* 1655–1664.

Ruggiero, S., Gralow, J., Marx, R.E., Hoff, A.O., Schubert, M.M., Huryn, J.M., et al. (2006). Practical guidelines for the prevention, diagnosis, and treatment of osteonecrosis of the jaw in patients with cancer. *Journal of Oncology Practice, 2,* 7–14.

Seymour, J.F., & Gagel, R.F. (1993). Calcitriol: The major humoral mediator of hypercalcemia in Hodgkin's disease and non-Hodgkin's lymphoma. *Blood, 82,* 1383–1394.

Sezer, O., Heider, U., Zavrski, I., Kuhne, C.A., & Hofbauer, L.C. (2003). RANK ligand and osteoprotegerin in myeloma bone disease. *Blood, 101,* 2094–2098.

Smith, W.J. (2000). Hypocalcemia/hypercalcemia. In D. Camp-Sorrell & R.A. Hawkins (Eds.), *Clinical manual for the oncology advanced practice nurse* (pp. 849–858). Pittsburgh, PA: Oncology Nursing Society.

Solimando, D.A. (2001). Overview of hypercalcemia of malignancy. *American Journal of Health-System Pharmacy, 58*(Suppl. 3), S4–S7.

Teitelbaum, S.L. (2000). Bone resorption by osteoclasts. *Science, 289,* 1504–1508.

Tummula, R. (1997). Hypercalcemia. In B. Djulbegovic & D.M. Sullivan (Eds.), *Decision making in oncology: Evidence-based management* (pp. 437–445). New York: Churchill Livingstone.

von Moos, R. (2005). Bisphosphonate treatment recommendations for oncologists. *Oncologist, 10*(Suppl. 1), 19–24.

Wilkes, G.M., Ingwersen, K., & Barton-Burke, M. (2001). *2001 oncology nursing drug handbook.* Sudbury, MA: Jones and Bartlett.

Wimalawansa, S.J. (1995). *Hypercalcemia of malignancy: Etiology, pathogenesis and clinical management.* Austin, TX: R.G. Landes.

Yeung, S.-C., & Gagel, R.F. (2003). Endocrine complications and paraneoplastic syndromes. In D.W. Kufe, R.E. Pollock, R.R. Weichselbaum, R.C. Bast, T. Gansler, J.F. Holland, et al. (Eds.), *Holland-Frei cancer medicine* (6th ed., pp. 2609–2622). Hamilton, Ontario, Canada: BC Decker.

Jeanne K. Clancey, RN, MSN, CNRN

Chapter 4

Increased Intracranial Pressure

Introduction

Increased intracranial pressure (ICP) is an oncologic emergency leading to neurologic complications that may be permanent or cause death. Both primary malignant brain tumors and metastatic brain tumors can cause increased ICP and result in neurologic deficits that affect patients' quality and length of life. Manifestations of increased ICP range from subtle behavioral changes to obvious expressive and receptive aphasia; the onset may be gradual or sudden; and the severity may be insignificant to severely disabling. Specific, localized symptoms depend on the intracranial location affected by the pressure injury and may be more devastating than the malignancy. Prompt intervention of increased ICP can interrupt the destructive cycle and preserve patients' cognitive and physical functioning. Untreated ICP can cause brain stem herniation, cessation of vital functions, and death (Belford, 2005; Wilkes, 2004). Oncology nurses are in an ideal position to recognize the subtle alterations in physical and cognitive functioning that are the earliest indicators of increased ICP. Prompt recognition and intervention of this oncologic emergency are key to limiting the consequences of increased ICP.

Incidence

The American Cancer Society estimates that 18,820 new cases of primary malignant brain tumors and 12,820 deaths will occur in 2006 (Jemal et al., 2006). Primary malignant brain tumors are not common for either adult males or females. The American Cancer Society (2006) did not include them in the leading sites of cancer in its *Cancer Facts and Figures, 2006*. Despite their infrequency, primary or metastatic brain tumors do occur and may affect patients' quality of life and lead to death. Adult brain tumors occur in the anterior and middle fossae (the supratentorial region). The cerebral cortex and the frontal, parietal, temporal, and occipital lobes of the brain comprise the supratentorial region of the brain. Gliomas, especially those from astrocytic cells, are the most common type of brain tumors and account for 40% of tumors. For unknown reasons, a recent increase has occurred in the number of primary malignant brain tumors in older adults, although other cancers are on the decline (Hickey, 2003a). Table 4-1 lists the common types of primary malignant and metastatic brain tumors.

Metastasis to the brain occurs in approximately 24% of all patients with cancer. The incidence of intracranial metastasis is highest with carcinomas of the lung (50%) and breast (15%–20%), unknown primary (10%–15%), melanoma (10%), and colon (5%) (Wilkes, 2004). Ninety percent of brain metastases develop in the cerebrum, and 10% in the posterior fossa. Fifty percent of patients with a brain metastasis have a single lesion, 20% have two lesions, and 10% have more than five lesions. Hematogenous spread is the most common mechanism of brain metastasis (McAllister, Ward, Schulman, & DeAngelis, 2002).

Table 4-1. Common Types of Primary and Metastatic Brain Tumors

Type of Tumor	Description	Location/Data	Treatment	Prognosis
Astrocytoma Grade I, II	Grade I—well-defined cells Grade II—less cell differentiation	Cerebral hemispheres Ages 20–40 years	Gross total resection recommended Radiation controversial; not usually for grade I	5–7 year median survival
Anaplastic astrocytoma Grade III	Cellular anaplastic	Cerebral hemispheres Ages 30–50 years	Gross total resection Radiation therapy Chemotherapy	18–24 months median survival
Glioblastoma multiforme Grade IV	Highly infiltrative Most common, fast growing Area of necrosis within tumor	Cerebral hemispheres Ages 50–70 years	Gross total resection Radiation therapy Chemotherapy	8–10 months median survival

(Continued on next page)

Table 4-1. Common Types of Primary and Metastatic Brain Tumors (Continued)

Type of Tumor	Description	Location/Data	Treatment	Prognosis
Oligoden-droglioma	Grade II–IV May be calcified Usually slow growing	Cerebral hemi-spheres Occur in adults	Gross total re-section Radiation ther-apy Chemotherapy	5–10 years median survival; de-pends upon grade
Ependy-moma	Slow growing from ependy-mal cells—lin-ing of the ventricular system	Occurs within ventricular system First two de-cades of life	Surgery if acces-sible Chemotherapy not helpful Radiation is controver-sial—may be craniospinal.	5–10 years; depends upon loca-tion
Meningioma	Slow growing From meningeal cells (menin-ges) Well circum-scribed Usually benign	Parasagittal sinus, sphe-noid ridge Adults, women more than men (3:2)	Gross total resection usu-ally Observation, depending upon size and location	"Cure" with total removal
Metastatic brain tumors	Spherical, con-trast-enhanc-ing with ne-crotic center Peritumoral edema Occurs in gray matter near major arteries	Common pri-mary sites: • Lung: 50% • Breast: 15%–20% • Melanoma: 10% • Unknown primary: 10% • GI tract: 5%	Surgery com-mon with single lesion Radiation ther-apy—often radiosensitive lesions	Depends on presence or absence of systemic disease

GI—gastrointestinal

Note. Based on information from DeVroom et al., 2004; Hickey, 2003b; Lindsay & Bone, 2004; Wilkes, 2004.

Risk Factors

Increased ICP is a common neurologic complication of patients with cancer. A variety of mechanisms may increase these patients' risk for developing increased ICP (see Table 4-2) Primary or metastatic cerebral lesions may create increasing pressure within the brain as they expand and occupy more space, or

Table 4-2. Factors Associated With the Development of Increased Intracranial Pressure

Factors	Explanation
Primary malignant brain tumors	
• Astrocytomas grade I–II	Grade I–II—benign; well differentiated; occurs primarily in the cerebral cortex
• Anaplastic astrocytoma grade III	Grade III—malignant; occurs primarily in the cerebral cortex
• Glioblastoma multiforme grade IV	Grade IV—rapidly growing; malignant; usually occurs in the cerebral cortex; accounts for 55% of all gliomas
Ependymoma	Occurs in the lining of the ventricles
Oligodendroglioma	May be well differentiated, low grade, or anaplastic, high grade; occurs in cerebral cortex; calcification within tumor is common.
Metastatic brain tumors	20%–40% of patients with cancer have brain metastasis, either single or multiple lesions; most frequently associated with cancers of the lung, breast, colon, and rectum.
Diffuse cerebral edema with leukemia	Attributable to leukostasis—blast counts > 4 x $10^5/\mu L$
Leptomeningeal metastasis	Often causes obstruction of flow of cerebrospinal fluid
Disseminated intravascular coagulation	Causes diffuse cerebral hemorrhages
Herpes simplex encephalitis	Causes extensive vasogenic edema
Opportunistic infections: cerebral toxoplasmosis, aspergillosis, candidiasis	Often present with signs of increased intracranial pressure
Syndrome of inappropriate antidiuretic hormone secretion	Causes an increase in the intracellular water and sodium content in the brain cells, resulting in cerebral edema
Cranial irradiation	Vasogenic edema caused by tissue damage from radiation therapy

Note. Based on information from Baehring, 2005; Hickey, 2003a.

they may cause intracranial or intratumoral hemorrhage. The risk of bleeding into the brain increases if disease-induced coagulopathies are present. Cerebral edema that develops around the tumor also is associated with increasing ICP, as is cytotoxic therapy, such as cranial irradiation used to treat benign or malignant brain lesions. Patients who are immunocompromised are at increased risk for brain abscesses secondary to bacterial, viral, or fungal opportunistic infections, meningitis, or encephalitis, all of which can cause increased ICP. Increased ICP also can result from obstruction to the flow of cerebrospinal fluid (CSF) by tumor cells or blood products that may impede the CSF reabsorption process, as may occur with leptomeningeal carcinomatosis. A tumor mass itself, especially if located at a "bottleneck" of spinal fluid pathways, such as the foramen of Monro or the aqueduct of Sylvius, also can obstruct the outflow of CSF from the brain, resulting in ICP (Baehring, 2005).

The blood-brain barrier (BBB) can contribute to increased risk for space-occupying intracranial metastases. The term *blood-brain barrier* describes the tight junctions between the endothelial cells and astrocytes within the brain (Slazinski & Littlejohns, 2004). Unlike capillaries in the rest of the body, capillaries in the brain do not have pores between adjacent epithelial cells. Therefore, the brain cannot derive molecules from blood plasma by a filtering process. Instead, active, highly selective processes transport molecules from the blood through the endothelial cells. One of the effects of the BBB is that it prevents the entrance of most chemotherapeutic agents into the brain tissue. The doses of chemotherapy necessary to reach the cerebral tissue through the BBB are often too toxic to use safely. Thus, this usually protective physiologic mechanism increases the potential for the growth of metastatic tumor deposits within the brain (Slazinski & Littlejohns).

Several actions, such as coughing, vomiting, hyperventilation, neck hyperextension, and the Valsalva maneuver, also can increase ICP. In addition, emotional upset, sexual excitement, pain, hyperthermia, and seizure activity will increase ICP (Hickey, 2003b).

Normal Brain Physiology

ICP is defined as "the pressure normally exerted by cerebrospinal fluid (CSF) that circulates around the brain and spinal cord and within the ventricular system" (Hickey, 2003b, p. 285). The normal range of ICP is 0–10 mm Hg, although 15 mm Hg often is considered high normal (Hickey, 2003b).

The Monro-Kellie hypothesis of ICP dynamics has been the basis for understanding ICP for more than two centuries. According to this hypothesis, ICP and volume are directly related. Thus, as the volume of brain and other tissue inside the rigid skull increases, the pressure inside the skull also increases because there is little room for expansion. The intracranial volume can be divided into three components: brain tissue (80%), blood (10%), and CSF (10%). In a healthy adult with an intact skull, the three components of the brain remain in a constant relationship (March & Wellwood, 2004). If the volume of any one component increases, another component must decrease to maintain this dynamic equilibrium. Without this relationship, increased ICP occurs (Hickey, 2003b). The human brain, which is confined within a rigid skull, can compensate for brief increases in ICP through several mechanisms to maintain the steady state of the intracranial volumes. These compensatory mechanisms are (a) displacement of venous blood through the jugular or scalp veins, (b) displacement of intracranial CSF into the spinal arachnoid space, and (c) decreased production of CSF. The displacement of CSF or blood is limited, and after the capacity of these mechanisms has been exceeded, increased ICP will occur (March & Wellwood).

Several concepts are involved in maintaining the dynamic volume-pressure relationships within the brain. Table 4-3 provides definitions of pertinent terms and formulas. *Compliance* refers to the adaptability of the brain to maintain this equilibrium. Compliance has been described as the brain's "stiffness" and is the ratio of change in volume to the resulting change in pressure (Hickey, 2003b). It is represented by the formula $C = \Delta V / \Delta P$. Small increases in volume are easier to accommodate than large volume increases, and if the increase is gradual over time, the brain can adapt more easily (March & Wellwood, 2004). Eventually a critical situation develops when the compensatory mechanisms are overwhelmed and an increase occurs in ICP. *Elastance* is the inverse of compliance and refers to the change in pressure observed for a given change in volume. Elastance is measured clinically through ICP monitoring (March & Wellwood). Figure 4-1 demonstrates the volume-pressure relationships within the brain.

To further comprehend the concept of ICP, one must understand the components related to cerebral hemodynamics. Cerebral hemodynamics includes

Table 4-3. Definitions of Terms and Formulas	
Terms and Formulas	**Definitions**
Intracranial pressure (ICP)	The pressure normally exerted by the cerebrospinal fluid, which circulates around the brain and spinal cord Normal range ICP = 0–10 mm Hg (15 = high normal)
Compliance	Adaptability of the brain to maintain equilibrium
$C = \Delta V / \Delta P$	Compliance: The ratio of change in cerebral volume to the resulting change in pressure
Elastance	Inverse of compliance—refers to pressure changes for a given change in volume
Cerebral blood flow	Cerebral perfusion pressure (CPP) divided by the cerebrovascular resistance
CVP	Central venous pressure
MAP	Mean arterial pressure
CPP	Blood pressure gradient of the brain Normal range = 70–100 mm Hg CPP is equal to the MAP minus the CVP (CPP = MAP – CVP)

Note. Based on information from Hickey, 2003b; March & Wellwood, 2004.

cerebral blood volume, cerebral blood flow, and the factors affecting them. Cerebral blood volume is the amount of blood in the brain at a given time. Blood normally occupies 10% (150 ml) of the intracranial space. Autoregulatory mechanisms affecting cerebral blood flow act to control and maintain this volume. Cerebral blood flow is defined as the cerebral perfusion pressure (CPP) divided by the cerebrovascular resistance. Normal cerebral blood flow is 50 ml/100 g/min in adults. Although the brain is only 2% of the body's weight, it consumes 15%–20% of the cardiac output. Cerebral blood flow is not constant. The gray matter of the brain receives six times as much as the white matter, and changes in cerebral activity will alter the blood flow. The brain depends upon its cerebral blood flow for its nutrients because it cannot store glucose. It utilizes 25% of the body's glucose supply as its only source of energy (Lindsay & Bone, 2004; March & Wellwood, 2004).

CPP, the blood pressure gradient of the brain, ranges between 70–100 mm Hg in an adult (Hickey, 2003b). CPP is calculated by the following formula: CPP = MAP (mean arterial pressure) – CVP (central venous pressure). CPP is an estimate of the cerebral circulation. The CVP can increase with positioning (flexion or rotation of the head), and hypotension (MAP < 50–70 mm Hg) can affect CPP.

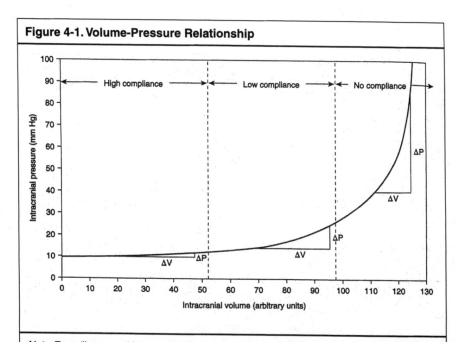

Figure 4-1. Volume-Pressure Relationship

Note. From "Increased Intracranial Pressure, Cerebral Edema, and Brain Herniation" (p. 2.3), by S.S. Rengachary and D.A. Duke in S.S. Rengachary and R.H. Wilkins (Eds.), *Principles of Neurosurgery*, 1994, St. Louis, MO: Mosby. Copyright 1994 by Elsevier. Reprinted with permission.

Autoregulatory mechanisms maintain the cerebral blood flow over varied blood pressure parameters by altering the diameters of the cerebral blood vessels. With a decrease in CPP, ischemia can occur; if this is not reversed, infarction results. As MAP increases, vasoconstriction occurs, and as it decreases, vasodilation occurs. Changes in partial pressure of oxygen (PaO_2) below 50 mm Hg (hypoxia) will cause vasodilation. A change of 1 mm Hg in the partial pressure of carbon dioxide ($PaCO_2$) results in a 2%–3% change in cerebral blood flow within a $PaCO_2$ range of 20–80 mm Hg (Hickey, 2003b; March & Wellwood, 2004). Under normal circumstances, the brain is a well-balanced organ with very stable relationships. It can maintain the equilibrium among the three compartments through slow and subtle changes, but once compliance is exhausted, the ICP will increase and symptoms will manifest.

Pathophysiology

The skull is a rigid structure and cannot accommodate expanding tumor masses or increases in the amount of CSF in the brain unless a corresponding decrease occurs in one of the other intracranial compartments. The volume and pressure increases that occur within the brain of patients with cancer are attributable to the presence of either primary or metastatic tumors or to cerebral edema that is either tumor-associated or the result of antineoplastic therapies.

Vasogenic edema is a type of extracellular edema that occurs in the white matter of the brain. It develops because of increased capillary permeability resulting from widening of tight endothelial junctions at the level of the BBB, allowing a plasma-like fluid to leak into the extracellular space. This type of edema occurs around brain tumors but also may occur with trauma or brain abscesses (Hickey, 2003b). *Cytotoxic edema* may develop as a result of oncologic treatments. Cytotoxic edema is an increase in the fluid in the neurons and glial and endothelial cells as a result of failure of the sodium-potassium active transport pump and accumulation of sodium within the cells. Diffuse brain swelling results. This form of edema also occurs with hyposmolarity conditions, such as water intoxication and the syndrome of inappropriate antidiuretic hormone secretion (SIADH) (Hickey, 2003b). See Chapter 7 for a full discussion of SIADH.

As ICP increases and the compensatory mechanisms are exhausted, evidence of mass effect will be present. This is the shifting of the cerebral tissue from an area of high pressure to an area of lower pressure and ultimately can lead to fatal herniation of the brain tissue into either the tentorium or the foramen magnum. Folds of dura mater divide the intracranial cavity into smaller compartments. The most important dural folds are falx cerebri, which divide the right and left supratentorial hemispheres of the brain. The tentorium cerebelli is a tent-shaped fold of dura between the cerebrum and the cerebellum. This dural fold divides the intracranial cavity into the supratentorium and the infratentorium (Hickey, 2003b; Plum & Posner, 1980).

Herniation of the brain refers to downward displacement of brain tissue that compresses brain structures and compromises blood flow, resulting in a sequence of neurologic compromise (Kirkness & March, 2004). Several different types of herniation can occur in the presence of increased ICP (Hickey, 2003b). The two most common types are central and uncal herniation. *Central herniation* results from a lesion in the cerebral cortex that produces a downward displacement of the cerebral hemispheres, basal ganglia, and midbrain through the small opening in the tentorium cerebelli. This herniation compresses the brain stem and begins the rapid neurologic decline to brain death (Kirkness & March; Lindsay & Bone, 2004). Figures 4-2 and 4-3 illustrate the progression of the neurologic deficits manifested with central and uncal herniation. *Uncal herniation* is the most common form and occurs when a cerebral mass in the temporal lobe area is displaced downward through the small hole in the tentorium cerebelli. The oculomotor nerve (the third cranial nerve, CN III) often catches on the tentorial notch, which leads to pressure on the nerve and the manifestation of ipsilateral pupillary dilatation (Kirkness & March; Lindsay & Bone). It is possible to reverse herniation, but

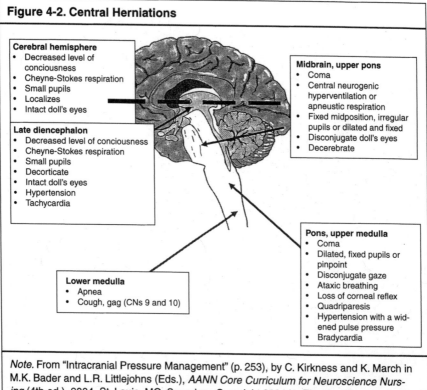

Figure 4-2. Central Herniations

Cerebral hemisphere
- Decreased level of conciousness
- Cheyne-Stokes respiration
- Small pupils
- Localizes
- Intact doll's eyes

Late diencephalon
- Decreased level of conciousness
- Cheyne-Stokes respiration
- Small pupils
- Decorticate
- Intact doll's eyes
- Hypertension
- Tachycardia

Midbrain, upper pons
- Coma
- Central neurogenic hyperventilation or apneustic respiration
- Fixed midposition, irregular pupils or dilated and fixed
- Disconjugate doll's eyes
- Decerebrate

Lower medulla
- Apnea
- Cough, gag (CNs 9 and 10)

Pons, upper medulla
- Coma
- Dilated, fixed pupils or pinpoint
- Disconjugate gaze
- Ataxic breathing
- Loss of corneal reflex
- Quadriparesis
- Hypertension with a widened pulse pressure
- Bradycardia

Note. From "Intracranial Pressure Management" (p. 253), by C. Kirkness and K. March in M.K. Bader and L.R. Littlejohns (Eds.), *AANN Core Curriculum for Neuroscience Nursing* (4th ed.), 2004, St. Louis, MO: Saunders. Copyright 2004 by Elsevier. Reprinted with permission.

Figure 4-3. Uncal Herniations

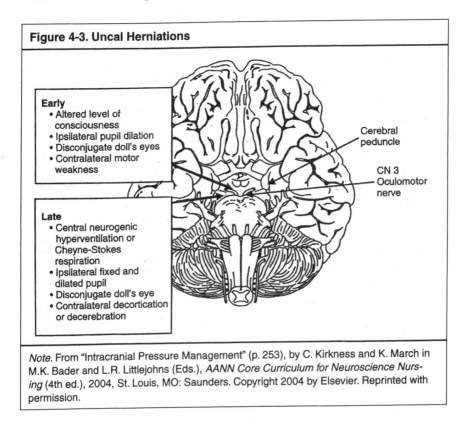

Early
- Altered level of consciousness
- Ipsilateral pupil dilation
- Disconjugate doll's eyes
- Contralateral motor weakness

Late
- Central neurogenic hyperventilation or Cheyne-Stokes respiration
- Ipsilateral fixed and dilated pupil
- Disconjugate doll's eye
- Contralateral decortication or decerebration

Cerebral peduncle

CN 3 Oculomotor nerve

Note. From "Intracranial Pressure Management" (p. 253), by C. Kirkness and K. March in M.K. Bader and L.R. Littlejohns (Eds.), *AANN Core Curriculum for Neuroscience Nursing* (4th ed.), 2004, St. Louis, MO: Saunders. Copyright 2004 by Elsevier. Reprinted with permission.

the time to do so is limited. Without prompt diagnosis and rapid treatment to interrupt the increases in ICP, irreversible brain damage, coma, and death will occur (Kirkness & March).

Clinical Manifestations

The clinical manifestations of increased ICP may vary depending on the location of the pressure-causing agent and the degree of increased ICP. Generalized neurologic symptoms include changes in the level of consciousness, such as drowsiness and lethargy; mental status changes; communication problems such as expressive and receptive aphasia; memory problems; personality changes; restlessness; headache with or without vomiting, which may be projectile; motor weakness; and coordination problems. Changes in the level of consciousness may differ depending on location. In comparison to the usual early manifestations of altered level of consciousness (drowsiness, confusion, lethargy), patients in the early stages of uncal herniation may be very wakeful. If the herniation continues, the neurologic deterioration will conclude with coma and death (Hickey, 2003b; Wilkes, 2004).

Headache is a common sign of increased ICP in adults. Waking up in the morning with a headache is a common clinical manifestation of increased ICP. The headache is severe, relentless, and resistant to most common analgesics. Often, patients will have complete relief from the headache after vomiting. The headache also may start as a migraine-type, nagging pain for several days. Visual abnormalities can occur early in the process of increasing ICP. Patients may report decreased visual acuity, blurred vision, diplopia, and a visual field cut. The change in visual acuity and blurring of vision occur because of early swelling in the cerebral hemisphere, and diplopia results from weakness of one or more of the extraocular muscles. Assessment of extraocular movements (EOMs) may determine which cranial nerves the increasing pressure affects. The cranial nerves involved in testing for EOMs are cranial nerves III, IV, and VI. The location of the cranial nerve origins provides information about brain stem functioning (Hickey, 2003b).

Motor weakness may develop in the leg and the arm on the side of the body opposite the intracranial mass because of pressure on the pyramidal tracts. As ICP continues to increase, hemiplegia, decortication, and decerebration can occur because of pressure on the brain stem from the herniation. Vomiting with increased ICP usually occurs because of an infratentorial lesion that produces pressure on the vomiting center, located on the floor of the fourth ventricle. This vomiting is projectile in nature and usually is not associated with nausea (Hickey, 2003b).

Vital signs can reflect an increase in ICP. Blood pressure is stable in the early stages, but as ICP increases, the blood pressure rises to compensate. This rise in blood pressure increases the cardiac output so that the heart pumps with more force, causing a widening pulse pressure. As ICP continues to increase, decompensation occurs and the blood pressure decreases. The pulse is stable in the early stages of increased ICP. As herniation occurs and the brain stem receives pressure, profound bradycardia develops from the pressure on the medulla. When decompensation occurs, the pulse becomes irregular, rapid, and thready and then ceases. The respiratory pattern also is indicative of pressure on the brain stem. Early increased ICP will be manifested by Cheyne-Stokes respirations because of pressure in the cerebral hemispheres. As ICP continues to increase, the respiratory pattern will change to ataxic or agonal respirations. The patient's temperature will remain normal unless hypothalamic damage occurs, which will be manifested by an elevated temperature. During the decompensatory phase, abnormally high temperatures are not unusual (Hickey, 2003b; Kirkness & March, 2004). Late signs of increased ICP are indicated by the Cushing triad and result from pressure on the medulla. The *Cushing triad* consists of hypertension with a widening pulse pressure, bradycardia, and abnormal respirations. This is a late sign of brain stem dysfunction and indicates low or loss of brain compliance. Often, cerebral herniation already has occurred (Hickey, 2003b).

Patient Assessment

History

Patients with primary malignant brain tumors are at risk for developing increased ICP. This could result from growth of the tumor, hemorrhage into the tumor increasing the mass effect, or obstruction of the normal flow and reabsorption of the CSF because of tumor cells or blood occluding the arachnoid villi. Metastatic brain tumors occur in approximately 24% of all patients with cancer, especially those with lung and breast cancers, cancers of unknown primary, melanoma, and colon cancer, placing them at risk for developing increased ICP (Wilkes, 2004).

Oncologic treatments also can cause increased ICP. Irradiation of a brain tumor, either primary or metastatic, will cause increased tumoral edema, which, if not treated, can cause increased ICP. Chemotherapeutic agents requiring aggressive hydration to prevent complications may lead to hyponatremia or SIADH, which may increase ICP (Wilkes, 2004).

Physical Assessment

Early detection of increased ICP is essential for a successful patient outcome. Increased ICP in the early stages usually is reversible; however, once brain stem involvement is evident, neurologic damage often is permanent. Nurses should utilize available tools to assess patients for signs of increased ICP. The Quick Neurologic Assessment for the Oncology Nurse (see Table 4-4) is a quick and structured tool to accomplish the neurologic assessment (Wilkes, 2004). An important aspect of the neurologic assessment is the effects on cranial nerves caused by increasing pressure on the brain stem. If the optic nerve (CN II) is compressed, patients will have evidence of decreased visual acuity and the presence of a visual field deficit. As ICP rises and pressure is exerted on the brain stem, pupillary changes become apparent.

Dysfunction of the oculomotor nerve (CN III) often is a classic sign of increased ICP. Check the pupils for size, shape, and symmetry. Normal pupils are round and 3–7 mm. Constricted pupils can indicate narcotic administration or damage to the pons in the brain stem. Dilated pupils can be from administration of an atropine-based medication or, if bilateral, can occur because of hypoxia. The oculomotor, trochlear (CN IV), and the abducens (CN VI) nerves are involved with EOMs (see Figure 4-4). Observe the patient's eyes for signs of nystagmus, a rapid, involuntary movement of the eyeball. Both eyes should move together; a disconjugate gaze results from pressure on the abducens nerve. Unequal pupils, with ipsilateral dilatation, are suggestive of herniation. Sluggishness of the pupillary response is an early sign of increased pressure. Observe the pupils for direct and consensual light response. Assessing the pupils' response to light evaluates the optic nerve,

Table 4-4. Quick Neurologic Assessment for the Oncology Nurse	
Areas to Assess	**Questions**
• Flow of speech • Orientation • Memory • Thought processes • Attention span	Ask what brings the patient to the hospital at this time. Ask what problems the patient has experienced and when they began. Note any restlessness, confusion, irritability, or if the patient loses interest.
• Short-term memory • Visual acuity	Tell the patient you are doing a memory test. Ask the patient to read his/her hospital number and to remember it. Ask the patient to repeat the number 5 minutes later.
• Gait • Lower extremity motor function, coordination • Ability to follow commands	Ask the patient, if able, to walk across the room—observe gait and posture. Ask the patient to sit in a chair, or on the side of the bed, and slide the right heel down the left leg—note coordination and smoothness of movement.
• Upper extremity motor function, coordination • Fine motor movement	Ask the patient to unbutton his/her shirt or unzip trousers or skirt. Ask the patient to pick up a dime from a flat surface.
• Cranial nerves III, IV, V, VI, VII (partial exam)	Ask the patient to smile, then clench his/her teeth. Observe the patient's pupils for size, equality, and reactivity to light when tested with your flashlight.

Note. From "Increased Intracranial Pressure" (p. 376), by G.M. Wilkes in C.H. Yarbro, M.H. Frogge, and M. Goodman (Eds.), *Cancer Symptom Management* (3rd ed.), 2004, Sudbury, MA: Jones and Bartlett. Copyright 2004 by Jones and Bartlett. Reprinted with permission.

which carries impulses from the eye to the brain, and the oculomotor nerve, which carries impulses from the brain to the eye. The direct response occurs when the light is shone into the pupil of one eye, and that pupil constricts. A consensual response occurs when the light is shone into one pupil, and both pupils constrict (Kazierad, 1998).

Motor function changes may range from mild weakness to a hemiparesis or hemiplegia (Wilkes, 2004). The Glasgow Coma Scale is a standardized numeric system for evaluating a patient's neurologic status (see Tables 4-5 and 4-6). It was designed for patients with head trauma but has been used with any patients with neurologic alteration. This scale provides a quick numeric report on the patient's neurologic status, demonstrating improvement or decline (Kazierad, 1998).

Patients at risk for increased ICP may demonstrate transient pressure signs with activities such as coughing, vomiting, hyperventilation, neck hyperextension, and the Valsalva maneuver. These activities may increase ICP for

Figure 4-4. Testing Extraocular Movements

1. Ask the patient to visually follow your finger as you move it through the six cardinal gazes.
2. Draw an "H" shape in the air with your finger, moving slowly as you change direction.
3. Pause during upward and lateral gazes to identify nystagmus.

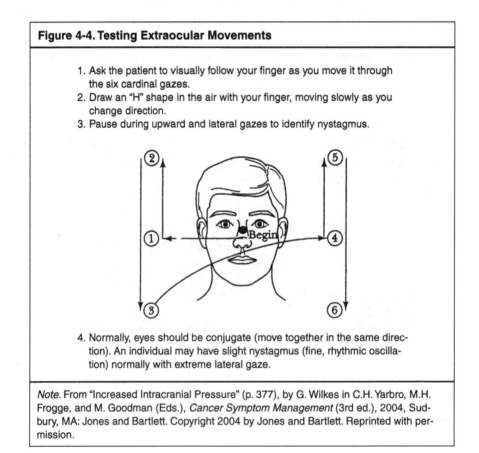

4. Normally, eyes should be conjugate (move together in the same direction). An individual may have slight nystagmus (fine, rhythmic oscillation) normally with extreme lateral gaze.

Note. From "Increased Intracranial Pressure" (p. 377), by G. Wilkes in C.H. Yarbro, M.H. Frogge, and M. Goodman (Eds.), *Cancer Symptom Management* (3rd ed.), 2004, Sudbury, MA: Jones and Bartlett. Copyright 2004 by Jones and Bartlett. Reprinted with permission.

brief periods as a result of interference in the CPP and may lead to transient cerebral ischemia. Transient pressure signs include pupillary abnormalities, change in level of consciousness, visual disturbance, motor dysfunction, complaints of headache, and speech difficulties. Although these manifestations may last only moments, they reflect the balance needed to maintain normal ICP (Hickey, 2003b).

Diagnostic Evaluation

Imaging Studies

Neuroradiology studies, such as computed tomography (CT) scans and magnetic resonance imaging (MRI), will provide information to assist with the diagnosis and establishment of treatment options. CT scans will show changes in brain structures indicative of increased pressure, such as effaced sulci and fissures, absent basal cisterns, loss of gray-white matter differentiation, and small or slit-like ventricles (Kirkness & March, 2004). MRI has surpassed the CT scan in the diagnosis of patients with increased ICP. Gadolinium-enhanced MRI has the ability to provide high definition to an area of increased cerebral edema with easier visualization of the lesion. Patients with cancer experiencing increased ICP often have lesions that have disrupted the BBB. The contrast-enhanced MRI assists the visualization of the edema and lesions (Baehring, 2005; Wilkes, 2004). Positron-emission tomography scan uses radiopharmaceuticals to map brain biochemistry. It complements the other neurodiagnostic tools, CT and MRI. It can determine cerebral blood flow to an area of the brain and often is used in research studies on this topic (Davis, Park, Darwich, Deveikis, & Rossini, 2004).

A lumbar puncture can be a useful diagnostic tool to determine the causative infectious agent of meningitis or to provide the diagnosis of carcinomatosis

Table 4-5. Glasgow Coma Scale	
Response	Score*
Eye opening	
Spontaneous	4
To sound	3
To pain	2
Never	1
Motor response	
Obeys commands	6
Localized pain	5
Normal flexion (withdrawal)	4
Abnormal flexion	3
Extension	2
Nil	1
Verbal response	
Oriented	5
Confused conversation	4
Inappropriate words	3
Incomprehensible sounds	2
None	1

* The highest possible score is 15.

Note. From "Appendix A: Scales for Disease Processes" (p. 965), in M.K. Bader and L.R. Littlejohns (Eds.), AANN Core Curriculum for Neuroscience Nursing (4th ed.), 2004, St. Louis, MO: Saunders. Copyright 2004 by Elsevier. Reprinted with permission.

Table 4-6. Glasgow Outcome Scale	
Score	**Description**
1	**Death**
2	**Persistent vegetative state** Patient exhibits no obvious cortical function.
3	**Severe disability** Conscious but disabled. Patient depends on others for daily support due to mental or physical disability or both.
4	**Moderate disability** Disabled but independent. Patient is independent as far as daily life is concerned. The disabilities found include varying degrees of dysphasia, hemiparesis, or ataxia, as well as intellectual and memory deficits and personality changes.
5	**Good recovery** Resumption of normal activities even though there may be minor neurologic or psychological deficits.
Total (1–5): ___.	

Note. From "Appendix A: Scales for Disease Processes" (p. 965), in M.K. Bader and L.R. Littlejohns (Eds.), *AANN Core Curriculum for Neuroscience Nursing* (4th ed.), 2004, St. Louis, MO: Saunders. Copyright 2004 by Elsevier. Reprinted with permission.

meningitis. However, for patients with suspected increased ICP, caution is advised. Performing a lumbar puncture on patients with increased ICP secondary to a space-occupying lesion may result in brain stem compression, herniation through the foramen magnum, and ultimately death (Hickey, 2003b). If ICP monitoring equipment is present, an ICP reading > 20 mm Hg lasting for longer than five minutes is considered to be intracranial hypertension and requires aggressive treatment (Kirkness & March, 2004).

Treatment Modalities

Treatment for increased ICP should begin aggressively with the early signs. Serial neurologic assessments will identify these early changes and prevent the compensatory mechanisms from changing into decompensation mechanisms.

Elevation of the Head of the Bed

The head of the bed should be elevated to at least 30° to facilitate jugular venous drainage, which will lower ICP. The venous system within the brain has no valves, so gravity will help to facilitate and increase venous drainage. Maintaining the head of the bed at 30° will help to achieve adequate intra-vascular volume, which is essential to sufficiently perfuse the brain (Hickey, 2003b).

Blood Pressure Maintenance

Hypotension can lead to cerebral ischemia and secondary brain injury. In contrast, hypertension has no effect on increasing the cerebral blood flow. The mean arterial blood pressure should be maintained above 90 mm Hg at all times. If hypotension occurs, administer a fluid bolus immediately (Hickey, 2003b; Kirkness & March, 2004).

Temperature Control

A 1°C increase in temperature will increase the cerebral blood flow by 5%–6%. This increased blood flow will increase the cerebral metabolic rate and, hence, will increase ICP. The patient's temperature should remain nor-mothermic with the use of antipyretics (Hickey, 2003b).

Intracranial Pressure Monitoring

ICP monitoring records patients' ICP readings and guides the therapy neces-sary to efficiently treat the condition. Trends in fluctuations of ICP pressures can be followed and can evaluate the effectiveness of the treatment. Several mechanisms are available to monitor ICP. The most commonly used are the intraventricular catheter, the subarachnoid bolt, and the subdural catheter. The purpose of inserting these devices is to have a mechanism to monitor ICP and pressure trends and to correlate them with the clinical neurologic presentation. These devices also provide a mechanism to drain off CSF to decrease ICP. Patients with ICP monitoring require close observation in a neurology intensive care unit (Hickey, 2003b).

Surgical Intervention

Surgical intervention via craniotomy is indicated if a resectable, localized mass, tumor, or hematoma is causing the increased ICP. A craniotomy is the surgical opening of the skull to provide access to the brain to remove a tumor or relieve the cerebral edema by resecting brain tissue. During the procedure, a ventriculostomy may be inserted to allow drainage of CSF and decrease the CSF pressure (Hickey, 2003b). Following a craniotomy, often the bone flap is not replaced to allow expansion of the brain during the period of increased pressure. The bone flap can be replaced later (Hickey, 2003b).

Fluid Management

Hypotension and dehydration can result in decreased CPP and cerebral ischemia. Hyponatremia can increase ICP by causing cerebral edema (Hickey, 2003b; Kirkness & March, 2004). The management goal for these patients is to attain normal fluid and electrolyte balance. Isotonic saline is used for fluid replacement to avoid hyponatremia and its complications.

Analgesics and Sedation

Pain, restlessness, and anxiety can exacerbate existing ICP. Narcotic analgesics are recommended to treat pain and for sedation. Morphine sulfate is the recommended analgesic agent for critically ill patients. Fentanyl may be used if patients are hemodynamically unstable. Midazolam and propofol are used for short-term treatment of anxiety. Lorazepam is recommended for long-term treatment of anxiety. Haloperidol is recommended for the treatment of delirium. Use of these drugs should be done cautiously with close monitoring of patients' neurologic status and potential side effects of the sedation (Hickey, 2003b).

Corticosteroids and Mannitol

Corticosteroids are effective in the treatment of the early signs of increased ICP caused by vasogenic edema. Studies have shown no benefit in using corticosteroids in the treatment of cytotoxic edema occurring secondary to cerebral infarction or intracranial hemorrhage. The normal dose is dexamethasone 6–10 mg every six hours. Research has not shown that higher doses increase the therapeutic benefit (Baehring, 2005).

Mannitol is an osmotic diuretic that does not cross the BBB but works on the principle of altering the osmotic pressure to draw water from the extracellular space in the edematous brain tissues. The normal dose of mannitol is a bolus of 0.25–0.5 g/kg and up to 1 g/kg every three to six hours. The maximal effect should be seen in 15–30 minutes and should last one to three hours. A rebound effect, with an increase in ICP, often occurs after a mannitol administration. Furosemide, a loop diuretic, may be given to manage the rebound effect. Side effects of mannitol include dehydration and electrolyte imbalance with hyponatremia and hypokalemia (Hickey, 2003b).

Seizure Control

Several factors may cause seizures in patients with cancer: meningitis and encephalitis from an opportunistic infection, a primary or metastatic brain tumor, or the delayed effects of cranial irradiation (Buelow, Long, Rossi, & Gilbert, 2004). Seizures increase the cerebral metabolic rate, which results in increased ICP. Patients with cancer with a known brain tumor, metastatic or primary, may or may not receive prophylactic therapy to prevent seizure activity. All anticonvulsants have adverse effects, and seizure prophylaxis has not always proved beneficial to patients (McAllister et al., 2002). Clinicians may institute seizure prophylaxis for patients with brain tumors accompanied by increased ICP or for those with a history of seizures. Anticonvulsants are administered, and drug levels should be followed to maintain a therapeutic serum level. The most common anticonvulsant is phenytoin. Phenytoin may be administered orally 100 mg three or four times a day (Hickey, 2003a).

Nursing Management

Prevention of Intracranial Pressure

Nurses should be aware that certain activities may increase ICP in patients with an intracranial lesion. Sneezing, coughing, straining, and the use of positive-end expiratory pressure will increase ICP. When being turned, patients may perform a Valsalva maneuver or isometric muscle contractions, such as gripping the side rail, and these actions may increase ICP (Belford, 2005). Nurses should establish a bowel regimen for patients to prevent constipation and straining. Straining while passing stool can cause increased intra-abdominal pressure and, hence, increased ICP. Patients should receive stool softeners and laxatives as needed (Hickey, 2003b). The daily nursing care of patients requires activities that can increase ICP as mentioned. Although combining nursing care activities, such as bathing, turning, and performing range of motion exercises, may seem productive, it may be detrimental to patients with increased ICP. Spacing out care activities will decrease the prolonged spikes of increased ICP (Belford). Often, patients with increased ICP require more aggressive pulmonary toilet to prevent pneumonia. Suctioning and repositioning with pulmonary toilet will increase ICP. These activities are essential for patients' well-being and cannot be eliminated but should be followed by a rest period to help to decrease ICP. Table 4-7 outlines the nursing management of patients with increased ICP.

Symptom Management

Headache is a common manifestation in patients with increased ICP. Analgesics are not often effective for pain management in headaches of this etiology; corticosteroids, which decrease cerebral edema, are more effective. As patients begin to manifest motor weakness, it is important to maintain proper positioning of the affected limbs to prevent contractures. Seizures may occur because of progressive increased ICP. Patients may require seizure prophylaxis with the diagnosis of a primary or metastatic brain tumor.

Table 4-7. Nursing Protocol for the Management of Increased Intracranial Pressure

Factor	Intervention
Airway/ adequate ventilation maintenance	Auscultate chest sounds q 4–8 hours. Monitor the administration of oxygen. Use suctioning if necessary only after preoxygenating with 100% FIO_2 for 1 minute. Suction should be intermittent and brief (< 15 seconds). Use opioids cautiously because they depress respirations. Monitor SaO_2 to keep saturation > 90%. Monitor blood gases. Keep PaO_2 > 60 mm Hg + $PaCO_2$ < 40 mm Hg.
Body positioning	Maintain bed rest. Make use of pressure-distributing mattresses (egg-crate or alternating-pressure mattresses), sheepskin paddings. Change position every 2 hours. Offer gentle body massage. Encourage patient to keep head in neutral position. Avoid rotated head positions, flexion or extension of neck, and extreme hip flexion. Keep head of bed elevated 30° to promote venous drainage. Side-lying position will decrease risk of aspiration in patients with an altered level of consciousness. Avoid prone position.
Physical stressors • Isometric muscle contractions • Cough • Vomiting • Constipation	Encourage patient to allow passive movement. Use pull sheets to turn and move patient. If the patient must move, encourage him to do so while exhaling. Avoid using restraints. Logroll patient. Determine etiology of the cough. A cough suppressant may be indicated. Assess etiology of vomiting. Administer antiemetics. Discourage straining. Maintain bowel regimen to prevent constipation. Avoid rectal route for medication administration and temperature assessment. No enemas.
Emotional stressors	Avoid emotional stress. Counsel family to maintain a calm atmosphere. Avoid disturbing conversations at patient's bedside. Help to maintain open channels of communication between patient, family, and interdisciplinary team. Cautious use of benzodiazepines, opioids, and neuroleptics for sedation.
Environmental factors • Excess stimulation	Explain the unavoidable hallway and equipment noises. Make attempts to minimize excess stimulation. Provide a quiet, darkened room. Discourage the use of television or radio. Restrict visitors to close family and friends. Make other hospital personnel (e.g., housekeeping, venipuncture team) aware of the need to avoid excess stimulation. Place sign in doorway.

(Continued on next page)

Table 4-7. Nursing Protocol for the Management of Increased Intracranial Pressure *(Continued)*

Factor	Intervention
• Stability of surroundings	Provide consistent nursing personnel. Develop a predictable daily care routine. Provide periods of uninterrupted rest. Avoid clustering of nursing activities because of risk for increasing intracranial pressure.
Safety factors	Observe frequently. Create a mechanism for patient to call the nurse if unable to use the call light/bell. Maintain all bed side rails in the elevated position. Supervise and/or assist with ambulation and activities of daily living. Minimize hazards of immobility. Assess skin integrity. Institute measures to maintain skin integrity. Assess for signs/symptoms of deep vein thrombosis. Apply pneumatic compression devices or elastic stockings as ordered. Institute seizure precautions if a history of seizures exists or if patient is at risk. Monitor for seizure activity. Administer anticonvulsant medications and monitor their blood level.
Treatment factors • Steroids	Establish baseline mental status and monitor for changes. Minimize risk for gastrointestinal disturbances. Steroids should be taken with meals, antacids, or milk. Avoid aspirin. Guaiac stool for occult blood. Minimize risk of infection. Avoid invasive procedures. Monitor complete blood count. Encourage all people who come in contact with the patient to wash hands. Maintain nutritional status. Institute a high-protein, high-calcium diet. Monitor for hyperglycemia and glucosuria. Monitor electrolytes, especially sodium and potassium. Weigh patient daily. Teach patient and family about visible changes (acne, abnormal fat distribution, facial changes, hirsutism). Advise them that these changes are reversible and will subside when steroid therapy is discontinued.
• Diuretics	Monitor serum electrolytes, glucose, and chemistries. Keep an accurate record of intake and output. Monitor blood pressure.

FIO_2—fraction of inspired oxygen; $PaCO_2$—partial pressure of arterial carbon dioxide; PaO_2—partial pressure of arterial oxygen; SaO_2—saturated arterial oxygen

Note. From "Obstructive Emergencies" (pp. 628–629), by D. Kazierad in B.L. Johnson and J. Gross (Eds.), *Handbook of Oncology Nursing* (3rd ed.), 1998, Sudbury, MA: Jones and Bartlett. Copyright 1998 by Jones and Bartlett. Reprinted with permission.

If seizure activity occurs, nurses should protect patients from harm, provide privacy, maintain an airway, and monitor them for the type of seizure activity, location of movement, and length of seizure as part of the basic nursing assessment for seizure.

Patient and Caregiver Education

The diagnosis of a primary or metastatic brain tumor begins a journey of uncertainty and fear for patients and caregivers. Patients who are conscious and aware may be anxious and frightened about the alteration in their thought processes and changes in their motor function. Nurses should inform the patients of the reason for these symptoms and the treatments planned to decrease ICP. Often, patients may not be aware of their neurologic decline. Their caregivers, however, will feel distressed. Keeping them informed of test results and treatment plans and providing reassurance and emotional support will help to decrease their anxiety.

With the manifestations of increased ICP, a neurosurgeon often will be consulted for diagnostic evaluation and to assist with the treatment plan. Surgeons often must resect intracranial tumors to treat increased ICP and diminish the neurologic deficits. However, this intracranial surgery is not without risk. The decision to proceed usually is a team decision based on the oncologist's assessment of the stability of the primary cancer and the neurosurgeon's assessment of the resectability of the lesion. Nurses should provide patients and caregivers with the opportunity and encouragement to ask questions and should clarify information related to the treatment plan to help the caregivers to arrive at an informed decision.

Conclusion

Increased ICP is an oncologic emergency requiring rapid and accurate neurologic assessment. Assessment and treatment of the early signs of increased ICP can prevent permanent neurologic deficits that can affect patients' quality of life or cause death. Once patients show evidence of brain stem dysfunction, the neurologic consequences may be irreversible. Managing increased ICP is a team effort between oncology and neurosurgery to identify, evaluate, assess, and treat patients in a timely fashion.

References

American Cancer Society. (2006). *Cancer facts and figures, 2006.* Atlanta, GA: Author.

Baehring, J.M. (2005). Increased intracranial pressure. In V.T. DeVita, S. Hellman, & S.A. Rosenberg (Eds.), *Cancer: Principles and practice of oncology* (7th ed., pp. 2281–2287). Philadelphia: Lippincott Williams & Wilkins.

Belford, K. (2005). Central nervous system cancers. In C.H. Yarbro, M.H. Frogge, & M. Goodman (Eds.), *Cancer nursing: Principles and practice* (6th ed., pp. 1089–1136). Sudbury, MA: Jones and Bartlett.

Buelow, J.M., Long, L., Rossi, A.M., & Gilbert, K.L. (2004). Epilepsy. In M.K. Bader & L.R. Littlejohns (Eds.), *AANN core curriculum for neuroscience nursing* (4th ed., pp. 586–587). St. Louis, MO: Saunders.

Davis, A.E., Park, S., Darwich, H., Deveikis, S., & Rossini, D. (2004). Neurodiagnostic tests. In M.K. Bader & L.R. Littlejohns (Eds.), *AANN core curriculum for neuroscience nursing* (4th ed., pp. 174–177). St. Louis, MO: Saunders.

DeVroom, H.L., Smith, R.K., Mogenson, K., & Clancey, J.K. (2004). Nervous system tumors. In M.K. Bader & L.R. Littlejohns (Eds.), *AANN core curriculum for neuroscience nursing* (4th ed., pp. 511–527). St. Louis, MO: Saunders.

Hickey, J.V. (2003a). Brain tumors. In J.V. Hickey (Ed.), *The clinical practice of neurological and neurosurgical nursing* (5th ed., pp. 483–508). Philadelphia: Lippincott Williams & Wilkins.

Hickey, J.V. (2003b). Intracranial hypertension: Theory and management of increases in intracranial pressure. In J.V. Hickey (Ed.), *The clinical practice of neurological and neurosurgical nursing* (5th ed., pp. 286–315). Philadelphia: Lippincott Williams & Wilkins.

Jemal, A., Siegel, R., Ward, E., Murray, T., Xu, J., Smigal, C., et al. (2006). Cancer statistics, 2006. *CA: A Cancer Journal for Clinicians, 56*, 106–130.

Kazierad, D. (1998). Obstructive emergencies. In B.L. Johnson & J. Gross (Eds.), *Handbook of oncology nursing* (3rd ed., pp. 617–630). Sudbury, MA: Jones and Bartlett.

Kirkness, C., & March, K. (2004). Intracranial pressure management. In M.K. Bader & L.R. Littlejohns (Eds.), *AANN core curriculum for neuroscience nursing* (4th ed., pp. 249–267). St. Louis, MO: Saunders.

Lindsay, K.W., & Bone, I. (2004). *Neurology and neurosurgery illustrated* (4th ed.). New York: Churchill Livingstone.

March, K., & Wellwood, J. (2004). Intracranial pressure concepts and cerebral blood flow. In M.K. Bader & L.R. Littlejohns (Eds.), *AANN core curriculum for neuroscience nursing* (4th ed., pp. 87–93). St. Louis, MO: Saunders.

McAllister, L.D., Ward, J.H., Schulman, S.F., & DeAngelis, L.M. (Eds.). (2002). *Practical neuro-oncology: A guide to patient care*. Boston: Butterworth-Heinemann.

Plum, F., & Posner, J.B. (1980). *The diagnosis of stupor and coma* (3rd ed.). Philadelphia: F.A. Davis.

Slazinski, T., & Littlejohns, L.R. (2004). Anatomy of the nervous system. In M.K. Bader & L.R. Littlejohns (Eds.), *AANN core curriculum for neuroscience nursing* (4th ed., pp. 52–53). St. Louis, MO: Saunders.

Wilkes, G.M. (2004). Increased intracranial pressure. In C.H. Yarbro, M.H. Frogge, & M. Goodman (Eds.), *Cancer symptom management* (3rd ed., pp. 374–385). Sudbury, MA: Jones and Bartlett.

Kristine Turner Story, RN, MSN, APRN

Chapter 5

Malignant Pleural Effusion

Introduction

Malignant pleural effusion (MPE), the abnormal collection of fluid in the pleural space, is a common complication in patients with cancer. Pleural effusions are life threatening because they affect respiratory function by restricting lung expansion, decreasing lung volume, and altering gas exchange. Although many pleural effusions are small and asymptomatic, many may present as or progress to massive size (see Figure 5-1). Over time, these abnormalities can lead to respiratory distress and respiratory and cardiac arrest. Nurses caring for patients with malignancies need to be vigilant about respiratory assessments so that they may detect pleural effusions early and implement interventions to maintain optimal cardiopulmonary function as long as possible.

Incidence

Many diseases can cause pleural effusions, but the most common causes in the United States are cancer, congestive heart failure (CHF), and pneumonia. More than one million cases of pleural effusion from all causes occur annually (Light, 2002). MPE is one of the leading causes of *exudative effusions,* an effusion with a high content of protein, cells, or solid materials, and accounts for 42%–77% of exudative effusions (American Thoracic Society [ATS], 2000; Chestnut & Prendergast, 2005). Approximately 50% of patients with cancer will develop MPE. It may be the first indication of disease, a complication of the disease or treatment, or a late finding.

The annual incidence of MPE in the United States is estimated at more than 150,000 cases (Marchi, Teixeira, & Vargas, 2003). Autopsy studies have shown pleural effusion in 15% of patients who died from cancer in which MPE was not previously diagnosed (Rodriguez-Panadero, Borderas Naranjo, & Lopez Mejias, 1989). Lung cancer is the most common cause of MPE, accounting for 30% of all cases. Breast cancer is second (25%), followed by tumors of the

123

Figure 5-1. Pleural Effusion

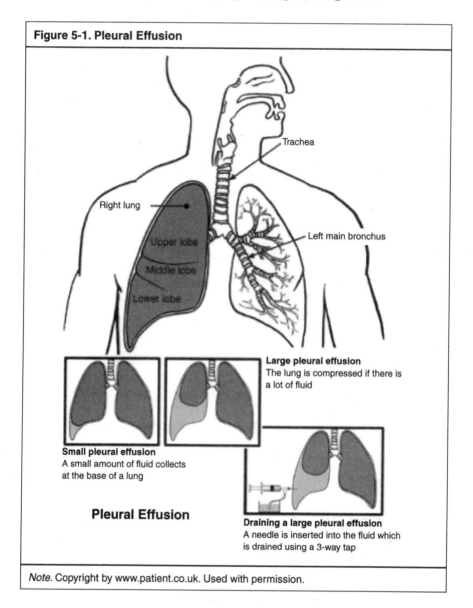

Trachea

Right lung

Left main bronchus

Upper lobe

Middle lobe

Lower lobe

Large pleural effusion
The lung is compressed if there is
a lot of fluid

Small pleural effusion
A small amount of fluid collects
at the base of a lung

Pleural Effusion

Draining a large pleural effusion
A needle is inserted into the fluid which
is drained using a 3-way tap

Note. Copyright by www.patient.co.uk. Used with permission.

lymphoma group, both Hodgkin disease and non-Hodgkin lymphoma (20%)
(ATS, 2000; Light, 2002). Other cancers less commonly associated with MPE
include leukemia, melanoma, mesothelioma, uterine, cervical, ovarian, and
gastric carcinomas, and sarcomas. Adenocarcinoma of unknown primary accounts for 5%–10% of MPE (ATS; Marchi et al.; Sahn, 1997). More women
than men experience MPE, primarily because of the high incidence rate in
breast cancer (Myers, 2001; Otto, 2001). Median survival from the time of

diagnosis of a pleural effusion varies based on tumor type. Median survival of one to two months has been reported in as many as 80% of people with MPE (Marchi et al.; Sahn). Other sources reported average median survivals following MPE as 6 months for patients with lung cancer, 14 months for patients with breast cancer, and 16 months for those with mesothelioma (Otto; Works & Maxwell, 2000). Pleural effusions of any kind in patients with lung cancer typically indicate locally advanced, incurable disease (Schrump & Nguyen, 2001).

Risk Factors

The presence of a malignancy that is associated with MPE is in itself a risk factor for development of an effusion. The occurrence of pleural metastases is a typical risk factor for MPE. Most pleural metastases result from tumor emboli on the visceral pleural surface, with secondary seeding to the parietal pleura. Other mechanisms include direct tumor invasion, lymphatic metastases, and hematogenous spread to the parietal pleura. Interference with the integrity of the lymphatic system anywhere between the parietal pleura and mediastinal lymph nodes can cause pleural fluid formation. Local inflammatory changes caused by the presence of malignant cells can increase capillary permeability, thus causing effusion (ATS, 2000; Chestnut & Prendergast, 2005; Marchi et al., 2003).

A *paramalignant effusion* is an effusion that is not caused by direct involvement of the pleura but is related to the effects of the primary tumor. Examples include postobstructive pneumonia, causing parapneumonic effusion; pulmonary embolism; and *transudative effusions* caused by postobstruction atelectasis and low plasma oncotic pressure because of cachexia. A chylothorax is a rare effusion containing chyle, a substance that is normally transported from the intestines to the systemic circulation via the thoracic duct. A chylothorax can occur because of obstruction of the thoracic duct by tumor (ATS, 2000; Chestnut & Prendergast, 2005). Other common nonmalignant causes of pleural effusion are CHF, pneumonia, pulmonary embolus, viral disease, pericarditis, tuberculosis, superior vena cava syndrome, hypoalbuminemia, nephrosis, coronary artery bypass surgery, and cirrhosis with ascites (Henke, 2000; Light, 2002; Marchi et al., 2003; Myers, 2001) (see Table 5-1).

Treatment of a primary tumor also can cause a pleural effusion. Radiation therapy to the mediastinum and chest increases the risk of MPE. Pleuritis can occur six weeks to six months after radiation therapy and can lead to MPE development. Later effects of radiation therapy include fibrosis of the mediastinum, constrictive pericarditis, and vena caval obstruction, which can occur months to years after treatment (Sahn, 1997). Chemotherapy agents such as methotrexate, procarbazine, cyclophosphamide, and bleomycin are associated with MPE (ATS, 2000; Marchi et al., 2003). The mechanism of chemotherapy-induced MPE usually is pleuritis or pleuropericarditis. Effects

Table 5-1. Differential Diagnosis of Pleural Effusion

Effusions	Cause
Transudative pleural	Congestive heart failure
	Pericardial disease
	Cirrhosis
	Nephrotic syndrome
	Peritoneal dialysis
	Superior vena cava obstruction
	Myxedema
	Pulmonary embolism
	Urinothorax
Exudative pleural	Metastatic malignancy
	Mesothelioma
	Infections
	• Bacterial/viral/fungal/parasitic
	• Tuberculosis
	Pulmonary embolism
	Gastrointestinal disorders
	• Esophageal perforation
	• Pancreatic disease
	• Intra-abdominal abscess
	• Diaphragmatic hernia
	Collagen-vascular diseases
	• Rheumatoid arthritis
	• Systemic lupus erythematosus
	• Sjögren syndrome
	• Wegener granulomatosis
	• Churg-Strauss syndrome
	Post-cardiac injury syndrome
	Asbestos exposure
	Sarcoidosis
	Uremia
	Meigs syndrome
	Yellow nail syndrome
	Drug-induced pleural disease
	• Nitrofurantoin
	• Dantrolene
	• Methysergide
	• Bromocriptine
	• Procarbazine
	• Amiodarone
	Trapped lung
	Radiation therapy
	Electrical burns
	Hemothorax
	Iatrogenic injury
	Ovarian hyperstimulation syndrome
	Chylothorax

Note. Based on information from Chester & Prendergast, 2005; Light, 2002; Myers, 2001; Weatherhead & Antunes, 2004.

of chemotherapeutic agents on the interstitium of the lung also may increase the risk of MPE (Sahn). Patients with late-stage MPE often have widespread metastases, physiologic deficits such as malnutrition or debilitation, and other comorbidities (Chestnut & Prendergast, 2005; Grannis, Wagman, Lai, & Curcio, 2002; Myers, 2001).

Pathophysiology

The pleura is a thin membrane that envelops the lungs and lines the thoracic cavity. The pleurae are dynamic and metabolically active membranes that are involved in maintaining the homeostasis of the pleural space and in responding to injury or inflammation (Schrump & Nguyen, 2001; Weatherhead & Antunes, 2004). The pleura has two layers—the visceral pleura and the parietal pleura. The visceral pleura adheres to and encases the lung and extends into the fissure separating the lobes of the lungs. Blood supply to the visceral pleura is supplied by the bronchial circulation, and lymphatic channels are present, but there are no nerve endings for pain. The parietal pleura lines the mediastinum, diaphragm, and chest wall. Blood supply to the parietal pleura comes from the intercostal arteries. Nerve endings are present and, if stimulated, will produce referred pain in the chest wall, shoulder, or abdomen (Myers, 2001; Works & Maxwell, 2000) (see Figure 5-1).

Between the two pleural layers is a potential space known as the pleural space. A small amount of fluid, 5–15 ml, normally is present in this space and serves as a lubricant, allowing the pleural surfaces to glide over each other without friction during inspiration and expiration. Fluid passes continuously through this space and is exchanged at a rate of approximately 100–200 ml per day (Henke, 2000; Otto, 2001; Works & Maxwell, 2000). The systemic capillaries of the parietal pleura produce fluid. The pulmonary capillaries of the visceral pleura absorb approximately 80%–90% of this fluid. The lymph channels of the visceral pleura reabsorb the remaining fluid (Myers, 2001; Weatherhead & Antunes, 2004). In a normal lung, no true pleural space exists, and if one develops, a pleural effusion has been created. Any condition in which fluid production exceeds fluid removal will lead to accumulation of fluid and subsequent pleural effusion. Pleural effusions reflect an imbalance in the production and clearance of fluid in the pleural space (Ruckdeschel & Jablons, 2001).

Normally, equilibrium exists between the osmotic and hydrostatic pressures that control secretion and absorption of pleural fluid. Five forces regulate equilibrium of fluid movement across the pleura: (a) capillary permeability, (b) hydrostatic pressure (capillary and interstitial), (c) colloidal osmotic pressure (plasma protein and interstitial protein), (d) negative intrapleural pressure, and (e) lymphatic drainage. Any alterations in these forces can cause a pleural effusion (Myers, 2001; Schrump & Nguyen, 2001). The pathologic mechanisms that account for most pleural effusions are (a) increased production of fluid in normal capillaries because of increased hydrostatic or decreased oncotic pressures, (b) increased production of fluid because of abnormal capillary permeability, (c) decreased lymphatic clearance of fluid from the pleural space, (d) infection in the pleural space, and (e) bleeding into the pleural space (Chestnut & Prendergast, 2005).

The most common etiologies of MPE are the obstruction of the pleural or pulmonary lymphatic system by tumor and pleural implants that cause inflammation and irritation, resulting in increased capillary permeability. Blockage of lymphatic channels or obstruction of venous circulation by tumor interferes with the drainage of fluid from the pleural space, causing an effusion. Impaired lymphatic drainage from the pleural space is the predominant mechanism for MPE development. A strong correlation exists between malignant infiltration of lymph nodes and development of MPE, whereas no relationship has been found between the extent of pleural metastasis and MPE development. Pleural effusions generally do not occur with pleural involvement by sarcomas because of a lack of lymphatic metastasis. Lymphatic obstruction exists most commonly with lymphoma and metastases from breast and lung cancers (Myers, 2001; Sahn, 1997; Weatherhead & Antunes, 2004).

Malignant cells may be shed from the pleura and grow freely in the pleural space, forming tumor cell suspensions, which demonstrate a greater number of cells on cytologic exam than pleural implants. Ovarian and lung cancers often are associated with tumor cell suspensions (Myers, 2001; Schrump & Nguyen, 2001). Direct invasion of a blood vessel, occlusion of venules, and tumor-induced angiogenesis may cause bloody MPE. Visceral pleural metastasis occurs through pulmonary artery invasion by tumor and embolization of malignant cells to the diaphragm and mediastinum initially and then spreads upward and outward. Adenocarcinoma of the lung is more likely to result in pleural effusion because of hematogenous spread of tumor. This is most common in the presence of bilateral pulmonary tumors and in the presence of metastasis to the liver (Sahn, 1997).

Vascular endothelial growth factor (VEGF) has been implicated in the development of MPE. VEGF can alter the permeability of the pleural membrane and is involved in angiogenesis. Metastatic cancers express VEGF locally and systemically, and VEGF receptors are present on pleural mesothelial cells. VEGF levels are significantly higher in pleural effusions in patients with non-small cell lung cancer, mesothelioma, and breast cancer. In the mouse model, inhibition of VEGF production decreased pleural effusion formation (Weatherhead & Antunes, 2004; Zebrowski et al., 1999). Further study in humans is necessary to determine the impact of VEGF on MPE development and treatment.

Clinical Manifestations

Symptoms associated with pleural effusion reflect the presence of abnormal fluid that expands the pleural space, leading to compression or collapse of the lung. Many patients are asymptomatic, and approximately 25% of MPEs are found incidentally (Myers, 2001; Works & Maxwell, 2000). The severity of symptoms is related to the volume and speed of development as well as underlying lung disease. Small effusions are less likely to be symptomatic compared to large or massive effusions. The progression of symptoms usually is linear and relatively predictable (Chestnut & Prendergast, 2005; Ruckdeschel & Jablons, 2001). However, it may be difficult to sort out the symptoms of MPE from underlying lung disease, the presence of generalized weakness, debilitation from advanced disease, and side effects of treatment (Works & Maxwell).

Most patients present with dyspnea at rest and on exertion, cough, and chest pain. Pulmonary compression, decreased lung expansion, and alveolar collapse cause dyspnea (Inzeo & Tyson, 2003). Dyspnea gradually increases with time and may progress to orthopnea and paroxysmal nocturnal dyspnea. Cough usually is dry and nonproductive. Patients may describe chest pain as pleuritic or sharp in nature when pleural inflammation is present or as dull, heavy, and continuous when parietal pleural metastasis is present. Patients may report anxiety and a fear of suffocation. They may experience general malaise and weight loss, may splint the area of the effusion, and may express a desire to lie on the affected side to improve comfort (Camp-Sorrell, 1999; Chestnut & Prendergast, 2005; Myers, 2001; Ruckdeschel & Jablons, 2001; Works & Maxwell, 2000).

Patient Assessment

Physical Examination

Physical findings usually are absent in small effusions. In larger effusions, clinicians may find dullness to percussion and decreased or absent breath sounds. Increased vocal fremitus, egophony, whispered pectoriloquy, and bronchial breath sounds may be present over the effusion (these terms are defined in Table 5-2). Decreased diaphragmatic excursion with percussion also may be present. Patients may complain of chest tenderness with palpation over the area of the effusion.

In more advanced cases, patients may experience tachypnea, labored breathing, use of accessory muscles, and restricted chest wall expansion. Cyanosis is rare but may be present in larger effusions where hypoxia is developing. The point of maximal impulse in the apex of the heart may have shifted to the left if the effusion is on the right. Lymphadenopathy is present in approximately one-third of patients at presentation. With massive effusions, increased intrapleural pressure will cause a contralateral shift of the trachea and bulging of intracostal spaces. Low cardiac output related to mediastinal compression also may occur (Chestnut & Prendergast, 2005; Henke, 2000; Myers, 2001; Sahn, 1997; Schrump & Nguyen, 2001; Works & Maxwell, 2000).

Other physical findings may point to causes other than malignancy for a pleural effusion and should be considered. The presence of an S3 gallop, jugular venous distention, and peripheral edema suggests CHF. A right ventricular heave or thrombophlebitis suggests pulmonary embolism. The presence of lymphadenopathy or hepatosplenomegaly suggests neoplastic disease, whereas ascites suggests a hepatic cause (Light, 2002). Other co-morbidities may confuse the picture, making it difficult to determine the cause of an effusion by physical findings alone (see Table 5-2 and Figure 5-2).

Table 5-2. Definitions of Common Physical Assessment Findings

Findings	Definition
Egophony	A change in transmitted sounds heard on auscultation of the chest when an effusion is present. The letter "e" spoken by the patient becomes higher pitched and sounds like the letter "a."
Vocal fremitus	A vibration in the chest wall produced by spoken word, felt on palpation of the chest when an effusion is present
Bronchial breath sounds	Breath sounds of a high-pitched, harsh, or blowing quality heard over a pleural effusion. The expiratory phase of respiration usually is as long as or longer than the inspiratory phase.
Whispered pecto-riloquy	The articulation of the sounds of a patient's voice, heard on auscultation of the chest when an effusion is present
S3 gallop	A third heart sound that immediately follows the second heart sound and is produced by blood flowing into an enlarged ventricle; usually seen with congestive heart failure
Ventricular heave	The visible upward movement of the chest wall over the apex of the heart in the case of an engorged ventricle; occasionally seen with congestive heart failure

Diagnostic Evaluation

Chest x-ray (CXR) generally first detects pleural effusions. Asymptomatic effusions may be diagnosed by routine CXR performed for follow-up of disease or as an incidental finding in patients without a diagnosis of malignancy. The lateral and decubitus views, an exposure obtained in a side-lying position, are most helpful and can show an effusion with as little as 75–100 ml of fluid. In general, 300 ml of fluid must be present to see an effusion on an upright anterior-posterior view. These effusions will appear as blunting of the costophrenic angle (see Figure 5-3). Massive effusions greater than 1,500 ml will appear as an opacification of one lung with a mediastinal shift

---

Figure 5-2. Clinical Features of Malignant Pleural Effusion

Symptoms
- May be asymptomatic
- Dyspnea on exertion or at rest
- Shortness of breath
- Dry, nonproductive cough
- Chest pain—may be achy and heavy or pleuritic
- Malaise
- Weight loss
- Anxiety, fear of suffocation
- Desire to lie on affected side

Signs
- Tachypnea
- Labored breathing
- Decreased or absent breath sounds
- Bronchial breath sounds
- Pleuritic rub over affected area
- Restricted chest wall expansion
- Decreased tactile fremitus
- Dullness to percussion
- Egophony
- Larger effusions also may exhibit
  - Splinting of chest
  - Cyanosis
  - Chest tenderness
  - Tracheal deviation to the unaffected side
  - Bulging of intercostal spaces
  - Lymphadenopathy
  - Shift in point of maximal impulse
  - Use of accessory muscles of breathing.

Note. Based on information from Camp-Sorrell, 1999; Chestnut & Prendergast, 2005; Henke, 2000; Myers, 2001; Sahn, 1997; Schrump & Nguyen, 2001; Works & Maxwell, 2000.

(Myers, 2001; Ruckdeschel & Jablons, 2001). Generally, in the case of lung cancer, a pleural effusion will be in the same lung as the primary tumor. When the primary tumor is not in the lung, effusions tend to be bilateral. Bilateral effusions with a normal heart size usually indicate malignancy (Sahn, 1997). Although large or massive effusions often indicate malignancy, clinicians also should consider parapneumonic effusions, empyema, and tuberculosis (Porcel & Vives, 2003).

Computed tomography (CT) scan of the chest can identify effusions with as little as 10 ml of fluid. They especially are helpful to identify a site for thoracentesis, to assess the mobility of fluid in the pleural space, and to confirm the presence or absence of loculations that might indicate fluid separation by adhesions (Chestnut & Prendergast, 2005; Myers, 2001). Chest CT also is

---

Figure 5-3. A Fairly Large Left Pleural Effusion

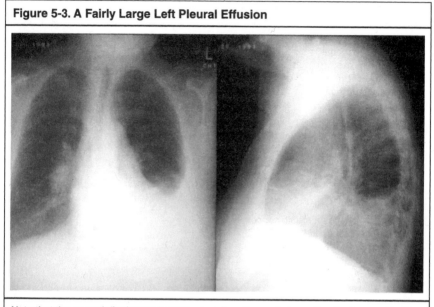

Note that the normal diaphragm border, as well as the posterior gutter, is obscured by the pleural effusion.

Note. Copyright by the author and the University of Iowa's Virtual Hospital, http://www .vh.org. Used with permission.

---

useful in diagnosing mesothelioma, defining pleural and parenchymal masses, and evaluating the mediastinum. It can rule out empyema, lymphangitic carcinomatosis, and benign asbestos pleural effusion (Sahn, 1997; Schrump & Nguyen, 2001; Works & Maxwell, 2001).

Ultrasound might be ordered to guide thoracentesis with small effusions and for evaluation in the presence of mesothelioma. Magnetic resonance imaging has limited use in MPE but may be helpful in evaluating the extent of chest wall involvement by tumor (ATS, 2000). Positron-emission tomography scans have not been used extensively in this situation but may play a role in evaluating the extent of disease in malignant mesothelioma (Bernard et al., 1998).

Performing thoracentesis can determine the characteristics of the effusion and provide symptom control. The indication for thoracentesis is the presence of a clinically significant pleural effusion of unknown cause (Light, 2002). Relative contraindications to thoracentesis are the presence of a minimal effusion, a coexisting bleeding abnormality, anticoagulation, and mechanical ventilation (ATS, 2000). Important complications of thoracentesis include pneumothorax, bleeding, infection, and spleen or liver laceration.

The initial thoracentesis usually is for diagnostic purposes and can be performed at the bedside. Following instillation of local anesthetic, a stab wound is made at the level of the sixth or seventh rib posteriorly, and a drainage tube is inserted. In general, 500–1,000 ml of fluid can be removed at one time, but if the effusion is large, it may be prudent to drain it gradually to avoid postexpansion pulmonary edema. Ultrasound or CT guidance may be necessary if the effusion is small or loculated, but ultrasound has not been shown to decrease the incidence of pneumothorax, a risk of this procedure. The experience of the clinician performing the thoracentesis probably is more important than the use of ultrasound (Light, 2002; Schrump & Nguyen, 2001). Routine post-thoracentesis CXR is not necessary unless patients have symptoms of cough, chest pain, or dyspnea, or if air is obtained during the procedure, or if tactile fremitus is lost over the upper part of the aspirated lung. Pneumothorax was found in 13 of 18 patients with one or more of these symptoms and in only 5 of 488 patients with none of these findings (Aleman et al., 1999).

Evaluation of the color and character of the pleural fluid removed via thoracentesis can help to determine the cause of the effusion. Purulent fluid indicates emphysema or infection; chylous (milky) fluid indicates a blockage of the thoracic duct with involvement of the mesenteric or retroperitoneal lymph nodes; and bloody fluid usually indicates malignancy. A prospective study of 715 patients with pleural effusion found that the most common cause of bloody effusions was cancer (47%), followed by trauma (12%) and pneumonia (10%). Most nonmalignant effusions were watery or serous (Villena, Lopez-Encuentra, Garcia-Lujan, Echave-Sustaeta, & Martinez, 2004). Pulmonary embolism also may cause a bloody effusion (Light, Erozan, & Ball, 1973). A pleural fluid hematocrit greater than 50% is more characteristic of hemothorax (Myers, 2001). The odor of an effusion also can narrow the diagnosis. A putrid odor usually indicates an infection caused by anaerobic bacteria. An odor of urine indicates a urinothorax, a rare type of pleural effusion defined as urine in the pleural space caused by urinary obstruction, failed tube nephrostomy, inflammatory or malignant process of the urinary tract, blunt renal trauma, shock wave lithotripsy, and posterior urethral valves (Light, 2002).

One of the major goals of thoracentesis is to determine whether an effusion is transudative or exudative. A transudate is clear fluid and usually means the effusion is nonmalignant but may indicate a malignancy in up to 20% of cases. It occurs when systemic factors that influence the formation or absorption of pleural fluid are altered (Ruckdeschel & Jablons, 2001). Common causes of transudates are CHF, cirrhosis, nephrotic syndrome, peritoneal dialysis, hypoalbuminemia, and constrictive pericarditis (Myers, 2001). Exudates are effusions that contain a high content of protein, cells, or solid materials derived from cells. They occur when local factors influence the formation and absorption of pleural fluid and are more indicative of a malignancy. Other causes of nonmalignant exudates are pneumonia, tuberculosis, chylothorax, sarcoidosis, systemic lupus erythematosus, pancreatitis, prior radiation therapy, and mesothelioma (Light, 2002; Myers; Sahn, 1997). A number of markers may indicate a malignant effusion (see Figure 5-4).

Cytologic evaluation of pleural fluid is the most specific test for malignancy. Tumor cells shed more rapidly than normal cells and should be detected in the pleural fluid in the presence of malignancy. Sixty percent to 80% of MPEs have positive cytology, but a negative cytology does not exclude cancer as the cause. An initial thoracentesis in a patient with a large pleural effusion may be negative for cytology because of the effect of dilution. A repeat thoracentesis several days later may improve the yield of malignant cells and result in a positive cytology. Negative cytology is most common with lymphoma. A pleural biopsy may be indicated, but usually a low yield results because this is a blind procedure, and significant complications can occur. Healthcare providers usually can make a diagnosis of MPE based on other factors, making pleural biopsy unnecessary (Myers, 2001; Ruckdeschel & Jablons, 2001; Sahn, 1997). If cytology and biopsy are both negative, clinicians should consider the existence of a paramalignant effusion and perform additional testing before attempting treatment (Marchi et al., 2003). Chromosomal analysis of pleural cells may prove useful in the future as another way to differentiate malignant from benign effusions, especially in cases of lymphoma, leukemia, and mesothelioma, but it is an expensive test and not widely available (Weatherhead & Antunes, 2004).

Additional tests may be necessary if the cause of the pleural effusion is not evident following thoracentesis or cytology or to provide more information regarding the extent of disease. These tests include bronchoscopy, thoracoscopy, transcutaneous needle biopsy, mediastinoscopy, video-assisted thoracic surgery (VATS), or open lung biopsy (Myers, 2001). Bronchoscopy may be helpful if an underlying lung cancer is suspected, especially with the presence

---

Figure 5-4. Characteristics of Exudative Effusions Caused by Malignancy

- Presence of Light's criteria (one or more of the following)
  - Ratio of pleural-fluid protein level to serum protein level > 0.5
  - Ratio of pleural-fluid LDH level to serum LDH level > 0.6
  - Pleural-fluid LDH level > two-thirds the upper limit of normal for serum LDH level
- Red blood cell count > 100,000/mm^3
- White blood cell count > 1,000/mm^3
- Low glucose (< 60 mg/dl)
- High specific gravity
- Low pH (< 7.3)
- High amylase
- Low adenosine deaminase
- Low C-reactive protein

LDH—lactate dehydrogenase

Note. Based on information from Chierakul et al., 2004; Light et al., 1972; Marchi et al., 2003; Myers, 2001; Porcel & Vives, 2003; Sahn, 1997.

of a lung lesion on CXR, atelectasis, hemoptysis, mediastinal shift, or a massive effusion. It is particularly useful in the case of MPE with no known primary site, but it requires the use of general anesthesia and should not be performed routinely (ATS, 2000; Grannis et al., 2002; Sahn, 1997).

Medical thoracoscopy, the placement of a fiberoptic scope into the pleural cavity, can be performed under local anesthesia or conscious sedation in an endoscopy suite, making it preferable over open surgical thoracotomy. It generally is indicated for evaluation of exudative effusions of unknown cause and for staging of malignant mesothelioma or lung cancer. After thoracoscopy, fewer than 10% of effusions remain undiagnosed. Thoracoscopy has a low complication rate, allows for visualization of the pleural cavity, and allows for pleural lavage and biopsy. The technique is similar to a chest tube insertion, with a scope placed to visualize the pleural cavity. Biopsies can be taken from all areas of the pleural cavity. Medical thoracoscopy also allows for immediate treatment by pleurodesis or pleurectomy (ATS, 2000; Grannis et al., 2002; Sahn, 1997).

VATS allows for a more extensive procedure than medical thoracoscopy and can combine diagnosis with treatment. It requires the use of general anesthesia and single-lung ventilation. VATS is contraindicated if patients cannot tolerate single-lung ventilation, if multiple pleural adhesions are present, or if the treatment team's expertise is insufficient to deal with potential complications (ATS, 2000).

Treatment Modalities

Healthcare providers should systematically evaluate all patients with pleural effusions before determining viability of treatment. Both the management and natural course of an effusion depend on the patient's status, the extent of clinical symptoms, the type and extent of the underlying malignancy, and the expected survival. Overall, 54% of patients with MPE die within one month of diagnosis; 84% live three months. Ideally, therapy should minimize discomfort and limit hospital time. The primary indication for treatment is relief of dyspnea (ATS, 2000; Schrump & Nguyen, 2001; Weatherhead & Antunes, 2004). Watchful waiting or treating the underlying cause may be appropriate care for patients who are asymptomatic. However, in 10%–30% of cases, if MPE is left untreated, the underlying lung may become encased by tumor and fibrous tissue, leading to trapped lung that is unresponsive to thoracentesis (Grannis et al., 2002). Table 5-3 presents an overview of treatment modalities used in the management of MPE.

Therapeutic Thoracentesis

The first line of treatment is therapeutic thoracentesis, which should be performed on all dyspneic patients to determine its effect on symptoms and

Table 5-3. Treatment of Malignant Pleural Effusion

Treatment	Indications	Methodology
Observation	Asymptomatic effusions; most will progress and require therapy.	Frequent reassessments with serial chest x-ray
Therapeutic thoracentesis	First line of treatment, rapid relief of dyspnea; obtain pleural fluid for analysis.	Catheter is inserted into pleural space, and fluid is withdrawn and sent to lab for analysis.
Chest tube drainage only	Loculated effusions, massive effusions, poor performance status, treatment failures	Large-bore chest tube or indwelling catheter is placed into the pleural space for long-term drainage.
Pleurodesis	Control of effusion; demonstrated benefit from therapeutic thoracentesis	Large-bore or small-bore chest tube is placed, fluid is drained, and sclerosant is administered into the tube. The tube is left in place until drainage volume is < 100 ml/day.
Thoracoscopy with talc poudrage	Control of effusion; demonstrated benefit from therapeutic thoracentesis	Thoracoscope is inserted into pleural space, fluid is drained, and talc is administered as a spray using an atomizer.
Pleuroperitoneal shunt	When other options have failed or are not indicated; may be useful with chylothorax	Denver® shunt is implanted into the abdomen with drainage catheters in the pleural and peritoneal space and drains fluid into the abdomen.
Indwelling pleural catheter	Control of effusion for outpatient management	Pleurx® or Tenckhoff® catheter is inserted into the pleural space and sutured in place; patient or caregiver can drain with special equipment. Implanted catheter may be intermittently accessed similar to other implanted ports.
Pleurectomy and pleural abrasion	Good performance status; used only if other measures have failed and good life expectancy	Requires thoracoscopy or thoracotomy; pleural membrane is resected and abraded; prevents reaccumulation of pleural fluid.

Note. Based on information from American Thoracic Society, 2000; Sahn, 1997; Weatherhead & Antunes, 2004.

to determine the rate and degree of recurrence (see Figure 5-1). Effusions recur within 30 days after initial thoracentesis in 97% of patients. Recurrence of an effusion within less than 30 days indicates the need for immediate treatment. If thoracentesis does not relieve dyspnea, the healthcare team should investigate other causes for the shortness of breath, such as atelectasis, thromboembolism, tumor embolism, and lymphangitic carcinomatosis (ATS, 2000; Schrump & Nguyen, 2001).

Therapeutic thoracentesis may serve as the primary treatment in patients who have advanced disease, poor performance status, and a low pleural fluid pH level. Periodic outpatient therapeutic thoracentesis may be preferable to hospitalization or more aggressive treatment, especially if patients have a Karnofsky performance score of less than 70 (see Table 5-4). However, recurrent effusions exist in up to 100% of patients with tube drainage alone (Marchi et al., 2003; Schrump & Nguyen, 2001). The amount of fluid that can safely be removed from the pleural space during therapeutic thoracentesis is not known. Generally, 1–1.5 L of fluid can be removed safely at one time, as long as patients do not develop chest pain, dyspnea, or severe cough (ATS, 2000). Alternatively, nurses can monitor the pleural fluid pressure, and if it does not drop below –20 cm H_2O, continued fluid removal probably is safe (Light, Jenkinson, Minh, & George, 1980).

In patients with massive effusions with or without mediastinal shift, the immediate placement of a chest tube may be appropriate. Long-term chest tube placement may be the preferred treatment in the case of trapped lung or if the lung expands less than two-thirds after thoracentesis. Chest tube drainage of recurrent effusions after therapeutic thoracentesis is necessary to ensure complete lung expansion before attempting pleurodesis (Marchi et al., 2003).

Table 5-4. Karnofsky Performance Score	
Score	Description
100	Normal, no complaints
90	Able to carry on normal activities. Minor signs or symptoms of disease
80	Normal activity with effort
70	Cares for self. Unable to carry on normal activity or do active work
60	Requires occasional assistance but able to care for most of own needs
50	Requires considerable assistance and frequent medical care
40	Disabled. Requires special care and assistance
30	Severely disabled. Hospitalization indicated, though death not imminent.
20	Very sick. Hospitalization and active supportive treatment are necessary.

Pleurodesis

Pleurodesis is a procedure that introduces a chemical agent into the pleural space in an effort to obliterate the space, thereby preventing recurrence of the effusion. The exact mechanism of action that causes obliteration of the pleural space is unknown and may vary based on the agent used. Talc and tetracycline have been shown to increase the presence of polymorphonuclear neutrophils followed by an influx of macrophages mediated by interleukin-8. Rapid deposition of pleural fibrin and fibroblast proliferation cause fibrosis of the pleural space. Intrapleural neutrophils release proteolytic enzymes and toxic oxygen radicals, damaging the mesothelial lining and causing fibrosis. Other agents may not act as sclerosants, but rather their cytotoxic effects may control pleural fluid turnover or induce apoptosis, intense necrosis, angiogenesis and inflammation, cell adhesion, and migration. Further study of the mechanism of pleurodesis will help to identify newer agents that may improve response rates (Marchi et al., 2003; Weatherhead & Antunes, 2004).

The initial use of pleurodesis as a treatment for pleural effusion dates back to the early 1900s when L. Spengler injected silver nitrate into the pleural cavity to control an effusion. Since then, several agents have been used, but the ideal sclerosing agent has yet to be found. The ideal agent should be cost effective, available worldwide, easily handled and sterilized, easy to administer, and 100% effective, and should produce no significant pain and no mortality or morbidity. To date, this agent does not exist (Marchi et al., 2003; Weatherhead & Antunes, 2004).

Patients selected for pleurodesis should have demonstrated symptom relief with thoracentesis before undergoing the procedure and should have a Karnofsky score greater than 70 to improve the chance of positive outcome (Martinez-Moragon et al., 1998). Complete reexpansion of the lung without evidence of bronchial obstruction or trapped lung is required. Pleural contact over a large surface area is necessary for sufficient fibrosis to occur to obliterate the space. The amount of tumor involvement also may be important, as pleurodesis is less effective with a larger tumor burden. In general, patients with a Karnofsky score greater than 70 will have the best long-term benefit from treatment; symptomatic and palliative treatment may be more appropriate for those with scores less than 70 (Marchi et al., 2003; Sahn, 1997; Weatherhead & Antunes, 2004).

Most pleurodesis is performed via standard chest tube. The chest tube is placed at the level of the sixth or seventh intercostal space laterally and is directed posteriorly to the most dependent portion of the pleural cavity. The tube then is connected to a water-seal drainage system under suction. This restores negative pressure in the pleural space, removes fluid, and allows the lung to reexpand. Prior to pleurodesis, clinicians should obtain CXR confirmation of complete lung expansion and administer IV narcotics and/or sedation to diminish the pain associated with sclerosing agents. The agent of choice then is instilled into the chest tube, usually in a solution of 50–100 cm³ of sterile saline, and the chest tube is clamped for one hour. The procedure does not require side-to-side rotation of patients. After one hour, the chest tube is reconnected to suction the fluid and remains that way until the 24-hour output from the tube is less than 150 cm³. This method of treatment usually requires hospitalization for four to six days (ATS, 2000; Sahn, 1997; Schrump & Nguyen, 2001; Weatherhead & Antunes, 2004). A recent study showed that removal of the chest tube after only two hours of drainage time may yield similar success rates as longer-term drainage and would have the advantage of lowered cost and reduced length of stay (Spiegler, Hurewitz, & Groth, 2003). Further study of this method is warranted.

Several studies have demonstrated that the use of small-bore catheters in place of traditional chest tubes for pleurodesis has produced similar efficacy rates (Marom et al., 1999; Patz et al., 1998). Small-bore catheters have the advantage of being less aggressive than a conventional chest tube and are better tolerated. They are easily placed using ultrasound guidance and can stay in place for weeks. Patients can learn to drain these devices at home and can receive sclerosis therapy as an outpatient. Disadvantages include more frequent obstruction of the catheters because of small lumen size and fibrin formation, and difficulty manipulating the catheter into the correct position during insertion (Brubacher & Gobel, 2003; Marchi et al., 2003; Patz, 1998; Patz et al.).

Sclerosing Agents

Several agents have been used to attempt pleurodesis (see Figure 5-5). Evaluating the efficacy of these agents is difficult, as most studies have used small sample sizes, different techniques and success criteria, and variable long-term follow-up. Few studies have compared one agent to another. The variability of disease progression among the more common cancers causing MPE adds to the uncertainty.

Tetracycline/Doxycycline

In the past, tetracycline was the agent of choice, but the powdered form is no longer available in the United States because the drug preparations did not meet U.S. Food and Drug Administration purity standards. Tetracycline as a sclerosing agent has an excellent record, with generally mild side effects (pain and fever being most common), and a single dose usually is sufficient to cause a positive response (Marchi et al., 2003; Schrump & Nguyen, 2001).

Doxycycline, a tetracycline analog, has replaced tetracycline. No direct studies comparing the two agents exist, but based on historical data, success rates using doxycycline are similar to tetracycline and range from 67%–92% in selected patients (Marchi et al., 2003; Patz et al., 1998; Pulsiripunya et al., 1996). The most common side effect of this agent is pain, which usually is mild and easily treated with non-narcotic pain relievers. Fever occurs infrequently

---

Figure 5-5. Sclerosing Agents Used in Managing Malignant Pleural Effusion

Commonly used sclerosing agents
- Doxycycline
- Bleomycin
- Mitoxantrone
- Talc poudrage: Used during thoracoscopy, talc is sprayed via atomizer into the pleural space.
- Talc slurry: Talc is mixed with sterile saline and instilled via chest tube.

Uncommon and novel sclerosing agents
- Tetracycline (not currently available because of impurities)
- Quinacrine
- Silver nitrate
- Sodium hydroxide
- OK-432
- Doxorubicin
- *Corynebacterium parvum*
- Iodopovidone
- Interferon alpha-2b
- Transforming growth factor-β2
- Matrix metalloproteinase inhibitors

---

in fewer than 10% of patients. Most studies recommend 500 mg of doxycycline mixed with 50–100 cm³ of sterile saline with preprocedure sedation or analgesia (Mansson, 1988; Patz et al.; Pulsiripunya et al.).

Bleomycin

Another agent commonly used for pleurodesis is bleomycin. Bleomycin inhibits DNA and protein synthesis, and local cytotoxic action may exist, but researchers do not fully understand the mechanism of pleurodesis (Weatherhead & Antunes, 2004). Several studies have directly compared bleomycin to tetracycline, showing success rates that are similar to slightly higher than with bleomycin (Hartman et al., 1993; Martinez-Moragon et al., 1997). Used in a dose of 60 IU of bleomycin mixed in 50–100 cm³ of sterile saline, patients systemically absorb approximately 40% of intrapleural bleomycin. Common side effects include pain, fever, and nausea. Hemoptysis, septic shock, diarrhea, alopecia, and lung fibrosis also have occurred (Ostrowski, 1986). A comparison of bleomycin to doxycycline using small-bore catheters yielded similar success rates—72% with bleomycin and 79% with doxycycline (Patz et al., 1998). Researchers also have compared bleomycin to talc slurry in 71 patients with MPE. They found no difference in success rates between the two agents, but the average cost of intervention was significantly lower for talc slurry (Haddad, Younes, Gross, & Deheinzelin, 2004). Bleomycin is more expensive than doxycycline or talc, costing more than $1,000 per 60 IU, but it has potential for cost-savings if the agent can be used with a small-bore catheter on an outpatient basis (ATS, 2000; Schrump & Nguyen, 2001).

Talc

Talc is an inexpensive and highly effective agent for pleurodesis. It is easy to handle and available worldwide. Talc that is used for pleurodesis is asbestos-free, but sterility is not required. Unsterilized talc contains *Bacillus* species, which generally are nonpathogenic, and the total bacterial count is limited based on U.S. Pharmacopeia standards. However, clinically significant disease from unsterilized talc has been reported, especially in immunocompromised hosts. Sterilization by prolonged heat exposure, ethylene oxide gas, or gamma irradiation is recommended (ATS, 2000; Sahn, 1997).

A recent review of published studies using talc pleurodesis for treatment of pleural effusions showed a 93% success rate in 165 patients with mostly malignant effusions (Walker-Renard, Vaughan, & Sahn, 1994). Success rates and long-term follow-up varied among the studies reviewed but generally were defined based on clinical and radiologic criteria. Doses ranged from 1–14 g, and researchers found little difference in outcome based on the method of talc administration (Walker-Renard et al.).

Two methods of instilling talc in the pleural space are available: talc poudrage and talc slurry. Poudrage is performed using thoracoscopy and involves spraying the pleural surface with talc. A thoracoscope is inserted into the pleural space, all fluid is removed, and the space is inspected for suspicious lesions. Biopsies may be performed, and adhesions can be removed, eliminating trapped lung. Approximately 5 g of talc is sprayed into the pleural space using an atomizer, and a repeat inspection ensures even distribution. A chest tube then is placed and suction applied and maintained until the amount of drainage in 24 hours is less than 100 ml. On average, the reported success rate with talc poudrage is greater than 90%, but definitions of success are not standard across studies. General anesthesia is required, thus limiting this procedure to patients in whom anesthesia is appropriate (Rodriguez-Panadero, 1985; Sanchez-Armengol & Rodriguez-Panadero, 1993; Weatherhead & Antunes, 2004).

Talc slurry is an effective pleurodesis agent in the treatment of MPE (Kennedy, Rusch, Strange, Ginsberg, & Sahn, 1994; Yin, Chan, Lee, Wan, & Ho, 1996). Talc slurring involves mixing 4–5 g of talc in 50 ml of sterile saline, which then is instilled via chest tube. The tube should be clamped for one hour after instillation. It is not clear whether talc slurry disperses as readily as tetracycline; therefore, rotating patients from side-to-side to distribute the talc throughout the pleural space is recommended until more is known (ATS, 2000; Weatherhead & Antunes, 2004). Both standard chest tubes and small-bore catheters have been successfully used with talc slurry, although it is more difficult to inject talc into small-bore catheters, and drainage may be more difficult because of fibrin clots (Marchi et al., 2003; Marom et al., 1999;

Thompson, Yau, Donnelly, Gowan, & Matzinger, 1998). Potential disadvantages of talc slurry include a lack of uniform distribution; accumulation in dependent areas of the pleural space, leading to incomplete sclerosis; and decreased contact time with the pleural space, causing lowered effectiveness.

The most common short-term adverse effects associated with talc are pain, ranging from nonexistent to severe, and fever. Fever up to 102.4°F has occurred in 16%–69% of patients. Fever generally occurs 4–12 hours after treatment and may last for 72 hours (Kennedy & Sahn, 1994). Other less common complications include empyema, local site infection, and cardiovascular complications such as arrhythmias, cardiac arrest, chest pain, myocardial infarction, or hypotension. Acute respiratory distress syndrome (ARDS), acute pneumonitis, and respiratory failure also have been rarely reported. In a study of 614 patients treated with talc poudrage, seven patients (1.2%) developed ARDS, which was fatal in three patients (de Campos et al., 2001). ARDS may be related to dose and particle size, reexpansion pulmonary edema, a local inflammatory response, or other factors related to instillation. The incidence is higher in patients with severe pulmonary disease, in patients with end-stage cancer, and after biopsy or other surgical procedures (Marchi et al., 2003; Rehse, Aye, & Florence, 1999; Weatherhead & Antunes, 2004). Serious adverse events tend to occur at higher dose ranges; therefore, dosages exceeding 5 g are not recommended, nor is unilateral pleurodesis in conjunction with pleural biopsy and bilateral simultaneous pleurodesis (ATS, 2000; Schrump & Nguyen, 2001).

Other Agents

Researchers also have studied other sclerosing agents to determine their efficacy in treating MPE. Quinacrine, an antimalarial agent, has been used for many years, primarily in Scandinavian countries, with good results and few side effects. Rare but serious neuropsychiatric side effects have occurred with this product (Weatherhead & Antunes, 2004). In a recent prospective study comparing quinacrine to talc slurry, primary success was no different between the two agents, and no difference in side effects was present, but significantly more patients needed repeat treatment with quinacrine (31%) versus talc (7%). The authors concluded that talc is the preferred agent, but quinacrine remains a good alternative (Ukale, Agrenius, Hillerdal, Mohlkert, & Widstrom, 2004). Another study comparing quinacrine to bleomycin showed greater efficacy with quinacrine and similar side effects (Koldsland, Svennevig, Lehne, & Johnson, 1993). Further study with this agent is necessary, but it currently is unavailable in North America and many European countries.

Mitoxantrone has been found to be effective in both breast and ovarian cancers. In one study, 114 patients with advanced breast cancer with a mean life expectancy of one month underwent pleurodesis with mitoxantrone. At 30 days, 56.3% of the patients had a complete response. At 60 days, complete response was 53.5%. Side effects were minimal and included fever, chest pain, and nausea and vomiting. Mean survival was 15.6 +/– 2 months. Patients with Karnofsky scores less than 30 had a significantly lower survival rate (Barbetakis, Antoniadis, & Tsilikas, 2004). Researchers have found similar results in patients with ovarian cancer. Sixty women with advanced ovarian cancer received mitoxantrone pleurodesis. There were 41 complete responses at 30 days, and 38 at 60 days. Side effects were minimal and were similar to those in the breast cancer study. Mean survival was 7.5 +/– 1.2 months (Barbetakis, Vassiliadis, Kaplanis, Valeri, & Tsilikas, 2004).

Silver nitrate, the original sclerosing agent, was used until the 1980s when talc and tetracycline replaced it. It generally produced good results, with success rates greater than 75%, but was associated with significant pain and longer hospital stays. Interest in silver nitrate has reemerged because of the incidence of ARDS with talc. A comparison study of silver nitrate to talc slurry showed talc to be effective in 21 of 24 patients (87.5%) and silver nitrate to be effective in 22 of 23 patients (95.6%), with similar side effects occurring in both groups (Paschoalini, Pereira, & Abdo, 1999). Silver nitrate tends to induce more damage to the lung than talc, which may be an advantage in ensuring sclerosis, but more study is needed with this agent.

Sodium hydroxide is a caustic agent that has been studied primarily in South American countries. Several studies of patients with a variety of cancers and MPE have shown success rates of 80%–100%, with survival ranging from 5–25 months, depending on the tumor type. Despite being strongly alkaline with a pH of greater than 11, sodium hydroxide seems to be well tolerated, with reports of only transitory and discrete pain. The amount of postprocedure drainage was low, with the possibility of early chest tube removal and early hospital discharge (Bezanilla, 1976; Marchi et al., 2003; Rioseco, 1980). The concomitant use of intrapleural lidocaine to control pain is contraindicated with sodium hydroxide because it appears to neutralize the agent and reduce its sclerosing effect (Teixeira et al., 1996).

Other novel agents studied in the treatment of MPE include OK-432, doxorubicin, *Corynebacterium parvum (C. parvum)*, iodopovidone, interferon (IFN) alfa-2b, transforming growth factor-β2 (TGF-β2), and matrix metalloproteinase (MMP) inhibitors. OK-432 increases neutrophils, macrophages, and lymphocyte counts and augments antitumor activity of large granular lymphocytes in ascites fluid. Both OK-432 (a preparation of *Streptococcus pyogenes*) and doxorubicin (30 mg) were instilled via chest tube in 20 patients with advanced lung cancer (Kishi et al., 2004). If the volume of chest tube drainage was more than 200 ml per 24 hours, additional OK-432 was instilled every three days. Sixteen patients had a complete response, two had a partial response, and two showed no response. Side effects were mild and included fever and pain that were easily treated with nonsteroidal anti-inflammatory drugs (NSAIDs) (Kishi et al.).

C. parvum, a gram-positive bacterium, appears to have tumoricidal and sclerosant properties. It produces an intense inflammatory response, with fever being a very common side effect and nausea and vomiting occurring less commonly. A small study comparing tetracycline and *C. parvum* showed similar efficacy but a higher incidence of side effects with *C. parvum* (Leahy et al., 1985; Schrump & Nguyen, 2001). The agent is no longer available in the United Kingdom. Iodopovidone, a topical antiseptic that is iodine-based, showed a 96% efficacy rate in 52 patients who underwent either thoracoscopy or chest tube pleurodesis (Olivares-Torres et al., 2002). Side effects were minimal, but caution is necessary because it is systemically absorbed and can lead to marked increases in serum iodine levels. It is contraindicated in patients with known iodine hypersensitivity or in people with active thyroid disease (Weatherhead & Antunes, 2004).

Researchers compared intrapleural IFN alpha-2b to bleomycin pleurodesis in 160 patients with rapidly recurrent MPE (Sartori et al., 2004). Bleomycin was administered as a single dose of 0.7 mg/kg. The dose was repeated in three days if fluid output was not less than 100 ml/day. IFN alpha-2b, 1 million units/10 kg, was administered for six courses at four-day intervals. The 30-day response was 84.3% for the bleomycin arm and 62.3% for the IFN arm (p = .002). Median time to progression was longer in the bleomycin group, as was median survival (Sartori et al.). IFN treatment is costly, requires more time than other treatment options, and will require more study to determine whether it is a viable treatment option.

Two other agents that have been studied in animal models hold promise for treatment of MPE. TGF-β2 is a potent stimulator of the production of extracellular matrix, has anti-inflammatory properties, and has demonstrated successful pleurodesis with a single dose (Light et al., 2000). Comparison of talc to TGF-β2 showed better results with TGF-β2 (Lee et al., 2001), but it is a recombinant product and is much more expensive than currently used products. MMPs are zinc atom-dependent endopeptides that are involved in the turnover and remodeling of extracellular matrix proteins. High levels of activated MMP inhibitors have been found in invasive and metastatic tumors. In a phase I study using intrapleural batimastat, an MMP inhibitor, patients with malignant effusions required significantly fewer pleural aspirations in the three months following administration compared to the three months before. Side effects were mild and included fever and reversible liver enzyme abnormalities (Macaulay et al., 1999). These agents hold promise, but further study is needed to determine their dose, safety, and efficacy.

Surgical Options

A pleuroperitoneal shunt (see Figure 5-6) is an option for patients who have failed pleurodesis or who have trapped lung, a condition that occurs when the visceral pleura becomes encased with a fibrous peel or rind, preventing the lung from expanding and from filling the thoracic cavity. A shunt may be particularly beneficial in patients who have a chylothorax, because it allows recirculation of the chyle into the circulation. Shunts can be placed in patients who are poor surgical candidates and have few complications. Palliation of

Figure 5-6. The Denver Pleuroperitoneal Shunt

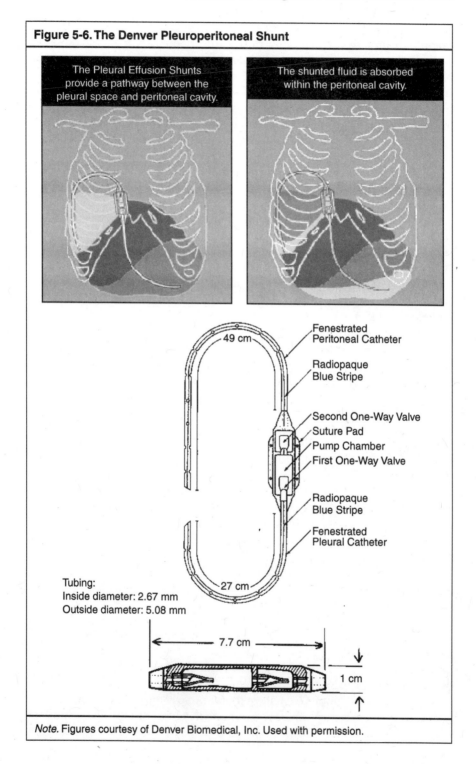

The Pleural Effusion Shunts provide a pathway between the pleural space and peritoneal cavity.

The shunted fluid is absorbed within the peritoneal cavity.

49 cm

Fenestrated Peritoneal Catheter

Radiopaque Blue Stripe

Second One-Way Valve
Suture Pad
Pump Chamber
First One-Way Valve

Radiopaque Blue Stripe

Fenestrated Pleural Catheter

Tubing:
Inside diameter: 2.67 mm
Outside diameter: 5.08 mm

27 cm

7.7 cm

1 cm

Note. Figures courtesy of Denver Biomedical, Inc. Used with permission.

symptoms occurs in 80%–90% of appropriately selected patients. The most commonly used device is a Denver® (Denver Biomedical, Inc., Golden, CO) pleuroperitoneal shunt. It consists of a unidirectional pump chamber connected to pleural and peritoneal catheters. The pumping chamber can be implanted subcutaneously. Manual compression of the chamber is required to move fluid from the pleural to peritoneal spaces and must be performed for 5–10 minutes four times per day, thus limiting its use to patients who have good performance status. More recent devices are heparinized systems that drain spontaneously by positive pressure created by the effusion. Significant fluid and protein loss with long-term drainage may be problematic in patients with nutritional deficiencies. The major problem with this method is shunt failure, which occurs in up to 12% of patients and is likely caused by occlusion of the catheter. Replacing the shunt can treat shunt occlusion, unless infection is confirmed. In that case, long-term chest tube drainage is indicated (ATS, 2000; Little et al., 1986; Myers, 2001; Ruckdeschel & Jablons, 2001; Sahn, 1997; Schrump & Nguyen, 2001; Works & Maxwell, 2000).

The placement of a simple pigtail catheter attached to a portable drainage system has been shown to be effective in MPE management. Two brands of catheters are available, the Pleurx® (Denver Biomedical, Inc.) catheter (see Figure 5-7) and the Tenckhoff® (Quinton Instrument, Seattle, WA) catheter. Both are silicone catheters that have numerous openings at the distal end and a polyester cuff to anchor the tube under the skin. Both tubes are placed similar to a chest tube and are sutured in place. The tube attaches to a closed drainage system that patients can empty, allowing for outpatient management. Both tubes can be capped off when not being drained, allowing for more mobility and independence in activities. Patients can be discharged immediately and can learn to care for the system at home. Typically, drainage subsides in two to three weeks, and sclerosis may occur without use of a sclerosing agent. Several studies have shown greater than 85% efficacy, with drainage subsiding in 30 days or less without additional pleurodesis (Putnam et al., 1999, 2000). Potential problems with this approach include patient discomfort from long-term catheter placement, the inconvenience of bulb drainage, and a small chance of infection (Brubacher & Gobel, 2003; Ruckdeschel & Jablons, 2001; Schrump & Nguyen, 2001; Works & Maxwell, 2000).

An implanted long-term access device also may be an option for long-term drainage. Intermittent drainage is accomplished by accessing the implanted port in a similar manner as ports used for vascular access. Use of an implanted port decreases the risk of pneumothorax and infection from repeated thoracentesis. The use of a noncoring needle to access the implanted port is less painful than repeat thoracentesis, and nurses in the outpatient or home setting can perform the drainage, thus reducing readmissions (Myers, 2001; Works & Maxwell, 2000).

Other surgical options include parietal pleurectomy, decortication, and pleuropneumonectomy. Surgical methods have not shown any advantage over chemical pleurodesis in MPE but are highly effective when unresectable

Figure 5-7. The Pleurx Pleural Catheter

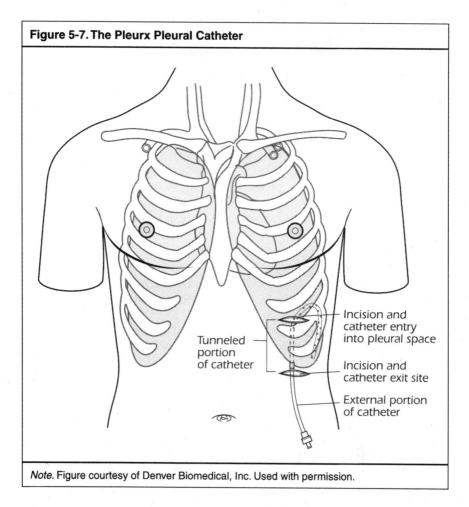

Tunneled portion of catheter

Incision and catheter entry into pleural space

Incision and catheter exit site

External portion of catheter

Note. Figure courtesy of Denver Biomedical, Inc. Used with permission.

tumor is found at the time of thoracotomy. In this case, surgical decortication—removal of the pleural lining—may be beneficial, but it is associated with severe complications, such as bronchopulmonary fistula and empyema, and generally is not recommended (Grannis et al., 2002). Pleuropneumonectomy, removal of the pleura and all or part of the lung, with or without pleural abrasion is nearly 100% effective in obliterating the pleural space. It is a major surgical procedure with high morbidity and mortality and should only be used in patients who have a reasonably long life expectancy, are in good condition, and have failed pleurodesis. It generally is not recommended in patients with MPE but may have a role in managing mesothelioma (ATS, 2000; Sahn, 1997; Schrump & Nguyen, 2001). Parietal pleurectomy using VATS may be an option and is associated with lower risk than open procedures. Not enough evidence exists to justify this procedure as a first-line option, however, and it should be reserved only for patients with good life expectancy who have failed less invasive and less expensive interventions (Schrump & Nguyen). An open thoracotomy for removal of malignant tissue covering the pleural surface may improve success with pleurodesis. Perioperative mortality is 12%, making patient selection critical (Fry & Khandekar, 1995).

Additional Therapies

Chemotherapy may be effective in decreasing MPE associated with lymphoma, small cell lung cancer, and breast cancer, but it generally is not as effective in treating MPE with other malignancies. Identification of hormone receptors in pleural fluid in patients with breast cancer may hold promise for hormone manipulation (ATS, 2000; Sahn, 1997). Systemic treatment should be started if no contraindications are present, and it can be combined with therapeutic thoracentesis and pleurodesis. Studies demonstrating the effectiveness of chemotherapy alone in MPE are somewhat lacking. A study of the effectiveness of platinum-based chemotherapy in patients with MPE with unknown primary showed a significant survival advantage, 12 months versus 5 months, in patients who received systemic chemotherapy (Ang et al., 2001).

Chemotherapy may be administered directly into the pleural space but requires high concentrations and carries the risk of systemic spread. Intrapleural chemotherapy generally is reserved for use in clinical trials only. To minimize systemic effects, antineoplastics have been combined with poly-L-lactic acid microspheres (Ike, Shimizu, Hitomi, Wada, & Ikada, 1991). Several studies using intrapleural chemotherapy have had mixed results. Intrapleural 5-fluorouracil and cisplatin were given weekly via an implanted port to 22 patients with MPE with a variety of primary tumors (Shoji, Tanaka, Yanagihara, Inui, & Wada, 2002). Median survival was 403 days, and the maximum was 792 days. The implanted port was involved with tumor in one patient. No adverse effect caused by intrapleural chemotherapy was observed in any case (Shoji et al.). In another study, intrapleural cisplatin (100 mg/m^2) and cytosine arabinoside ($600–1,200 \text{ mg/m}^2$) produced complete response in only 27% of patients, and significant side effects suggesting systemic absorption occurred in 76% of the patients (Rusch, Figlin, Godwin, & Piantadosi, 1991). Desai and Figueredo (1979) found that intrapleural doxorubicin produced complete response in only 22% of evaluable patients with frequent systemic side effects. Other studies using intrapleural chemotherapy have shown similar results (Schrump & Nguyen, 2001).

Active cytokines may be instilled directly into the pleural space. The use of IFN-β, IFN-γ, and interleukin-2 has produced variable results. It is not clear whether the response is due to sclerosing activity or to an immunologic effect. Further study is needed (ATS, 2000). Radiation therapy to mediastinal lymph nodes in lymphoma and small cell lung cancer may decrease an obstructive effusion. One study showed that close to 90% of malignant lymphoma effusions were controlled by mediastinal and hemithorax radiation in doses of

1.4–2.3 Gy (Schrump & Nguyen, 2001). Radiation therapy to the hemithorax generally is contraindicated in MPE arising from lung cancer, as the risk of radiation pneumonitis outweighs the benefits (Sahn, 1997).

Medical Management

Additional medical management of the patient with a pleural effusion involves preservation of optimal pulmonary function. Mild effusions may be cautiously treated with diuretics such as furosemide (Lasix®, Aventis Pharmaceuticals Inc., Bridgewater, NJ) or spironolactone (Aldactone®, G.D. Searle LLC, Chicago, IL), observing for fluid volume compromise. Healthcare providers should coadminister antibiotics if infection is present. Patients also may receive high-dose steroids or NSAIDs, although some concerns exist regarding the use of steroids. Pleurodesis depends on producing a robust fibrotic pleural reaction, and concurrent administration of corticosteroids has been hypothesized to reduce this effect. Studies in animals have shown decreased efficacy of talc and tetracycline when corticosteroids are coadministered. Because of these findings, corticosteroid use should be minimized around the time of pleurodesis using these agents. The effect of corticosteroids with other agents is not known (Weatherhead & Antunes, 2004).

Administration of saline, plasma, and blood products will expand circulatory volume but must be monitored closely because volume infusion may worsen the pleural effusion and increase dyspnea. Oxygen therapy via nasal prongs or a mask will improve saturation and decrease dyspnea. Aggressive pulmonary toilet measures may be necessary, including incentive spirometry, nebulizer treatments, and chest physical therapy. Bronchodilators and opioids may help to improve respiratory function. Mechanical ventilation with positive airway pressure may be necessary in patients with massive effusions to prevent hypoxia and respiratory arrest (Inzeo & Tyson, 2003; Myers, 2001).

A possible role for thrombolytic therapy exists in patients with loculated effusions in whom tube drainage and pleurodesis would not be successful. Thrombolytic therapy has been used in pleural effusions caused by infection and appears to be safe. Ten patients with multiloculated malignant effusions who received 500,000–1,500,000 U of streptokinase demonstrated satisfactory radiographic improvement (Davies, Traili, Gleeson, & Davies, 1999). Larger prospective trials are needed to evaluate response and safety, particularly the risk of hemorrhage.

Nursing Management

The nursing approach to patients with a pleural effusion depends on the size of the effusion, the patients' symptoms, and underlying lung function. Because many effusions are asymptomatic, a high degree of suspicion, coupled with excellent assessment skills, is important in identifying a possible effusion early before it becomes a true emergency. Figure 5-8 provides an overview of nursing management in the care of patients with MPE.

Frequent assessment of the pulmonary system is paramount to identification and early intervention in MPE. The nurse has a crucial role in assessing the patient's respiratory rate, rhythm, and depth and auscultating the lungs for decreased or absent breath sounds, rales, rhonchi, bronchial breath sounds, egophony, or increased vocal fremitus. Nurses also observe the patency of the airway, use of accessory muscles, difficulty speaking, change in sputum color, hemoptysis, clubbing of fingernails, change in skin color and temperature, and cyanosis. The patient is questioned about dyspnea, shortness of breath, orthopnea, paroxysmal nocturnal dyspnea, cough, decreased activity toler-ance, headache, and chest pain. The chest is palpated for decreased tactile fremitus, crepitance, and asymmetric chest expansion and is percussed for dullness or hyperresonance. Pulse oximetry is assessed at rest and with exercise

---

Figure 5-8. Nursing Management of Patients With a Pleural Effusion

Frequent assessment of cardiac, respiratory, and nervous systems
- Monitor vital signs and pulse oximetry.
- Perform auscultation of heart and lung sounds.
- Assess for sputum characteristics, cough, dyspnea, use of accessory muscles, and cyanosis.
- Assess for chest pain, decreased activity tolerance, clubbing, and cyanosis.
- Assess for headache, change in mental status, and level of consciousness.

Maintenance of optimal pulmonary status
- Administer oxygen to keep saturation > 92%.
- Position patients with head of the bed up or in forward-leaning position.
- Encourage energy conservation/frequent rest periods.
- Initiate deep breathing, coughing, pursed-lip breathing, postural drainage, and suctioning.

Comfort measures
- Administer analgesics as ordered.
- Administer antianxiety medications as ordered.
- Implement relaxation techniques.

Preparation for invasive procedures

Care of chest tubes, drainage tubes and other devices as indicated

Patient and caregiver education
- Recognize signs and symptoms of effusion recurrence.
- Provide instruction in breathing techniques (e.g., pursed lip, diaphragmatic, alternating rhythm).
- Provide catheter care for indwelling catheter.
- Emphasize the importance of adequate hydration, nutrition, smoking cessation, and measures to allay anxiety.

Discharge planning

to determine the degree of hypoxia. Nurses observe for changes in mental status and level of consciousness and monitor laboratory and test results, paying close attention to complete blood count, electrolytes, arterial blood gases, oximetry, CXR, pulmonary function studies, and other tests, and notify the physician immediately of any changes in the patient's status (Camp-Sorrell, 1999; Henke, 2000; Inzeo & Tyson, 2003; Myers, 2001).

Implementing measures to maintain optimal respiratory status is an important nursing function. Oxygen is administered to keep saturation levels greater than 92% and to prepare the patient for mechanical ventilation as ordered. The patient is positioned with the head of the bed elevated or in a forward-leaning position, if this is more comfortable. Nurses should encourage frequent deep breathing, coughing, and the use of pursed-lip breathing. They also provide frequent mouth care, postural drainage, and suctioning, if necessary. Patients require assistance with all activities to conserve energy, and nurses should schedule frequent rest periods. Instituting comfort measures, such as analgesics, antianxiety medications, and relaxation techniques, can decrease the workload on the heart and lungs. However, nurses must observe and report any adverse effects of analgesics on respiratory function so that, if indicated, the dose can be adjusted. If ordered, bronchodilators, diuretics, and steroids are administered (Camp-Sorrell, 1999; Inzeo & Tyson, 2003; Myers, 2001).

Other important nursing actions in the care of patients with MPE include preparing patients for all invasive procedures or transfers to the operating room and providing education to patients and families regarding each procedure, including sensations that might be experienced, the type of equipment that may be used, and expected outcomes of each procedure. Providing simple explanations and allowing patients to discuss concerns may help to allay their anxiety and reduce psychosocial distress, which also may decrease workload on the heart and lungs. Nurses also ensure that informed consent is obtained prior to all procedures, procure all equipment needed for bedside procedures, including emergency resuscitation equipment, and ensure IV access. In addition, nurses confirm that all necessary monitoring equipment is present and in working order. Analgesics or sedation are administered as ordered, and the patient is positioned appropriately. During the procedure, nurses monitor the respiratory rate, vital signs, and hemodynamic status and maintain aseptic technique throughout. They also observe for complications, monitor the amount and characteristics of any drainage, and ensure that any specimens obtained are sent to the laboratory for analysis as ordered (Works & Maxwell, 2000). In the case of pleurodesis, patient rotation generally is not necessary unless the pleurodesis agent is talc slurry. If the agent is talc slurry, nurses must ensure that the patient is rotated every 10–15 minutes while the chest tube is clamped (ATS, 2000).

Once the procedure is completed, nurses must assess for complications, including bleeding, signs of infection, increasing dyspnea, absent or decreased breath sounds, which may indicate pneumothorax, and evidence of reaccumulation of pleural fluid as evidenced by worsening respiratory status. Performing pulmonary toilet prevents atelectasis and pneumonia. Pain management, oral hygiene, skin care, nutrition, and passive and active exercise are all important areas of postprocedure nursing focus.

Chest tube and drainage tube management is important following thoracentesis, pleurodesis, or chest surgery. Once a chest tube is inserted, it is connected to underwater seal drainage to prevent air from going back up the tube and into the pleural cavity. Negative pressure is exerted on the tube, usually at 20 cm H_2O. If the patient has a pleural effusion, bubbling in the water-seal chamber could indicate a leak in the system. If the bubbling stops when the chest tube is clamped near the patient, a leak probably exists at the insertion site or inside the pleural cavity. If the bubbling does not stop when the tube is clamped, the leak is likely between the chest tube and the drainage system. This area always should be secured with adhesive tape to reduce the risk of air leakage. It rarely is necessary to clamp a chest tube, unless the patient is experiencing acute pulmonary edema from rapid drainage of fluid. If a chest tube is inadvertently left clamped, a tension pneumothorax could occur. Stripping and milking a chest tube is almost never indicated, unless a blood clot or other material is obstructing the tube (Camp-Sorrell, 1999; Otto, 2001). The amount and characteristics of any tube drainage are monitored, and care is provided for tubes according to hospital protocol. Postprocedure wound assessment and wound care are performed using sterile technique (Myers, 2001; Works & Maxwell, 2000).

Pleurx or Tenckhoff catheters require care similar to standard chest tubes. The manufacturers provide special kits used to drain these catheters. Each kit contains a vacuum bottle with an attached drainage line, a new cap for the end of the catheter, and supplies for changing the dressing. While the patient is hospitalized, drainage and dressing changes should be done using sterile technique. Prior to discharge, patients and caregivers must learn the appropriate care of these catheters and should receive a home healthcare referral. Once patients are home, clean technique may be used for dressing changes and tube drainage. Patients may shower as long as a transparent dressing is in place but should change the dressing if it becomes damp (Brubacher & Gobel, 2003). Implanted pleural catheters require the same care as any implanted port, and nursing measures should follow established hospital protocol.

Patient and Caregiver Education

Once patients are stabilized and ready to be discharged home, nurses should teach the patients and caregivers how to recognize the signs and symptoms that may indicate recurrence of an effusion. Some patients may be asymptomatic and only require periodic office visits to monitor their status. Patient education should include pursed-lip breathing, diaphragmatic breathing, and alteration of the breathing rhythm. Education also should stress the importance of adequate hydration and nutrition, scheduled rest periods, and measures to decrease anxiety. Efforts at smoking cessation are important, and referral to a cessation program may be appropriate. If patients have an indwelling catheter, they need to learn catheter care and maintenance. A home healthcare referral should be made to assess for nursing needs and to reinforce the teaching. Other patients may require short-term or long-term care in an extended care facility or a hospice referral. Patients and their families should be aware of the prognosis associated with MPE and should identify plans and goals in the event of recurrence. Nurses should assess and support patients' and caregivers' coping skills along with providing emotional support and appropriate referrals.

Conclusion

MPE is a life-threatening oncologic emergency that requires rapid identification and intervention to avoid respiratory collapse and death. Patients may be asymptomatic or may present with massive effusions, requiring astute observation skills and rapid intervention on the part of nurses. MPE is associated with advanced disease and shortened life expectancy, but the use of therapeutic thoracentesis or pleurodesis may improve both life expectancy and quality of life and should be considered for most patients. More extensive surgical procedures generally are reserved for patients with longer life expectancy because of the inherent risks and complications of these procedures. Chemotherapy, biotherapy, and radiation therapy may have a role in managing MPE with lymphoma, small cell lung cancer, and breast cancer but generally are disappointing in treating MPE with other malignancies. Nursing care should focus on maintaining optimal cardiopulmonary function, providing comfort measures, caring for chest tubes and other devices, and providing patient education and support.

References

Aleman, C., Alegre, J., Armadans, L., Andreu, J., Falco, V., Recio, J., et al. (1999). The value of chest roentgenography in the diagnosis of pneumothorax after thoracentesis. *American Journal of Medicine, 107*, 340–343.

American Thoracic Society. (2000). Management of malignant pleural effusions. *American Journal of Respiratory and Critical Care Medicine, 162*, 1987–2001.

Ang, P., Tan, E.-H., Leong, S.-S., Koh, L., Eng, P., Agasthian, T., et al. (2001). Primary intrathoracic malignant effusion: A descriptive study. *Chest, 120*, 50–54.

Barbetakis, N., Antoniadis, T., & Tsilikas, C. (2004). Results of chemical pleurodesis with mitoxantrone in malignant pleural effusion from breast cancer. *World Journal of Surgical Oncology, 2*, 16.

Barbetakis, N., Vassiliadis, M., Kaplanis, K., Valeri, R., & Tsilikas, C. (2004). Mitoxantrone pleurodesis to palliate malignant pleural effusions secondary to ovarian cancer. *BMC Palliative Care, 3*, 4.

Bernard, F., Sterman, D., Smith, R.J., Kaiser, L.R., Albelda, S.M., & Alavi, A. (1998). Metabolic imaging of malignant pleural mesothelioma with fluorodeoxyglucose positron emission tomography. *Chest, 144*, 713–722.

Bezanilla, A.R. (1976). Treatment for malignant pleural effusions [Letter]. *Chest, 70,* 408–409.

Brubacher, S., & Gobel, B.H. (2003). Use of the Pleurx Pleural Catheter for the management of malignant pleural effusions. *Clinical Journal of Oncology Nursing, 7,* 35–38.

Camp-Sorrell, D. (1999). Malignant pleural effusion. *Clinical Journal of Oncology Nursing, 3,* 36–39.

Chestnut, M.S., & Prendergast, T.J. (2005). Pleural effusion. In L.M. Tierney, S.J. McPhee, & M.A. Papadakis (Eds.), *Current medical diagnosis and treatment, 2005* (44th ed., pp. 296–299). New York: Lange Medical Books/McGraw-Hill.

Chierakul, N., Kanitsap, A., Chaiprasert, A., & Viriyataveekul, R. (2004). A simple C-reactive protein measurement for the differentiation between tuberculosis and malignant pleural effusion. *Respirology, 9,* 66–69.

Davies, C.W., Traili, Z.C., Gleeson, F.V., & Davies, R.J. (1999). Intrapleural streptokinase in the management of malignant multiloculated pleural effusions. *Chest, 115,* 729–733.

de Campos, J.R., Vargas, F.S., de Campos Werebe, E., Cardoso, P., Teixeira, L.R., Jatene, F.B., et al. (2001). Thoracoscopy talc poudrage: A 15-year experience. *Chest, 119,* 801–806.

Desai, S.D., & Figueredo, A. (1979). Intracavitary doxorubicin in malignant effusions [Letter]. *Lancet, 1,* 872.

Fry, W.A., & Khandekar, J.D. (1995). Parietal pleurectomy for malignant pleural effusion. *Annals of Surgical Oncology, 2,* 160–164.

Grannis, F.W., Wagman, L.D., Lai, L., & Curcio, L.D. (2002). Fluid complications. In R. Pazdur, L.R. Coia, W.J. Hoskins, & L.D. Wagman (Eds.), *Cancer management: A multidisciplinary approach* (pp. 943–958). Melville, NY: PRR.

Haddad, F.J., Younes, R.N., Gross, J.L., & Deheinzelin, D. (2004). Pleurodesis in patients with malignant pleural effusions: Talc slurry or bleomycin? Results of a prospective randomized trial. *World Journal of Surgery, 28,* 749–753.

Hartman, D.L., Gaither, J.M., Kesler, K.A., Mylet, D.M., Brown, J.W., & Mathur, P.N. (1993). Comparison of insufflated talc under thoracoscopic guidance with standard tetracycline and bleomycin pleurodesis for control of malignant pleural effusions. *Journal of Thoracic and Cardiovascular Surgery, 105,* 743–748.

Henke, S. (2000). Pleural effusion. In D. Camp-Sorrell & R.A. Hawkins (Eds.), *Clinical manual for the oncology advanced practice nurse* (pp. 161–166). Pittsburgh, PA: Oncology Nursing Society.

Ike, O., Shimizu, Y., Hitomi, S., Wada, R., & Ikada, Y. (1991). Treatment of malignant pleural effusions with doxorubicin hydrochloride-containing poly(L-lactic acid) microspheres. *Chest, 99,* 911–915.

Inzeo, D., & Tyson, L. (2003). Nursing assessment and management of dyspneic patients with lung cancer. *Clinical Journal of Oncology Nursing, 7,* 332–333.

Kennedy, L., Rusch, V.W., Strange, C., Ginsberg, R.J., & Sahn, S.A. (1994). Pleurodesis using talc slurry. *Chest, 106,* 342–346.

Kennedy, L., & Sahn, S.A. (1994). Talc pleurodesis for the treatment of pneumothorax and pleural effusion. *Chest, 106,* 1215–1222.

Kishi, K., Homma, S., Sakamoto, S., Kawabata, M., Tsuboi, E., Nakata, K., et al. (2004). Efficacious pleurodesis with OK-432 and doxorubicin against malignant pleural effusions. *European Respiratory Journal, 24,* 263–266.

Koldsland, S., Svennevig, J.L., Lehne, G., & Johnson, E. (1993). Chemical pleurodesis in malignant pleural effusions: A randomised prospective study of mepacrine versus bleomycin. *Thorax, 48,* 790–793.

Leahy, B.C., Honeybourne, D., Brear, S.G., Carroll, K.B., Thatcher, N., & Stretton, T.B. (1985). Treatment of malignant pleural effusions with intrapleural *Corynebacterium parvum* or tetracycline. *European Journal of Respiratory Disease, 66,* 50–64.

Lee, Y.C.G., Teixeira, L.R., Devin, C.J., Vaz, M.A.C., Vargas, F.S., Thompson, P.J., et al. (2001). Transforming growth factor-b2 induces pleurodesis significantly faster than talc. *American Journal of Respiratory and Critical Care Medicine, 163,* 640–644.

Light, R.W. (2002). Pleural effusions. *New England Journal of Medicine, 346,* 1971–1977.

Light, R.W., Cheng, D.S., Lee, Y.C., Rogers, J., Davidson, J., & Lane, K.B. (2000). A single intrapleural injection of transforming growth factor-b2 produces an excellent pleurodesis in rabbits. *American Journal of Respiratory and Critical Care Medicine, 162,* 98–104.

Light, R.W., Erozan, Y.S., & Ball, W.C. (1973). Cells in pleural fluid: Their value in differential diagnosis. *Archives of Internal Medicine, 132,* 854–860.

Light, R.W., Jenkinson, S.G., Minh, V., & George, R.B. (1980). Observations on pleural pressures as fluid is withdrawn during thoracentesis. *American Review of Respiratory Disease, 121,* 799–804.

Light, R.W., MacGregor, M.I., Luchsinger, P.C., & Ball, W.C. (1972). Pleural effusion: The diagnostic separation of transudates and exudates. *Annals of Internal Medicine, 77,* 507–513.

Little, A.G., Ferguson, M.K., Golomb, H.M., Hoffman, P.C., Vogelzang, N.J., & Skinner, D.B. (1986). Pleuroperitoneal shunting for malignant pleural effusions. *Cancer, 58,* 2740–2743.

Macaulay, V.M., O'Byrne, K.J., Saunders, M.P., Braybrooke, J.P., Long, L., Gleeson, F., et al. (1999). Phase I study of intrapleural batimastat (BB-94), a matrix metalloproteinase inhibitor, in the treatment of malignant pleural effusions. *Clinical Cancer Research, 5,* 513–520.

Mansson, T. (1988). Treatment of malignant pleural effusion with doxycycline. *Scandinavian Journal of Infectious Diseases Supplementum, 53,* 29–34.

Marchi, E., Teixeira, L.R., & Vargas, F.S. (2003). Management of malignancy-associated pleural effusion: Current and future treatment strategies. *American Journal of Respiratory Medicine, 2,* 261–273.

Marom, E.M., Patz, E.F., Erasmus, J.J., McAdams, H.P., Goodman, P.C., & Herndon, J.E. (1999). Malignant pleural effusions: Treatment with small-bore-catheter thoracostomy and talc pleurodesis. *Radiology, 210,* 277–281.

Martinez-Moragon, E., Aparicio, J., Rogado, M.C., Sanchis, J., Sanchis, F., & Gil-Suay, V. (1997). Pleurodesis in malignant pleural effusions: A randomized study of tetracycline versus bleomycin. *European Respiratory Journal, 10,* 2380–2382.

Martinez-Moragon, E., Aparicio, J., Sanchis, J., Menendez, R., Rogado, C., & Sanchis, F. (1998). Malignant pleural effusion: Prognostic factors for survival and response to chemical pleurodesis in a series of 120 cases. *Respiration, 65,* 108–113.

Myers, J. (2001). Oncologic complications. In S. Otto (Ed.), *Oncology nursing* (4th ed., pp. 548–588). St. Louis, MO: Mosby.

Olivares-Torres, C., Laniado-Laborin, R., Chavez-Garcia, C., Leon-Gastelum, C., Reyes-Escamilla, A., & Light, R.W. (2002). Iodopovidone pleurodesis for recurrent pleural effusions. *Chest, 122,* 581–583.

Ostrowski, M.J. (1986). An assessment of long-term results of controlling the reaccumulation of malignant effusions using intracavitary bleomycin. *Cancer, 57,* 721–727.

Otto, S.E. (2001). Lung cancers. In S. Otto (Ed.), *Oncology nursing* (4th ed., pp. 380–415). St. Louis, MO: Mosby.

Paschoalini, M.S., Pereira, J.R., & Abdo, E.F. (1999). Sliver nitrate versus talc slurry for pleurodesis in patients with malignant pleural effusions [Abstract]. *American Journal of Respiratory and Critical Care Medicine, 159,* A384.

Patz, E.F., Jr. (1998). Malignant pleural effusions: Recent advances and ambulatory sclerotherapy. *Chest, 113*(Suppl. 1), 74S–77S.

Patz, E.F., Jr., McAdams, H.P., Erasmus, J.J., Goodman, P.C., Culhane, D.K., Gilkeson, R.C., et al. (1998). Sclerotherapy for malignant pleural effusions: A prospective trial of bleomycin vs. doxycycline with small-bore catheter drainage. *Chest, 113,* 1305–1311.

Porcel, J.M., & Vives, M. (2003). Etiology and pleural fluid characteristics of large and massive effusions. *Chest, 124,* 978–983.

Pulsiripunya, C., Youngchaiyud, P., Pushpakom, R., Maranetra, N., Nana, A., & Charoenratanakul, S. (1996). The efficacy of doxycycline as a pleural sclerosing agent in malignant pleural effusion: A prospective study. *Respirology, 1,* 69–72.

Putnam, J.B., Light, R.W., Rodriguez, R.M., Ponn, R., Olak, J., Pollak, J.S., et al. (1999). A randomized comparison of indwelling pleural catheter and doxycycline pleurodesis in the management of malignant pleural effusion. *Cancer, 86,* 1992–1999.

Putnam, J.B., Walsh, G.L., Swisher, S.G., Roth, J.A., Suell, D.M., Vaporciyan, A.A., et al. (2000). Outpatient management of malignant pleural effusion by a chronic indwelling pleural catheter. *Annals of Thoracic Surgery, 69,* 369–375.

Rehse, D.H., Aye, R.W., & Florence, M.G. (1999). Respiratory failure following talc pleurodesis. *American Journal of Surgery, 177,* 437–440.

Rioseco, A. (1980). More about NaOH in the management of malignant pleural effusions. *Chest, 77,* 813–814.

Rodriguez-Panadero, F. (1985). Talc pleurodesis for treating malignant pleural effusions. *Chest, 108,* 1178–1179.

Rodriguez-Panadero, F., Borderas Naranjo, R., & Lopez Mejias, J. (1989). Pleural metastatic tumours and effusions: Frequency and pathogenic mechanisms in a post-mortem series. *European Respiratory Journal, 2,* 366–369.

Ruckdeschel, J.C., & Jablons, D. (2001). Malignant effusions in the chest. In J.M. Kirkwood, M.T. Lotze, & J.M. Yasko (Eds.), *Current cancer therapeutics* (4th ed., pp. 334–339). Philadelphia: Current Medicine.

Rusch, V.W., Figlin, R., Godwin, D., & Piantadosi, S. (1991). Intrapleural cisplatin and cytarabine in the management of malignant pleural effusions: A Lung Cancer Study Group trial. *Journal of Clinical Oncology, 9,* 313–319.

Sahn, S.A. (1997). Pleural diseases related to metastatic malignancies. *European Respiratory Journal, 10,* 1907–1913.

Sanchez-Armengol, A., & Rodriguez-Panadero, F. (1993). Survival and talc pleurodesis in metastatic pleural carcinoma, revisited: Report of 125 cases. *Chest, 104,* 1482–1485.

Sartori, S., Tassinari, D., Ceccotti, P., Tombesi, P., Nielsen, I., Trevisani, L., et al. (2004). Prospective randomized trial of intrapleural bleomycin versus interferon alfa-2b via ultrasound-guided small-bore chest tube in the palliative treatment of malignant pleural effusion. *Journal of Clinical Oncology, 22,* 1228–1233.

Schrump, D.S., & Nguyen, D.A. (2001). Malignant pleural and pericardial effusions. In V.T. DeVita, S. Hellman, & S.A. Rosenberg (Eds.), *Cancer: Principles and practice of oncology* (6th ed., pp. 2729–2744). Philadelphia: Lippincott Williams & Wilkins.

Shoji, T., Tanaka, F., Yanagihara, F., Inui, K., & Wada, H. (2002). Phase II study of repeated intrapleural chemotherapy using implantable access system for management of malignant pleural effusion. *Chest, 121,* 821–824.

Spiegler, P.A., Hurewitz, A.N., & Groth, M.L. (2003). Rapid pleurodesis for malignant pleural effusions. *Chest, 123,* 1895–1898.

Teixeira, L.R., Vargas, F.S., Carmo, A.O., Cukier, A., Silva, L.M., & Light, R.W. (1996). Effectiveness of sodium hydroxide as a pleural sclerosing agent in rabbits: Influence of concomitant intrapleural lidocaine. *Lung, 174,* 325–332.

Thompson, R.L., Yau, J.C., Donnelly, R.F., Gowan, D.J., & Matzinger, F.R. (1998). Pleurodesis with iodized talc for malignant effusions using pigtail catheters. *Annals of Pharmacotherapy, 32,* 739–742.

Ukale, V., Agrenius, V., Hillerdal, G., Mohlkert, D., & Widstrom, O. (2004). Pleurodesis in recurrent pleural effusions: A randomized comparison of a classical and a currently popular drug. *Lung Cancer, 43,* 323–328.

Villena, V., Lopez-Encuentra, A., Garcia-Lujan, R., Echave-Sustaeta, J., & Martinez, C.J. (2004). Clinical implications of appearance of pleural fluid at thoracentesis. *Chest, 125,* 156–159.

Walker-Renard, P., Vaughan, L.M., & Sahn, S.A. (1994). Chemical pleurodesis for malignant pleural effusions. *Annals of Internal Medicine, 120,* 56–64.

Weatherhead, M., & Antunes, G. (2004). Chemotherapeutic management of malignant pleural effusion. *Expert Opinion in Pharmacotherapy, 5,* 1233–1242.

Works, C., & Maxwell, M.B. (2000). Malignant effusions and edemas. In C.H. Yarbro, M.H. Frogge, M. Goodman, & S.L. Groenwald (Eds.), *Cancer nursing: Principles and practice* (5th ed., pp. 816–821). Sudbury, MA: Jones and Bartlett.

Yin, A.C., Chan, A.T., Lee, T.W., Wan, I.Y., & Ho, K.K. (1996). Thoracoscopic talc insufflation versus talc slurry for symptomatic malignant pleural effusion. *Annals of Thoracic Surgery, 62,* 1655–1658.

Zebrowski, B.K., Yano, S., Liu, W., Shaheen, R.M., Hicklin, D.J., Putnam, J.B., et al. (1999). Vascular endothelial growth factor levels and induction of permeability in malignant pleural effusions. *Cancer Research, 5,* 3364–3368.

Barbara Holmes Gobel, RN, MS, AOCN®, and
Glen J. Peterson, RN, OCN®, ACNP

⊃ **Chapter** **6**

Sepsis and Septic Shock

Introduction

Sepsis and septic shock are both potentially life-threatening oncologic emergencies. Septic shock is one stage in a clinical continuum of infection and systemic inflammatory mechanisms progressing from sepsis to severe sepsis and finally to septic shock. These stages make up a syndrome referred to as *systemic inflammatory response syndrome* (SIRS) (Muckart & Bhagwanjee, 1997). Septic shock is manifested by hemodynamic instability and alterations in cellular metabolism caused by sepsis. Septic shock is characterized by fever, chills, tachycardia, tachypnea, mental status changes, and hypotension/hypoperfusion that persist despite aggressive fluid challenge. This disorder occurs when the body fails to initiate an adequate immune response to bacterial, viral, or fungal infection. Management of this syndrome requires prompt assessment and treatment. Early detection and intervention related to sepsis and septic shock increase patients' chances of a positive outcome. Patients with cancer who are granulocytopenic are at risk for the development of sepsis and septic shock, particularly patients with hematologic malignancies. Nursing management of sepsis and septic shock requires knowledge of the risk factors for development of this syndrome, measures to prevent infection and sepsis, and knowledge of the many various medications that are used to treat sepsis and septic shock. Early hemodynamic assessment of patients suspected of sepsis is critical for definitive recognition and treatment to provide maximal benefit in terms of a positive outcome.

Definitions

Bone et al. (1992) published definitions related to SIRS, which were standardized by the American College of Chest Physicians/Society of Critical Care Medicine. The phases of SIRS represent a progressive state of this pathologic process. These standardized definitions (see Table 6-1) progress from infection, bacteremia, SIRS, sepsis, severe sepsis, septic shock, and multiple organ dysfunction syndrome (MODS) (Bone et al.).

Table 6-1. Definitions of Sepsis

Term	Definition
Infection/bacteremia	Presence of bacteria or fungi in the blood as evidenced by positive blood cultures or positive catheter culture
Systemic inflammatory response syndrome (SIRS)	Indicated by the presence of two or more of the following criteria: • Oral temperature > 100.4°F (38°C) • Heart rate > 90 beats/minute • Respiratory rate > 20 breaths/minute • White blood cell count > 12,000 cells/mm³, < 4,000 cells/mm³, or > 10% bands in the peripheral blood
Sepsis	Documented infection with the presence of two or more of the SIRS criteria
Severe sepsis	Presence of sepsis with one or more of the following: organ dysfunction, hypotension, or hypoperfusion
Septic shock	Presence of sepsis with hemodynamic instability that persists despite aggressive fluid challenge
Multiple organ dysfunction syndrome	Dysfunction of more than one organ; homeostasis must be maintained with immediate intervention.

Note. Based on information from Bone et al., 1992.

Sepsis is a systemic inflammatory response to pathogenic microorganisms and associated endotoxins in the blood. Sepsis generally presents with two or more of the following parameters: an oral temperature greater than 100.4°F (38°C); a heart rate greater than 90 beats/minute; a respiratory rate greater than 20 breaths per minute; and a white blood cell count greater than 12,000, less than 4,000, or more than 10% bands in the blood. A state of organ dysfunction, hypotension, or hypoperfusion demonstrates *severe sepsis. Septic shock* is manifested by hemodynamic instability and is characterized by fever, chills, tachycardia, tachypnea, mental status changes, and hypotension/hypoperfusion that persist despite aggressive fluid challenge. MODS is a state of dysfunction of more than one organ that requires intervention (Bone et al., 1992). MODS is so severe that homeostasis cannot be maintained without prompt and precise intervention (Segal, Walsh, & Holland, 2001).

Incidence

The incidence of sepsis is significant. In the United States, approximately 750,000 cases of sepsis and 210,000 deaths related to sepsis are estimated to occur annually (Angus et al., 2001; Martin, Mannino, Eaton, & Moss, 2003). The mortality rate of severe sepsis and septic shock remains unacceptably high in most centers (Dellinger et al., 2004; Friedman, Silva, & Vincent, 1998). Hematologic malignancies have been shown to have a higher association with severe sepsis than do solid tumors. An analysis of hospitalized patients with cancer demonstrated that the incidence of severe sepsis was 66.4 per 1,000 for hematologic malignancies and 7.6 per 1,000 for solid tumor malignancies. Compared to patients without malignancies, the risk of developing severe sepsis was 15 times greater for patients with hematologic tumors and 1.8 times greater for those with solid tumors. Mortality rates were similar for both types of malignancies (Williams et al., 2004).

Bacterial organisms are the most common source of sepsis (see Table 6-2). Historically, gram-negative bacterias, such as *Escherichia coli, Klebsiella pneumoniae,* and *Pseudomonas aeruginosa,* were responsible for 50%–60% of all cases of septic shock (Rangel-Frausto & Wenzel, 1997), but gram-negative bacterias now account for 40% of cases (Pelletier, 2003). The incidence of septic shock caused by gram-positive organisms, such as *Streptococcus pneumoniae* and *Staphylococcus aureus,* has been increasing rapidly in recent years, in part because of the extensive use of vascular access devices and the mucosal toxicity of cytotoxic regimens (Marchetti, Cometta, & Calandra, 2001). Currently, gram-positive bacterias account for 5%–10% of septic shock cases (Filbin & Stapczynski, 2002). Other causative organisms implicated in the development of septic shock include viruses, fungi, such as *Candida* and *Aspergillus,* anaerobes, and protozoa. Fungal infections are associated with significant mortality (Gobel, 2005). In approximately 20% of all cases of septic shock, the specific causative organism is never identified (Martin et al., 2003).

Table 6-2. Most Common Infectious Organisms Associated With Sepsis	
Type of Organism	**Examples**
Bacterial	Gram-negative organisms: *Escherichia coli, Klebsiella pneumoniae, Pseudomonas aeruginosa* Gram-positive organisms: *Streptococcus pneumoniae, Staphylococcus aureus*
Viral	Herpes simplex, respiratory syncytial virus, influenza A and B, cytomegalovirus, adenovirus
Fungal	*Candida, Aspergillus*

Risk Factors

Granulocytopenia is the single most important risk factor in the development of sepsis in patients with cancer (Sachdeva, 2002; Safdar & Armstrong, 2001). Increased duration and severity of granulocytopenia elevates the risk for sepsis (Safdar & Armstrong). Granulocytopenia can result from several factors, including disease, such as leukemia and lymphoma; treatment with chemotherapy and biotherapy or radiation therapy that involves sites of marrow development; and infiltration of bone marrow by solid tumors (Moore, 2005).

Another risk factor for the development of sepsis and septic shock is the presence of malignancy-related immunosuppression. Humoral immunity, in which B lymphocytes produce antibodies to foreign antigens, is modified in patients with multiple myeloma, chronic lymphocytic leukemia, Waldenström macroglobulinemia, and in patients who are asplenic and receiving cytotoxic chemotherapy (Gobel, 2005; Moore, 2005). Patients with humoral immune deficiencies are at greater risk for fulminant infections caused by *Streptococcus pneumoniae* and other encapsulated organisms. Cellular immunity, which serves to eliminate pathogens, malignant cells, and viruses via monocytes, macrophages, and T lymphocytes, is modified in patients with Hodgkin disease, acute leukemia, advanced lung cancer, intravascular tumors, and those undergoing stem cell transplants (Ellerhorst-Ryan, 2000). Patients with relapsed or refractory hematologic malignancies have impaired T lymphocytes (Safdar & Armstrong, 2001).

Other risk factors in the development of sepsis and septic shock include age younger than 1 year or older than 65 years (Filbin & Stapczynski, 2002); loss of skin or mucosal injury; long intensive care stays (Alberti et al., 2002); central vascular access devices (Hachem & Raad, 2002); indwelling devices such as urinary catheters and feeding tubes; diabetes; and organ-related diseases, including renal, hepatic, cardiovascular, pulmonary, and gastrointestinal (Shelton, 1999). Table 6-3 provides an overview of the risk factors related to the development of sepsis and septic shock.

Pathophysiology

Infection

Infection occurs when an organism or microbe enters the bloodstream and is able to colonize and reproduce within a host. Disease results if the infectious organism, such as gram-negative bacteria, causes injury, pathologic changes, or organ dysfunction in the host (see Figure 6-1).

Sepsis

In the presence of infection, the body mounts an inflammatory response. If a localized inflammatory response is insufficient to manage the infection,

Table 6-3. Risk Factors in the Development of Sepsis and Septic Shock

Risk Factor	Comments
Granulocytopenia	Single most important risk factor (Sachdeva, 2002) Duration and severity increase the risk for sepsis (Safdar & Armstrong, 2001). Related to disease (leukemia, lymphoma), treatment (chemotherapy, biotherapy, radiation therapy), and bone marrow infiltration by solid tumors (Moore, 2005)
Malignancy-related immunosuppression	Humoral immunity modified in patients with multiple myeloma, chronic lymphocytic leukemia, Waldenström macroglobulinemia, and in asplenic patients (Gobel, 2005; Moore, 2005) Cellular immunity modified in patients with Hodgkin disease, acute leukemia, advanced lung cancer, and intravascular tumors and in patients undergoing stem cell transplant (Ellerhorst-Ryan, 2000)
Age	Older than 65 or younger than 1 (Filbin & Stapczynski, 2002)
Loss of skin or mucosal injury	–
Long intensive care stays	–
Central vascular access devices	Increasing incidence of gram-positive bacterial infections associated with increasing use of central vascular access devices (Hachem & Raad, 2002)
Indwelling devices	Foley catheters, feeding tubes, tracheostomy tubes
Diabetes	–
Organ-related diseases	Renal, hepatic, cardiovascular, pulmonary, and gastrointestinal diseases (Shelton, 1999)

sepsis occurs. Sepsis is defined as a systemic response to infection. Substances such as endotoxins (released from gram-negative bacteria) and exotoxins (released from gram-positive bacteria) are released from the cell walls of dead bacteria after they have been phagocytized by neutrophils (Gobel, 2005). These toxins activate the coagulation cascade and the complement systems (Peterson, 1998). The activation of the complement system causes a release of vasoactive mediators such as kinins, histamine, interleukins, and tumor necrosis factor-alpha (TNF-α), all of which lead to vasodilation and potentially to capillary leak syndrome. These vasoactive mediators further activate the coagulation cascade, which leads to the aggregation of platelets and formation of fibrin, resulting in the coagulopathies seen in sepsis. Initially, increases in inflammatory mediators may characterize sepsis, but as sepsis persists, a shift toward an

Figure 6-1. Pathophysiology of Septic Shock

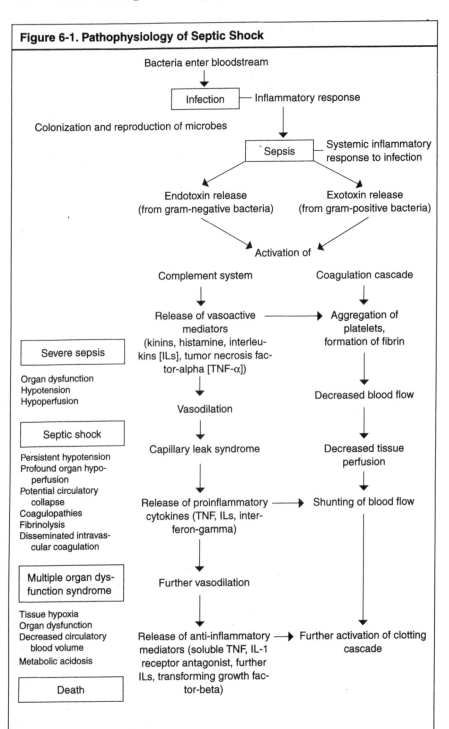

anti-inflammatory immunosuppressive state occurs (Oberholzer, Oberholzer, & Moldawer, 2001). Patients with sepsis who are immunosuppressed have a loss of delayed hypersensitivity, an inability to clear infection, and a predisposition to nosocomial infections (Oberholzer et al.).

A high cardiac output with widespread vasodilation and normal or slightly elevated blood pressure usually characterize the early stage of sepsis. Vasodilation increases if sepsis continues without adequate treatment, and a capillary leak may develop, resulting in significant edema. Without adequate treatment, the blood pressure falls, cardiac function becomes further depressed, and severe sepsis occurs. In severe sepsis, decreased blood flow occurs because of the continuation of fibrin formation and aggregation of platelets. This decreased blood flow leads to decreased tissue perfusion and a state of organ dysfunction.

Septic Shock

Septic shock represents an uncontrolled inflammatory response to bacterial toxins (Hotchkiss & Karl, 2003). Septic shock is associated with persistent systemic hypotension and profound organ hypoperfusion, accompanied by abnormal shunting of blood flow in the microcirculation that compromises delivery of nutrients to the tissues. Septic shock is the most common cause of circulatory collapse in patients with cancer (Bogolioubov, Keefe, & Groeger, 2001). In septic shock, further release of proinflammatory cytokines such as TNF, interleukin (IL)-1, IL-8, and interferon-gamma occurs because of the presence of bacterial toxins in the bloodstream. Higher levels of these bloodstream toxins generally correlate with increased severity of septic shock. TNF and IL-1 are potent vasodilators and pyrogens. IL-8 may play a role in perpetuating tissue inflammation (Dinarello, 1997). There also is a release of counter-regulatory molecules such as soluble TNF receptor, IL-1 receptor antagonist, IL-4, IL-10, IL-13, and transforming growth factor-beta (TGF-β) (Bogolioubov et al.). IL-4, IL-10, IL-13, and TGF-β provide anti-inflammatory effects by suppressing gene function and synthesis of IL-1 and TNF. These cytokines interact extensively with neutrophils and endothelial cells. This process of extensive cytokine release further promotes cell-leukocyte adhesion, release of proteases and arachidonate metabolites, and activation of the clotting cascade. As septic shock continues, further coagulopathies, fibrinolysis, and disseminated intravascular coagulation may occur (Nimah & Brilli, 2003).

Clinical Manifestations

Septic shock generally progresses from the hyperdynamic phase to the hypodynamic phase of shock. The hyperdynamic phase of septic shock occurs after initial fluid resuscitation for a septic event. During this phase, the cardiac output usually is elevated, but cardiac performance is depressed. Further vasodilation within the vascular system occurs, and hypotension and tachycardia result. Without adequate intervention, the hypodynamic phase of septic shock follows, in which the mediators of sepsis (e.g., endotoxins, exotoxins, related cytokines) increase vascular permeability, and fluid leaks from the vascular space into the interstitial space (Stoll, 2001). Venous pooling and maldistribution of blood volume are present, thereby decreasing the circulating blood volume. The decreased circulating blood volume results in tissue hypoxia and metabolic acidosis. Organ dysfunction and multisystem organ failure may be the sequelae of septic shock.

Vital signs provide invaluable information about the potential for the presence of septic shock. Vital sign changes that indicate septic shock include increased or decreased temperature (> 100.4°F [38°C] or < 96.4°F [36°C]), tachycardia, tachypnea, and persistent hypotension that do not respond to fluid resuscitation. Central nervous system alterations that may reflect septic shock include significant confusion and disorientation progressing to obtundation and coma. These effects arise from cerebral hypoxia, cerebral edema, and metabolic abnormalities (Moore, 2005). Cardiovascular manifestations of septic shock include tachycardia, cyanosis, hypovolemia, dysrhythmias, widened pulse pressure, persistent hypotension that is unresponsive to fluid resuscitation, and a decreased ejection fraction (Dellinger et al., 2004). Septic shock generally is defined as being present when the systolic blood pressure is less than 90 mm Hg, being unresponsive to fluid resuscitation, and requiring vasoactive drugs (Bone et al., 1992).

One of the earliest changes seen in the development of septic shock is tachypnea with associated dyspnea, which may result in respiratory alkalosis (Martin & Bernard, 2001). Other pulmonary manifestations of septic shock include bilateral rales, severe hypoxemia, pulmonary edema and hypertension, and acute respiratory distress syndrome (ARDS). Respiratory failure occurs if septic shock is not immediately and aggressively managed. Alterations of the gastrointestinal system that may be seen with septic shock include decreased gastric motility, ileus, and gastrointestinal bleeding. The effects of septic shock on the renal system most often include transient oliguria related to the hypotension of sepsis, but anuria also may develop, and the blood urea nitrogen and creatinine levels may increase. Acute renal failure also may ensue if septic shock is not reversed. Skin changes caused by septic shock are related to a lack of tissue oxygenation and may include cold and clammy skin, cyanosis, and acrocyanosis (persistent, painless, symmetric cyanosis of the hands and, less commonly, of the feet). Jaundice of the skin or sclera may develop and reflect hyperbilirubinemia and elevation of serum liver transaminases (Wheeler & Bernard, 1999). See Table 6-4 for an overview of the clinical manifestations of septic shock.

Patient Assessment

Patient History

At the onset of a septic incident, obtaining a thorough patient history is critical. The history may be the single most significant determinant of the septic

Table 6-4. Clinical Manifestations of Septic Shock

Organ System	Clinical Signs and Symptoms
Vital signs	Temperature > 100.4°F (38°C) or < 96.4°F (36°C) Tachycardia, tachypnea, and persistent hypotension (< 90 mm Hg) or reduction of ≥ 40 mm Hg from the patient's baseline that does not respond to fluid resuscitation
Central nervous system	Significant confusion and disorientation Obtundation and coma
Cardiovascular	Cyanosis Tachycardia Hypovolemia Dysrhythmias Metabolic acidosis Widened pulse pressure Cardiac output normal or elevated in the hyperdynamic phase of septic shock Decreased systemic vascular resistance in the hyperdynamic phase of septic shock Cardiac output depressed in the hypodynamic phase of septic shock Persistent hypotension not responsive to fluid resuscitation Increased systemic vascular resistance
Pulmonary	Tachypnea with associated dyspnea, resulting in respiratory alkalosis Bilateral rales Severe hypoxemia Pulmonary edema and hypertension Acute respiratory distress syndrome Respiratory failure
Gastrointestinal	Decreased gastric motility Ileus Gastrointestinal bleeding
Renal	Transient oliguria Anuria Increased blood urea nitrogen and creatinine levels Acute renal failure
Hepatic	Jaundice of skin or sclera Hyperbilirubinemia Elevation of serum liver transaminases
Skin	Cyanosis Acrocyanosis Cold, clammy skin

cause, or at least of the contributing factors related to sepsis, and should be gathered from a variety of sources, including the patient, family, and medical record. Nurses should focus on the history of burns, trauma, infection, nutritional status, recent blood product administration, surgical procedures (including insertion of invasive devices), presence and type of malignancy, immunosuppression, and any recent illness or infection (Stoll, 2001). Information also should include recent cancer treatments, including chemotherapy and radiation therapy, organ or stem cell transplant, concomitant illnesses such as HIV or diabetes, and the patient's medication regimen, including herbal and nutritional supplements and over-the-counter drugs. The history of prior infections and antibiotic use can provide useful information about potentially resistant organisms and secondary infections.

Physical Examination

In addition to a thorough history, a complete physical examination is critical in the assessment of patients with suspected or actual sepsis. The patient's vital signs can provide invaluable information regarding the presence or progression of a septic condition, as well as clues to poor tissue perfusion. Tachycardia, tachypnea, decreases in blood pressure, decreased oxygen saturation, and febrile or subfebrile states provide significant clues to a septic event (Moore, 2005). Immunosuppressed patients may not be able to mount a normal immune response because of neutropenia, and fever may be the primary clue regarding the presence of infection.

Central nervous system dysfunction or mental status changes, even subtle ones, may indicate an infection or impending sepsis. Unusual somnolence, agitation, anxiety, confusion, apprehension, cranial nerve deficits, photophobia, papilledema, and nuchal rigidity all may be symptoms of overwhelming infection (Shelton, 1999).

Inspection of the head and neck may reveal signs of infection, such as orbital and sinus tenderness, ocular redness and drainage, proptosis (bulging eyes), and/or signs of trauma. Oral thrush, mucositis, and signs and symptoms of esophagitis may be present in patients with cancer, all of which may lead to sepsis. Inspection and palpation of the neck may demonstrate lymphadenopathy related to infection.

Cardiopulmonary exam includes inspection, auscultation, palpation, and percussion of the heart and lungs. Chest pain, edema, tachypnea, tachycardia, orthopnea, hypotension, cyanosis, arrhythmias, onset of productive cough, shortness of breath, pulsus paradoxus, and decreased oxygen saturation may indicate infectious processes such as abscesses, pneumonia, pericarditis, and pericardial or pleural effusions.

A thorough abdominal exam is critical when assessing patients with cancer for sepsis, as the abdomen is a common site of infection in this patient population. Hypoactive bowel sounds may provide clues to peritonitis or a localized abdominal infection. Tenderness identified on palpation or general abdominal pain may reveal pathology secondary to neutropenic typhlitis (inflammation of the cecum), *Clostridium difficile* infection, bowel obstruction, ileus or perforation, or hemorrhage. Tenderness or pain also may indicate spleen or liver abnormalities caused by infection or organ enlargement. The gallbladder, pancreas, and appendix all should be suspect in the presence of abdominal pain. The gastrointestinal and urinary tracts are common sites of infection in patients with cancer. Diarrhea may indicate infection, particularly with clostridium, and nausea and vomiting may occur secondary to infection or obstruction. Common signs of infection of the urinary tract include pain, burning, urgency, and frequency with urination, microscopic or frank hematuria, and cloudy, dark urine. Careful monitoring of the patient's intake and output is important because a decrease in urine output may be a sign of impending sepsis (Gobel, 2005). Fever, flank pain, nausea and vomiting, and costovertebral angle tenderness are possible signs of pyelonephritis and may indicate a septic event.

The skin also is a common site of infection in patients with cancer; therefore, healthcare providers should conduct a thorough inspection of the skin. Pain, rashes, wounds, drainage, swelling, cyanosis, pallor, jaundice, and cellulitis may be further indicators of infection or organ compromise (Shelton, 1999). Nurses should closely examine any indwelling catheters, especially central vascular access devices, as these are a major source of infection (Segal et al., 2001). Table 6-5 provides a review of the physical examination of patients with known or suspected sepsis.

Diagnostic Evaluation

Laboratory Studies

A number of laboratory studies may assist in the diagnosis of sepsis or evaluate the severity of septic shock (see Table 6-6). A complete blood count with differential may provide clues as to an infectious process. A white blood cell count greater than 12,000 cells/mm^3 or less than 4,000 cells/mm^3 or a differential with greater than 10% bands is indicative of infection. A complete metabolic panel with liver function tests may help to determine organ function status. Elevated blood urea nitrogen and creatinine levels may indicate decreased kidney function, and elevated liver transaminases may indicate liver pathology related to sepsis. Elevated prothrombin time and activated partial thromboplastin times, decreased fibrinogen, decreased platelet count, and an elevated D-dimer assay may demonstrate coagulation abnormalities seen in sepsis. Disseminated intravascular coagulation is rare in sepsis; however, the development of this condition doubles the risk of death caused by sepsis (Fisher & Yan, 2000). Elevated blood glucose levels may be present in sepsis and septic shock, or, conversely, hypoglycemia may be present with prolonged septic shock because of hepatic failure and loss of compensatory mechanisms.

Table 6-5. Physical Examination of Patients With Known or Suspected Sepsis

System	Assessment Parameters That May Indicate Infection or Sepsis
Vital signs	Fever may be the only sign of infection in an immunosuppressed patient. Tachycardia, tachypnea, decrease in blood pressure, subfebrile states (< 96°F [36°C]), decreased oxygen saturation
Central nervous system	Changes in mental status, including somnolence, agitation, anxiety, confusion, and apprehension Cranial nerve deficits, photophobia, papilledema, nuchal rigidity
Head and neck	Orbital/sinus tenderness Redness and drainage from nose Proptosis Mucositis, oral thrush, signs or symptoms of esophagitis Lymphadenopathy
Cardiopulmonary	Chest pain, edema, tachypnea, tachycardia, orthopnea, hypotension, cyanosis, arrhythmias, and pulsus paradoxus Dyspnea, onset of cough with sputum, and decreased oxygen saturation
Abdominal	Hypoactive bowel sounds, tenderness on palpation, general abdominal pain
Gastrointestinal	Diarrhea, nausea and vomiting
Urinary tract	Pain, burning, urgency, frequency of urination, cloudy and dark urine, and microscopic or frank hematuria Close monitoring of intake/output and weight Fever, flank pain, nausea and vomiting, and costovertebral angle tenderness
Skin	Pain, rashes, wounds, drainage, swelling, cyanosis, pallor, jaundice, and cellulitis Monitoring of exit site of all indwelling catheters

Elevated lactate levels (lactic acidosis) indicate the tissue hypoperfusion that is seen prior to hypotension (Dellinger et al., 2004).

Biochemical markers such as IL-6, C-reactive protein, procalcitonin, and high mobility group box 1 (HMGB1, an abundant chromatin protein) all indicate the presence of severe systemic inflammation and sepsis, and their levels may correlate with patient outcomes (Luzzani et al., 2003; Oberhoffer et al., 1999; Sama, D'Amore, Ward, Chen, & Wang, 2004).

Table 6-6. Diagnostic Evaluation of Septic Patients

Diagnostic Study	Rationale
Complete blood count with differential	White blood cell count > 12,000 cells/mm^3, < 4,000 cells/mm^3, or > 10% bands indicates an infection.
Complete metabolic panel including liver function tests	Elevated blood urea nitrogen/creatinine levels may reflect dehydration and/or decreased renal function. Elevated liver transaminases and bilirubin may reflect liver changes from infection/sepsis.
Coagulation tests	Prolonged PT and PTT, elevated D-dimer assay, and decreased fibrinogen and platelet count may reflect fibrinolysis and/or disseminated intravascular coagulation. Decreased PT may indicate hepatic failure.
Blood glucose level	Hyperglycemia may be present in sepsis and septic shock. Hypoglycemia may be seen in prolonged septic shock.
Serum lactate	Elevated serum lactate indicates tissue hypoperfusion; helpful in evaluating metabolic acidosis
Biochemical markers (interleukin-6, CRP, PCT, HMGB1)	Elevations are correlated with the presence of sepsis.
Blood cultures	To be obtained before initiating antimicrobial therapy At least two sets of cultures should be drawn initially, one set from the vascular access catheter and one drawn percutaneously. An additional set of blood cultures should be drawn 24 hours after the onset of fever or further signs of infection. Repeat blood cultures should be done every 24 hours or based on the clinical findings.
Cultures of body fluids, including urine, stool, and throat, wound, sputum, and spinal fluids	To be obtained before initiating antimicrobial therapy Specific specimens are collected based on clinical findings.
Arterial blood gases	Assess oxygenation of patient; helpful in evaluating respiratory alkalosis and metabolic acidosis.
Miscellaneous diagnostic tests • Chest radiographs • Chest CT	Done to further diagnose sources of infection or further evaluate organ function • Rule out lung infection • Done based on suspicious x-ray or unresolved symptoms of infection

(Continued on next page)

Table 6-6. Diagnostic Evaluation of Septic Patients *(Continued)*	
Diagnostic Study	Rationale
Miscellaneous diagnostic tests *(cont.)*	
• Abdominal ultrasound	• Done based on complaints of abdominal symptoms
• Doppler ultrasound	• Diagnostic for venous thrombosis based on fever
• Venogram or spiral CT	• Diagnostic for pulmonary embolus based on fever and symptoms
• Thoracentesis	• Assists in isolating a source of bacterial infection
• Bronchoscopy/endoscopy	• May be considered in patients who continue to show signs of infection despite treatment
• Electrocardiogram/ echocardiogram	• Done based on suspicion for a cardiac source of infection to evaluate rate and rhythm
• Lumbar puncture	• Done if neurologic infection is suspected

CRP—C-reactive protein; CT—computed tomography; HMGB1—high mobility group box 1; PCT—procalcitonin; PT—prothrombin time; PTT—partial thromboplastin time

Note. Based on information from Dellinger et al., 2004; Fisher & Yan, 2000; Luzzani et al., 2003; Oberhoffer et al., 1999; Sama et al., 2004.

Blood cultures determine the pathogenic organisms responsible for the septic condition. At least two sets of cultures should be drawn initially, one from the vascular access catheter and one drawn percutaneously. According to the Surviving Sepsis Campaign guidelines (Dellinger et al., 2004), ideally one set of blood cultures should be drawn from each lumen of the vascular access catheter. An additional set of blood cultures should be drawn 24 hours after the onset of fever or further signs of infection. Healthcare providers collect cultures of body fluids such as urine, stool, throat, wound, sputum, and spinal fluid based on clinical findings before initiating antibiotics. The frequency of culturing depends on patients' clinical features, not solely on the presence of fever. Arterial blood gases may be drawn to assess oxygenation and to determine whether patients are in a state of respiratory alkalosis, which is seen with hyperventilation and gram-negative bacteremia (Martin et al., 2003).

Other Diagnostic Studies

Healthcare providers often perform additional diagnostic tests to identify sources of infection or to further evaluate organ function, especially when culture results are negative or if infection persists after appropriate treatment has been initiated. Chest radiographs can rule out lung infection. Suspicious chest x-ray results or unresolved symptoms of infection may necessitate chest computed tomography (CT). Abdominal symptoms such as pain, tenderness, or distention may warrant an abdominal ultrasound. Doppler ultrasound often is the first choice of procedures for diagnosing venous thrombosis as a suspected cause of fever (Bernardi et al., 1998). A venogram or a spiral chest CT is ordered for diagnosing a pulmonary embolus as the source of fever. Thoracentesis can help to manage a symptomatic pleural effusion by evacuating the fluid and also can assist in isolating a source of bacterial infection. Bronchoscopy and endoscopy may be useful in patients who continue to show signs of infection despite appropriate therapeutic interventions. Clinicians use electrocardiograms and echocardiograms when they suspect a cardiac source of infection. Suspicion of neurologic infection indicates the use of lumbar puncture.

Treatment Modalities

Several objectives exist regarding the management of severe sepsis in patients with cancer. These include initial resuscitation with early goal-directed therapy (EGDT), cardiovascular support, pulmonary support, antibiotics, and antisepsis interventions, including administering activated protein C, replacement dose steroids, and investigational therapies.

Initial Resuscitation

Once healthcare professionals have made a diagnosis of severe sepsis/SIRS based on the accepted criteria, it is extremely important to immediately initiate intensive therapy. They should not delay therapy pending transfer or admission to the intensive care unit (ICU), although a move to a monitored environment should be done in a timely manner to provide appropriate monitoring and resuscitation support (Dellinger et al., 2004). A central venous catheter is placed if one is not already present, and an arterial catheter also may be beneficial upon admission to the ICU (Connors et al., 1996). Once patients are in the ICU, supportive monitoring of blood pressure, mean arterial pressure (MAP), central venous pressure (CVP), venous oxygen saturation ($ScvO_2$), arterial saturation (SpO_2, O_2 saturation), and arterial blood gases is imperative (Rivers et al., 2001).

The treatment team should accomplish initial resuscitation within the first six hours after the diagnosis of severe sepsis (see Figure 6-2). The goals of initial resuscitation include maintaining a CVP of 8–12 mm Hg, MAP greater than or equal to 65 mm Hg, urine output greater than or equal to 0.5 ml/kg/hour, and central venous or mixed venous oxygen saturation greater than or equal to 70%. Serum lactate levels also are useful to quantify tissue hypoxia. If supplemental oxygen cannot maintain adequate oxygenation, patients should receive mechanical ventilation prior to their PaO_2 level falling below 60 mm Hg (Dellinger et al., 2004).

Figure 6-2. Goals for Initial Resuscitation of Sepsis*

- Maintain a central venous pressure of 8–12 mm Hg.
- Maintain a mean arterial pressure ≥ 65 mm Hg.
- Maintain a urine output ≥ 0.5 ml/kg/hour.
- Maintain a central venous or mixed venous oxygen saturation ≥ 70%.
- Initiate mechanical ventilation if PaO_2 falls below 60 mm Hg.

PaO_2—partial pressure of arterial oxygen

* Goals are to be accomplished within first six hours after the diagnosis of severe sepsis.

Early Goal-Directed Therapy

The key to survival in the management of septic patients with cancer is prompt intervention at the first sign of sepsis. The sooner that therapy is initiated for these acutely ill patients, the greater the potential that stabilization can occur and the progression to severe sepsis and SIRS is prevented. The goal of EGDT (see Table 6-7) is to identify and maximize treatment to minimize sepsis-induced hypoxia. In a study investigating the potential benefit of EGDT, 263 severely septic patients admitted to a hospital emergency room were randomized into the EGDT group or to the standard therapy (control) group (Rivers et al., 2001). The EGDT group spent a mandatory six hours in the emergency department completing an EGDT protocol, whereas members of the control group were admitted to the ICU as beds became available. EGDT consisted of the administration of IV fluids, vasopressors, blood transfusions based on venous oxygen saturation ($ScvO_2$), and inotropic agents if the $ScvO_2$ did not respond after transfusion. The end results of this study showed lower in-hospital mortality, decreased length of stay, higher $ScvO_2$, lower lactate levels, lower base deficit, and higher pH for the EGDT group compared to the standard therapy group. The results in the EGDT group may be attributed to early identification of high-risk patients, earlier resuscitation, and prompt management of hypovolemia, myocardial dysfunction, and disturbed vasoregulation and maintenance of organ perfusion (Rivers et al.).

Cardiovascular Support

Volume Resuscitation

Cardiovascular response to sepsis includes decreased vascular tone, myocardial depression, and a shift of plasma volume into the interstitial space resulting in decreased intravascular volume and hypotension. These processes result in decreased organ perfusion and potential dysfunction. The initial goal regarding cardiovascular support is to immediately replace intravascular volume to replenish organ perfusion. Typical fluid replacement consists of

Table 6-7. Early Goal-Directed Therapy

Therapy	Implications
Antibiotic initiation (within one hour of fever onset)	Directed to most likely microbes
Central venous access as quickly as possible	Continuous SaO_2 monitoring
Step 1: What is central venous pressure?	< 8–12 mm Hg requires 500 cc crystalloid bolus. Continue boluses until > 8–12 mm Hg.
Step 2: What is the mean arterial pressure?	< 65 mm Hg requires increased vasopressor use (e.g., norepinephrine). Titrate until > 65 mm Hg.
Step 3: What is the central venous O_2 saturation?	< 70%—maintain with oxygen therapy. Initiate mechanical ventilation if PaO_2 falls below 60 mm Hg.
What is the HCT?	< 30% HCT requires transfusion until > 30% HCT. > 30% HCT—can add and titrate dobutamine.
Decision to initiate: Steroids Activated protein C Insulin	

HCT—hematocrit; PaO_2—partial pressure of arterial oxygen; SaO_2—oxygen saturation

Note. Based on information from Rivers et al., 2001.

crystalloids (e.g., normal saline, lactated ringers) infused in large volumes at a rapid rate. Some patients may require upwards of 10 L to restore intravascular volume and blood pressure (Ognibene, 1996). Colloids, such as albumin, also may be infused, usually in smaller volumes. No evidence exists to support the use of one fluid type over another (Dellinger et al., 2004; Finfer et al., 2004). During fluid resuscitation, it is very important to monitor fluid balance and progression to overload and pulmonary edema, especially in patients with a history of cardiovascular disease. Nurses should ensure that patients' fluid volume is restored prior to initiation of vasopressor agents to enhance their efficacy.

Initial fluid resuscitation typically does not involve the use of blood products, but it does have therapeutic value under certain conditions. Clinicians should use fresh frozen plasma only if patients are bleeding or for the correction of coagulation factors in preparation for an invasive procedure. Healthcare professionals should administer platelets to patients with a platelet count < 5,000 cells/mm³ with or without bleeding, patients with a count of 5,000–30,000 cells/mm³ if they have potential to bleed, patients whose platelet count is > 50,000 cells/mm³ prior to invasive procedures, or anytime a patient is thrombocytopenic and bleeding (Dellinger et al., 2004). Several circumstances indicate the need for administration of packed red blood cells: hemoglobin is < 7 g/dl (goal is 7–9 g/dl), acute bleeding, ischemia or myocardial dysfunction, or when patients with a hematocrit < 30 g/dl are receiving EGDT (Rivers et al., 2001). The literature has discussed erythropoietin as a treatment to increase oxygen delivery, but because of its delayed action (7–10 days), it likely is not effective during the acute phase of sepsis.

Vasopressors and Inotropic Drugs

The decreased vascular tone seen in sepsis results in excessive peripheral hypotension, vasodilation, and impaired organ perfusion. If fluid resuscitation does not effectively correct this clinical situation or if fluid overload occurs, causing heart failure and altered tissue perfusion, then patients require vasopressor drugs such as dopamine or norepinephrine (Dellinger et al., 2004). Table 6-8 provides a review of vasopressor and inotropic drugs used in sepsis management. These drugs are adrenergic agonists and cause increased cardiac contractility and vasoconstriction in high doses, resulting in increased perfusion and blood pressure. Healthcare providers also may administer epinephrine and phenylephrine for their adrenergic effect, but these are used less frequently to maintain blood pressure. However, patients may receive epinephrine to maintain blood pressure if other first-line drugs are deemed ineffective, and phenylephrine also may be used for this reason because it produces less tachycardia than dopamine (Turkoski, Lance, & Bonfiglio, 2004). Vasopressin (antidiuretic hormone) may be useful for refractory hypotension in patients who do not respond to first-line agents (Patel, Chittock, Russell, & Walley, 2002). All of these drugs are best administered through a central line because of the potential for extravasation (Turkoski et al.).

Treatment involves inotropic drugs in the case of severely refractory septic patients who do not respond to fluids and high-dose vasopressors. Dobutamine is the inotropic drug of choice because of its strong adrenergic effect on beta-1 receptors in the heart, causing a large increase in contractility and heart rate. In the face of sepsis, patients may receive inotropic agents in combination with vasopressors in an attempt to maintain blood pressure and perfusion (Dellinger et al., 2004).

Arterial catheter placement is useful in septic patients to closely monitor blood pressures and obtain accurate readings; manual blood pressures may be much lower than actual intra-arterial pressures in the presence of severe peripheral vasoconstriction or septic shock. Controversial data exist regarding the benefit of using pulmonary artery catheters in severely septic patients (Richard et al., 2003). Pulmonary arterial catheters may be useful in determining the cause of shock, volume status, cardiac output, cardiac index, mixed $ScvO_2$, left ventricular end-diastolic pressure, and continuous end-diastolic

Table 6-8. Vasopressor and Inotropic Drugs for the Management of Sepsis		
Agent	**Dose**	**Effect**
First-line drug		
Norepinephrine	0.01–3 mcg/kg/min	Vasoconstriction, increased MAP with little change in heart rate or cardiac output
Dopamine	< 5 mcg/kg/min	Vasodilation causing increased glomerular filtration rate and sodium excretion
	5–10 mcg/kg/min	Increases cardiac contractility and heart rate
	> 10 mcg/kg/min	Vasoconstriction and increased blood pressure
Second-line drug		
Phenylephrine	0.4–9.1 mcg/kg/min	Vasoconstriction, increased blood pressure
Epinephrine	0.1–1 mcg/kg/min	Increased MAP by increased cardiac index and stroke volume
Vasopressin	0.01–0.04 units/min	Vasoconstriction, increased cAMP levels, causing decreased urine volume and increased osmolality and water retention
Dobutamine	2.5–20 mcg/kg/min	Increased cardiac contractility and heart rate

cAMP—cyclic adenosine monophosphate; MAP—mean arterial pressure

Note. Based on information from Hollenberg et al., 2004; Turkoski et al., 2004.

volume. However, clinicians must weigh the risks of insertion against the potential benefit of the information gained from the catheter (Procaccini & Clementi, 2004).

Pulmonary Support

Acute Respiratory Distress Syndrome and Acute Lung Injury

The inflammatory cytokines involved in sepsis may cause acute lung injury and ARDS because of their actions on the endothelium and epithelium of the alveolar-capillary wall. The insult to the alveolar-capillary wall causes alveolar fluid retention, resulting in pulmonary edema and decreased production and activity of surfactant. Neutrophils sequestered in the lung secondary to the initial inflammatory response also stimulate release of additional inflammatory mediators, contributing to further lung damage that may resolve quickly or progress to fibrotic lung injury. Severe inflammation of the lungs may lead to extreme ventilation/perfusion mismatching, hypoxia, and the need for intubation and mechanical ventilation (Ware & Matthay, 2000).

Mechanical Ventilation

Once the decision is made to intubate patients because of hypoxemia and respiratory failure, the treatment team immediately initiates mechanical ventilation. For patients who develop ARDS, the ventilation strategy consists of low tidal volumes (6 ml/kg/ideal body weight) and positive end-expiratory pressure (PEEP) of at least 5–10 cm/H_2O to prevent lung collapse at end expiration and resultant lung injury (Dellinger et al., 2004). Placing severely hypoxic septic patients in the prone position may improve oxygenation, but only experienced facilities should attempt "proning" because of the potential for life-threatening complications, such as accidental dislodgment of the endotracheal tube and/or central venous catheters (Dellinger et al.). All ventilated patients should be placed in a semirecumbent position at an elevation of 45°, as tolerated, to aid in the prevention of ventilator-associated pneumonia (Drakulovic et al., 1999). According to reports in the literature, mechanically ventilated patients may not be weaned as promptly as warranted following stabilization. As many as half of the patients who spontaneously extubate themselves do not require reintubation (Estaban et al., 1999). Healthcare providers should conduct a spontaneous breathing trial to assess patients' readiness for weaning from the ventilator when they demonstrate improvement evidenced by increased mental status and arousability, hemodynamic stability without vasopressor support, low ventilator and PEEP requirements, and low oxygen requirements. Daily trials of spontaneous breathing should be conducted on these patients as their stability permits. Research has shown that interventions to appropriately wean patients decrease the number of days of mechanical ventilation, the need for reintubation, complications, the need for tracheostomy, and healthcare costs (Estaban et al.).

Sedation, Analgesia, and Neuromuscular Blockade

Effective sedation and analgesia are important to provide comfort and to decrease the strenuous work of breathing by reducing oxygen consumption and elevated CO_2 levels in septic patients maintained on mechanical ventilation (Shelly, 1999). Several types of medication have a useful therapeutic effect in mechanically ventilated patients and are divided into three main drug classes: analgesics, sedatives, and neuromuscular blockers. Analgesic drugs of choice are fentanyl and morphine. Fentanyl is used more frequently in unstable patients because of its modest positive effects on hemodynamic stability. Use of the sedatives propofol, midazolam, and lorazepam typically decreases agitation during ventilation. Patients usually receive propofol and midazolam during the initial 24 hours of sedation, whereas lorazepam may be used for a longer duration (Shapiro et al., 1995).

In patients who continue to be agitated or if pain persists while on appropriate sedation and analgesic regimens, a neuromuscular blockade may be beneficial. The drugs pancuronium, vecuronium, or cisatracurium primarily maintain neuromuscular blockade. Cisatracurium is useful in hemodynamically unstable patients, especially those with cardiac disease or at risk for histamine release (Shapiro et al., 1995). However, neuromuscular blockade is avoided whenever possible because of the possibility of prolonged paralysis after the drug is discontinued. Healthcare providers should take caution to limit blockade use to the initial hours of sedation and to not prolong administration (Rossiter, Souney, McGowan, & Carvajal, 1991). Excessive sedation in ventilated patients can lead to longer ICU stays, polyneuropathy, and mental status impairment necessitating additional diagnostic testing and increased healthcare costs. Current data support the use of nursing-implemented protocols to determine appropriate sedation delivery, with daily periods of interrupted sedation to promote patient wakefulness. Guidelines from the Surviving Sepsis Campaign (Dellinger et al., 2004) state that such a protocol has been shown to reduce ventilation duration, hospital length of stay, and the need for tracheostomy placement (Kress, Pohlman, O'Connor, & Hall, 2000).

Antibiotics and Infection Source Control

Bacteria is the primary source of infection contributing to the development of severe sepsis and septic shock. However, sepsis also can develop secondary to infection with viral and fungal pathogens or other organisms. Early detection of the causal organism and potential source and the immediate initiation of appropriate antibiotic therapy are crucial to an improved outcome for septic patients. A retrospective study evaluating the adequacy of antibiotic coverage for 492 patients admitted to hospital ICUs with known bloodstream infections demonstrated that patients who received adequate antibiotic treatment had a lower mortality rate (28.4%) than those who were inadequately treated with antibiotics (61.9%) (Ibrahim, Sherman, Ward, Fraser, & Kollef, 2000).

Initially, the most useful tool to determine the presence and source of infection is a thorough history and physical examination, paying particular attention to the most frequent sites of infection associated with sepsis—the lungs, abdomen, and urinary tract, followed by the skin, soft tissue, and central nervous system. The history and physical exam can provide clues to a probable source of infection. Sources of infection may include, but are not limited to, infected catheters (e.g., venous, arterial, urinary), pleural abscess or empyema, pericardial effusion, and wounds. Cultures should be obtained from all potential sources prior to antibiotic administration, which should not be delayed. Antibiotics are administered as soon as possible but no later than one hour after the recognition of severe sepsis, using broad-spectrum antibiotics empirically targeted toward the most likely bacterial and fungal pathogens. Current susceptibility patterns in the community and institution and the ability of the antibiotic to penetrate the potential source are considerations when choosing a broad-spectrum antibiotic. Focused therapy, using narrow-spectrum antibiotics, begins once the pathogen is identified. Patient factors such as allergy, drug intolerance, underlying disease, organ function, and clinical situation also are considerations when determining the appropriate antibiotics (Dellinger et al., 2004).

Specific antibiotic therapy will be based on the factors discussed previously and requires frequent reevaluation to assess its effectiveness, any expansion or narrowing of coverage, patient tolerance and toxicity, and the current clinical status of patients. The management of septic infection involves the use of a great variety of antibiotics, of which a full discussion is beyond the scope of this chapter. See Table 6-9 for an overview of antibiotics appropriate for different infected sites.

The most common bacterias causing infection in sepsis are gram-negative types; however, gram-positive bacteremia is becoming more prevalent. *Escherichia coli*, *Klebsiella* species, and *Pseudomonas aeruginosa* are the most common gram-negative pathogens, whereas coagulase-negative staphylococci, *Staphylococcus aureus*, viridans group streptococci, and enterococci are the primary gram-positive bacterias causing pathology. Viral suspects will likely be herpes simplex, respiratory syncytial virus, parainfluenza, and influenza A and B; however, cytomegalovirus and adenovirus may present as serious viral infections in immunocompromised individuals. Fungal causes are almost always *Candida* and *Aspergillus* species (National Comprehensive Cancer Network [NCCN], 2004).

Initial antibiotic therapy based on a monotherapy approach should consist of IV carbapenem (imipenem-cilastatin or meropenem) or an extended-spectrum cephalosporin (ceftazidime or cefepime). Other options with expanded double coverage include an aminoglycoside plus an antipseudomonal penicillin or an extended-spectrum cephalosporin; ciprofloxacin and an antipseudomonal penicillin; or a double beta-lactam consisting of an extended-spectrum cephalosporin plus antipseudomonal penicillin or monobactam. Patients at high risk for sepsis or those exhibiting signs of sepsis should immediately begin double coverage regimens. Expanded antibiotic coverage will be based on the patient's clinical appearance, infection site and commonly infecting organisms, pending cultures, and specific diagnostic tests indicative of infection (NCCN, 2004).

It may seem rational to prevent antimicrobial resistance by using narrow-spectrum antibiotics to treat infection; however, in the case of critically

Table 6-9. Antibiotic Considerations by Potentially Infected Site

Site of Infection	Antibiotic Considerations
Skin	
Cellulitis	Vancomycin
Wound	Vancomycin
Vesicles	Acyclovir, famciclovir, valacyclovir
Disseminated papules/lesions	Vancomycin and antifungal
Urinary tract	Coverage appropriate on initial therapy pending culture
Central nervous system	
Bacterial	Cefepime, ceftazidime, imipenem, meropenem Vancomycin
Viral	High-dose acyclovir
Gastrointestinal tract	
Mouth	Anaerobic coverage Antiviral (acyclovir) Topical or systemic antifungal (fluconazole, topical nystatin)
Esophagus	Antifungal (fluconazole, caspofungin, amphotericin) Acyclovir Ganciclovir or foscarnet if suspect cytomegalovirus (CMV)
Abdomen (intestinal, rectal, liver)	Anaerobic coverage (metronidazole if diarrhea) Enterococcal coverage (antipseudomonal penicillin) Antifungal coverage if liver involvement (voriconazole or amphotericin)
Sinus/nasal	Amphotericin or voriconazole Vancomycin (periorbital cellulitis)
Lung	
Pneumonia (with focal lesions on x-ray)	Atypical coverage (fluoroquinolone, macrolide, doxycycline) Antifungal therapy (voriconazole)
Interstitial infiltrates (on x-ray)	Atypical coverage (fluoroquinolone, macrolide, doxycycline) Anti–*Pneumocystis carinii* pneumonia coverage (trimethoprim/sulfamethoxazole) Influenza A and B coverage (oseltamivir) Ganciclovir or foscarnet if suspect CMV
Venous access device	Vancomycin

Note. Based on information from Gilbert et al., 2004; National Comprehensive Cancer Network, 2004.

ill septic patients, restriction of antibiotics until the organism is identified may adversely affect patient outcomes. Prompt, aggressive, broad-spectrum antibiotic coverage is pertinent initially, with subsequent evaluation and microbe identification leading to narrow coverage as infection stabilizes (Dellinger et al., 2004; Ibrahim et al., 2000). Source infection control in severely septic patients may involve many disciplines.

Intestinal ischemia or perforation, cholangitis, and intra-abdominal abscesses are of concern in this population and may require specialty assistance. Interventions should begin immediately when infectious sources are identified; however, the risks of certain procedures, such as surgery, must be weighed against their potential benefits, especially for immunocompromised or thrombocytopenic patients who are at increased risk for infection and bleeding (Dellinger et al., 2004).

Steroid Use

The pathology of severe sepsis is mostly the result of an intense host inflammatory response. In the face of a severe acute illness such as severe sepsis and SIRS, relative adrenal insufficiency with a reduction of cortisol reserves may occur, as seen in approximately half of all patients in septic shock (Meduri & Chrousos, 1998). Relative adrenal insufficiency results from the suppressive effect of cytokines on adrenocorticotropic hormone (ACTH) and cortisol resistance of tissues (Annane & Cavaillon, 2003). Because of their actions, glucocorticoid steroids have shown at least mild effectiveness in treating the inflammatory response of sepsis and aiding in correction of illness-related adrenal insufficiency (Annane et al., 2004). The use of steroids, however, is somewhat controversial, and varying opinions exist as to their effectiveness. Initial studies using high-dose regimens of approximately 30 mg/kg of methylprednisolone for short periods of time showed mostly no benefit (Lefering & Neugebauer, 1995). More recently, renewed interest in the use of steroids has emerged. A systematic review and meta-analysis of 16 clinical trials with a total of 2,063 patients revealed several benefits to extended duration (longer than five days) of low-dose steroids using less than 300 mg of hydrocortisone per day (Annane et al., 2004). Results showed that the use of corticosteroids reduced mortality in ICUs, increased the reversal of shock at 7 days and again at 28 days, decreased mortality from all causes at 28 days, and decreased hospital mortality related to septic shock (Annane et al., 2004).

According to the Surviving Sepsis Campaign (Dellinger et al., 2004), hydrocortisone in doses of 200–300 mg, delivered in three or four divided doses daily or by continuous infusion, is recommended for patients who require vasopressor therapy to maintain blood pressure. Recommendations suggest performing an ACTH stimulation test to determine the ability of the adrenal cortex to respond to ACTH with a rebound increase in cortisol. This test entails administering 250 mcg of ACTH and then measuring cortisol levels 30–60 minutes later. Patients whose cortisol levels increase more than 9 mcg/dl are considered *responders* and are not likely to benefit from exogenous steroids and therefore should not receive steroid therapy (Annane et al., 2002). If the ACTH stimulation test reveals a *nonresponder*, defined as a cortisol level below 9 mcg/dl, replacement dose steroids should be given 30–60 minutes after ACTH administration (Dellinger et al.).

Activated Protein C

The pathophysiologic processes seen with severe sepsis and SIRS include varying degrees of inflammation, increased coagulation, and lack of fibrinolysis and endothelial cell dysfunction in response to toxins or trauma. Protein C, an antithrombotic/profibrinolytic plasma protease, plays an important role in maintaining normal hemostasis and thrombosis. Its activated form, activated protein C, participates in modulating the body's response to inflammation and to systemic sepsis and the resulting intravascular coagulation. The main effect of protein C is to reduce the production of thrombin, which has proinflammatory, procoagulant, and antifibrinolytic actions. It also inhibits the influence of tissue factors in stimulating the clotting system and has anti-inflammatory properties (Tazbir, 2004). Protein C is consumed in states of sepsis and systemic inflammation, resulting in loss of inhibition of coagulation and inflammatory processes. Recent evidence suggests that replacement therapy with exogenous activated protein C can improve the clinical outcome of patients with severe sepsis (Grinnell & Joyce, 2001).

A relatively new targeted drug therapy, drotrecogin alfa (activated), a recombinant human version of activated protein C, has shown positive outcomes in the treatment of severely septic patients who have a high risk of death. An outcome prediction model called the Acute Physiology and Chronic Health Evaluation II (APACHE II) is used to categorize mortality risk and to determine justification for administering drotrecogin alfa. In the Protein C Worldwide Evaluation in Severe Sepsis (PROWESS) trial, 1,690 subjects with severe sepsis were randomized into either a placebo group or the drotrecogin alfa treatment group. Results were significant for the drotrecogin alfa group, showing a reduction of 19.4% in the relative risk of death and a 6.1% reduction in the absolute risk of death compared to the placebo group (Bernard et al., 2001). Indications for using drotrecogin alfa depend on the severity of the septic situation and the patient's risk of death as determined by the APACHE II score, preferably within the first 24 hours after recognition of severe sepsis. Drotrecogin alfa is given via IV infusion at a dose of 24 mcg/kg/hr over 96 hours (Eli Lilly and Co., 2004). The most serious and common adverse reaction of the drug is bleeding. Because of the increased risk for bleeding, healthcare providers should use drotrecogin alfa with caution in patients with an international normalized ratio > 3 or a platelet count < 30,000 cells/mm³. Figure 6-3 reviews precautions for the administration of drotrecogin alfa.

Figure 6-3. Precautions for the Administration of Drotrecogin Alfa

- International normalized ratio > 3
- Known bleeding tendency (diathesis)
- Chronic severe hepatic disease
- Platelet count < 30,000 cells/mm^3
- Concurrent therapeutic dosing of heparin
- Recent history (within three months) of ischemic stroke
- Recent history (within three days) of thrombolytic therapy
- Recent history (within six weeks) of gastrointestinal bleed
- Intracranial arteriovenous malformation or aneurysm
- Recent administration (within seven days) of aspirin (> 650 mg/day) or other platelet inhibitor
- Recent administration (within seven days) of oral anticoagulants or glycoprotein IIb/IIIa inhibitors

Note. Based on information from Eli Lilly and Co., 2004.

Investigational Therapies

A number of investigational therapies currently are under study for the treatment of sepsis that have demonstrated potential for improved patient outcomes.

Monoclonal Antibodies

TNF-α is an inflammatory cytokine that is implicated in the pathogenesis of sepsis and SIRS. Studies of patients experiencing a severe inflammatory response have demonstrated survival benefits when TNF-α is antagonized by monoclonal antibodies such as afelimomab and CDP571 (Pittet et al., 1999). Positive responses also have occurred with use of the TNF neutralizing receptor fusion protein (p55-IgG) that binds to human immunoglobulin G (IgG) antibody. A clinical trial that enrolled 498 patients with refractory shock or severe sepsis demonstrated that over a 28-day period, treatment with p55-IgG (lenercept) was associated with a trend toward reduced mortality, decreased new organ dysfunction, and decreased incidence and duration of organ failure in comparison to placebo. The p55-IgG group also had a shorter need for mechanical ventilatory support and decreased length of stay (Pittet et al.).

Anticytokine Agents

Several cytokines are involved in the pathogenesis of sepsis and inflammation, and the effects of cytokine inhibition on sepsis outcomes are the subjects of much investigation. In addition to TNF-α, other cytokines that play a role in the proinflammatory response of sepsis are migration inhibitory factor, complement (C5a and others), HMGB1, IL, and interferon (Rendon-Mitchell et al., 2003; Riedemann et al., 2004). Studies have demonstrated that inhibition of these cytokines could potentially decrease the inflammatory response in sepsis (Huber-Lang et al., 2001). Other studies of the actions of natural coagulants, such as antithrombin (AT) (Baudo et al., 1998), tissue factor pathway inhibitor, and protein C (discussed earlier), in treating or reversing the hypercoagulation abnormalities seen in sepsis mostly have not demonstrated a benefit to support their use.

Nursing Management

Prevention and Early Detection

Early detection and intervention are critical in preventing the progression of infection to septic shock. Providing meticulous nursing care to immuno-suppressed patients is of utmost importance because granulocytopenia is the single most important risk factor in the development of sepsis in patients with cancer (Sachdeva, 2002; Safdar & Armstrong, 2001). Nurses must be able to identify and report the early signs and symptoms of infection and sepsis to the primary care provider immediately (Reigle & Dienger, 2003).

Asepsis and Antisepsis

Patients with cancer are inherently immunocompromised and are at much higher risk for infection because of their treatment and underlying disease. Therefore, the focus for prevention of sepsis involves control and prevention of infection in these individuals. Proper hand-hygiene procedures according to institutional policies are the most important infection control strategy (Eggimann et al., 2000). Nurses should be diligent in advocating for an aseptic environment for all patients. The nursing staff should implement strict policies to prevent infectious transmission to patients via visitors, medical professionals, and ancillary staff. Nurses should wear gloves anytime there is risk of contact with blood or body fluids. When working with patients, they should remove and replace gloves when moving from a contaminated body part to a clean body part. Gloves are removed in the patient care room and discarded between patients. Artificial nails are discouraged, and natural nails should be kept less than one-fourth inch in length (Boyce & Pittet, 2002).

Respiratory Infections—Pneumonia

Pneumonia contributes to sepsis in critically ill patients with cancer. It often is associated with invasive therapies such as intubation with mechanical ventilation, aspiration secondary to enteral nutrition, or atelectasis caused by prolonged periods of immobility. The use of endotracheal or tracheostomy tubes and nasogastric tubes predisposes patients to infection, so these should be used only as long as medically necessary. Patients should be weaned from mechanical ventilation as soon as tolerated and noninvasive ventilation attempted. Keeping the head of the bed elevated to 30°–45° and providing endotracheal suctioning, especially above the cuff, and stringent mouth care are very important nursing measures for patients receiving mechanical ventilation and enteral nutrition (Schleder, Stott, & Lloyd, 2002). Proper enteral tube placement should be verified frequently to prevent aspiration of stomach contents and resultant pneumonia (McClave et al., 2002). Dysphasic patients who are unable to tolerate secretions or oral feeding require close monitoring to prevent aspiration. Ambulation and deep breathing exercises (i.e., incentive spirometry) are encouraged in all patients as physical and mental status permits (Chumillas, Ponce, Delgado, Viciano, & Mateu, 1998). Nursing intervention in the prevention and early detection of clinical signs of pneumonia is of utmost importance and is extremely influential in decreasing morbidity related to pneumonia complications.

Intravascular Catheter-Related Infections

Any invasive line passing through the skin creates a serious infection risk in immunocompromised patients. It often is not feasible to limit the number of IV catheters placed during a patient's stay, but using aseptic technique is important and can significantly decrease infection rates. Close monitoring of IV sites for redness, tenderness, infiltration, and drainage helps to prevent infectious complications. Documentation of IV insertion dates also is very important to prevent prolonged placement and subsequent contamination and tissue disruption. Clean or sterile gloves are to be worn when inserting an IV catheter, and sterile gloves are required for the insertion of arterial and central catheters (O'Grady et al., 2002). Catheter site care requires cutaneous antisepsis with an appropriate antiseptic before catheter insertion and during dressing changes. Peripheral catheters can be cleaned with a 2% chlorhexidine-based preparation (preferred), tincture of iodine, an iodophor, or 70% alcohol (Little, Murray, Traynor, & Spitznagel, 1999). Multiple studies have found chlorhexidine gluconate to significantly reduce the number of bloodstream infections in patients with vascular access devices (Chaiyakunapruk, Veenstra, Lipsky, & Saint, 2002). Institutional policies determine the replacement of IV administration sets, tubing, stopcocks, and caps.

Indwelling Urinary Catheters

Indwelling urinary catheters pose a great risk of infection to patients with cancer and are to be used only if absolutely necessary and removed as soon as possible. The longer the catheter is in place, the more likely infection will arise. Intermittent catheterization, condom catheters, and suprapubic catheters are safer alternatives to indwelling urethral catheters in immunocompromised patients. Aseptic sterile technique is required throughout the catheter insertion procedure, and the smallest lumen is recommended to allow adequate drainage and prevent urethral trauma. A closed drainage system is important to maintain a sterile environment. Catheter irrigation should be minimized and aseptic technique used if any irrigation is required. Close nursing assessment of urine consistency, color, volume, and clarity, in addition to urethral or pelvic complaints, is necessary to prevent and disclose urinary tract complications and infection.

Wound Care

Any break in the skin presents a risk of infection. Wounds require close monitoring and surveillance for any change in condition. Standard precautions, in addition to sterile technique with sterile dressings, are required. Disposal of all supplies, gloves, etc., in their appropriate location helps to prevent cross-contamination of infectious material to other patients. Wound-care nurses are helpful in determining the appropriate care and treatment for specific wounds (Mangram, Horan, Pearson, Silver, & Jarvis, 1999).

Other Supportive Nursing Care

Supportive nursing measures are crucial to preventing complications that could adversely affect patient outcomes. Nursing interventions in many of the following areas can positively influence morbidity and mortality of patients with severe sepsis and septic shock.

Stress Ulcer Prophylaxis

Ulceration of the gastrointestinal tract can occur during periods of critical illness. Septic patients are at increased risk for ulceration because of decreased blood flow to the gut with tissue ischemia and resultant injury to the mucosal lining. These patients also experience a reduction in cytoprotectant prostaglandins and an inability to protect the mucosa from damage because of the presence of gastric acid, bile, and other digestive enzymes. Risk factors for gastrointestinal bleeding include respiratory failure, especially with prolonged ventilation, coagulopathies, hypotension, and liver and kidney failure. Stress ulcer prophylaxis should be instituted in all patients with sepsis. Commonly used medications include H_2-receptor blockers, proton pump inhibitors, and sucralfate. Studies show that H_2-receptor blockers are more effective and are preferable over sucralfate in patients requiring ICU therapy (Cook et al., 1998).

Deep Venous Thrombosis Prophylaxis

Septic patients, especially those being treated in an ICU, are at high risk for thrombus formation secondary to venous stasis resulting from immobility, vessel injury caused by invasive therapies, and sepsis-induced hypercoagulopathy. It is critical for nurses to maintain prophylaxis for deep venous thrombosis

(DVT). Low-molecular-weight heparin or low-dose unfractionated heparin is used unless contraindications to heparin exist, including thrombocytopenia, severe coagulopathies, and active or recent bleeding episodes, such as intracerebral hemorrhage. Sequential compression devices should be used if heparin is contraindicated or should be used in combination with heparin in those patients who are at very high risk for developing thrombosis (Dellinger et al., 2004). Bedside nursing input is crucial in determining the patient's mobility status and need for DVT prophylaxis and ambulation. A thorough nursing assessment is often the first clue to the development of a thrombosis.

Renal Replacement Therapy

Transient renal insufficiency is not uncommon in septic patients and usually results because of periods of hypotension with poor renal perfusion. Although the incidence of renal failure requiring renal replacement therapy (RRT) in critically ill patients is less than 5% and renal function usually recovers over time, these patients have significantly higher mortality rates compared to those without renal failure (Metnitz et al., 2002). Adequate fluid volume and vasopressor support are important to maintain renal perfusion. A variety of RRTs are available for patients based on their needs. Traditional intermittent dialysis may be used, but hemodynamically unstable septic patients often do not tolerate this treatment. Continuous hemofiltration may be more appropriate and much better tolerated because of the smaller volume exchanges over an extended period of time (Meyer, 2000).

Nutritional Support

Patients with sepsis are forced into a hypermetabolic state that requires high calorie, protein, and electrolyte replacement. Enteral nutrition is the preferred route for nutritional support in most patients and is associated with preservation of gut integrity, barrier and immune functions, and resultant reduction in infectious complications. Adequate nutrition also improves wound healing, decreases infection rates, and shortens hospital stays. Parenteral nutrition can be used alternatively when the enteral route is contraindicated, but it is associated with an increased risk of infection (Cerra et al., 1997). Nursing assessment of nutritional intake and suggestions for nutritional sources that are well-tolerated or palatable for patients are highly beneficial in maintaining adequate nutritional requirements. See Table 6-10 for a description of nutritional requirements for septic patients.

Glycemic Control

Critically ill patients often have increased insulin resistance with hyperglycemia preceding hypoglycemia. Recent studies recommend maintaining blood glucose levels below 150 mg/dl without inducing hypoglycemia. A large

Table 6-10. Nutritional Requirements for Septic Patients	
Element	**Supplement Requirements**
Macronutrients	
Calories	25–30 kcal/kg/usual body weight/day
Protein	1.3–2 grams/kg/day
Glucose	30%–70% of daily caloric intake
Lipids	15%–30% of daily caloric intake
Micronutrients	
Potassium, magnesium, zinc, phosphate	All should be supplemented to maintain normal serum levels.

Note. Based on information from Cerra et al., 1997.

randomized controlled trial demonstrated the benefits of intensive insulin therapy. Patients randomized into the intensive insulin treatment group, in which the blood glucose was maintained between 80–110 mg/dl, showed a significant decrease in mortality (4.6%) compared to the conventional treatment group (8%), in which blood glucose was maintained at approximately 180–200 mg/dl. For those patients who remained in the ICU more than five days, the mortality rate for the intensive insulin group was 10.6%, compared to 20.2% for the conventional treatment group (van den Berghe et al., 2001).

Delirium Intervention

A large percentage of septic patients treated in the ICU, especially if intubated, will suffer from delirium. Altered cognition in the form of confusion, anxiety, agitation, and lethargy can begin early in therapy and last days to weeks. These effects typically relate to prolonged sedation with narcotics and benzodiazepines during and after mechanical ventilation. Delirium also is associated with prolonged hospital stays; results of one study showed that it was the strongest predictor of prolonged length of stay in the ICU (Ely et al., 2001). Intervention for delirium begins with discontinuing or minimizing the cause. Limiting sedation by decreasing the use of narcotics and benzodiazepines, depending on the clinical situation, often will decrease delirium. Providing a safe environment during the period of confusion and altered cognition is of utmost importance. During this time, restraints may be necessary to prevent patient injury. Frequent reorientation of patients to the environment and increased sensory stimulation through measures such as opening window shades, providing clocks and calendars, making available the patients' eyeglasses and hearing aids, and allowing objects from home and visits from family and friends are all appropriate interventions for delirium. Intervention by a clinical psychologist or psychiatrist also may be beneficial. Haloperidol may be used to decrease agitation and anxiety associated with delirium. Haloperidol is the agent of choice for the management of delirium in patients with cancer because of its useful sedating effects and relatively low cardiovascular and anticholinergic effects (Abrahm, 2000). Relatively low doses, initially 0.5–1 mg orally or parenterally, can be given for treating agitation, paranoia, and fear (Morrison, 2003). Doses may be repeated every 45–60 minutes.

Patient and Caregiver Support

Holistic health care involves not only the patients but also the loved ones who care for them. During an acute illness such as sepsis, caregivers have to cope with many difficult decisions and emotions, including fear, guilt, sorrow, alienation, and grief. Many patients who experience sepsis and septic shock are transferred from an oncology care setting to an ICU. Patients and caregivers are likely to become frightened and anxious during this time. The supportive environment provided by the nurse during this stressful time is critical to their well-being and ability to cope. Nurses can serve as knowledgeable advocates and provide emotional support and listening skills as patients and caregivers face potential end-of-life issues. Referrals to multidisciplinary sources of support such as spiritual support through a chaplaincy program, counseling from a psychologist or social worker, case management assistance, and patient or family support groups may be beneficial. Nurses should provide ongoing, detailed information as appropriate to each patient's situation and foster open communication with patients and their caregivers. If patients and caregivers are well informed and able to voice their questions and concerns, they are less likely to be anxious and fearful and are more satisfied with their care (Gobel, 2005).

Patient and Caregiver Education

Because granulocytopenia is the single most important risk factor in the development of sepsis in patients with cancer (Sachdeva, 2002), it is critical to educate patients and caregivers on the importance of preventing infection during periods of immunocompromise. Nurses should encourage patients to turn, cough, and deep breathe to help to prevent respiratory compromise and to ambulate to decrease coagulopathy risk. Personal hygiene is stressed to decrease the colonization of bacteria on the skin. Caregivers also need to understand the importance of good hand hygiene during periods of immunocompromise of patients. Although the nutritional requirements for patients with sepsis increase, patients may not have a good appetite or may be too tired to eat. Nurses are in a key position to emphasize the importance of nutrition and to offer high-calorie/high-protein supplements. If food and fluids do not meet patients' nutritional needs, patients may require enteral or parenteral nutrition. It is important to educate patients and caregivers that this type of nutrition is intended as a short-term solution to provide much-needed calories, proteins, and electrolytes.

As patients become critically ill, providing patients and their caregivers with information about the potential transfer to an ICU setting, the need for additional medications, such as antibiotics and vasopressors, and the possibility of mechanical ventilation is an important nursing task. Patients and caregivers also should be informed of the various consultants they may come into contact with during the course of managing sepsis and septic shock, such as infectious disease specialists, cardiologists, pulmonologists, and intensive care specialists.

Conclusion

Sepsis and septic shock are life-threatening oncologic emergencies that can occur very quickly after the onset of infection. Because of the rapidity and severity of these conditions, early detection and intervention are essential for better patient outcomes. A number of malignancies can modify immunity in patients with cancer and cause granulocytopenia, the single most important risk factor in the development of sepsis. Oncology nurses play a pivotal role in promptly recognizing and reporting aberrant vital signs or other signs of infection so that appropriate therapies can be immediately initiated.

Although much is understood about the development and treatment of sepsis and septic shock, more investigation is needed to provide new insights into this complex syndrome and to develop more effective targeted therapies. Oncology nurses are in a key position to conduct research on optimal evidence-based nursing care of immunosuppressed patients with cancer.

References

Abrahm, J.L. (2000). *A physician's guide to pain and symptom management in cancer patients.* Baltimore: Johns Hopkins University Press.

Alberti, C., Brun-Buisson, C., Burchardi, H., Martin, C., Goodman, S., Artigas, A., et al. (2002). Epidemiology of sepsis and infection in ICU patients from an international multicentre cohort study. *Intensive Care Medicine, 28,* 108–121.

Angus, D.C., Linde-Zwirble, W.T., Lidicker, J., Clermont, G., Carcillo, J., & Pinsky, M.R. (2001). Epidemiology of severe sepsis in the United States: Analysis of incidence, outcome, and associated costs of care. *Critical Care Clinics, 16,* 1303–1310.

Annane, D., Bellissant, E., Bollaert, P.E., Briegel, J., Keh, D., & Kupfer, Y. (2004). Corticosteroids for severe sepsis and septic shock: A systematic review and meta-analysis. *BMJ, 329, 4*

Annane, D., & Cavaillon, J.M. (2003). Corticosteroids in sepsis: From bench to bed. *Shock, 20,* 197–207.

Annane, D., Sebille, V., Charpentier, C., Bollaert, P.E., Francois, B., Korach, J.M. (2002). Effect of treatment with low doses of hydrocortisone and fludrocorti mortality in patients with septic shock. *JAMA, 288,* 862–871.

Baudo, F., Caimi, T.M., de Cataldo, F., Ravizza, A., Arlati, S., Casella, G., et al. (1 tithrombin III (ATIII) replacement therapy in patients with sepsis and/or p complications: A controlled double-blind, randomized, multicenter study. *Intensive Care Medicine, 24,* 336–342.

Bernard, G.R., Vincent, J.L., Laterre, P.F., LaRosa, S.P., Dhainaut, J.F., Lopez-Rodriguez, A., et al. (2001). Efficacy and safety of recombinant human activated protein C for severe sepsis. *New England Journal of Medicine, 344,* 699–709.

Bernardi, E., Prandoni, P., Lensing, A.W.A., Agnelli, G., Guazzaloca, G., Scannapieco, G., et al. (1998). D-dimer testing as an adjunct to ultrasonography in patients with clinically suspected deep vein thrombosis: Prospective cohort study. *BMJ, 317,* 1037–1040.

Bogolioubov, A., Keefe, D.L., & Groeger, J.S. (2001). Circulatory shock. *Critical Care Clinics, 17,* 697–719.

Bone, R.C., Balk, R.A., Cerra, F.B., Dellinger, R.P., Fein, A.M., Knaus, W.A., et al. (1992). The American College of Chest Physicians/Society of Critical Care Medicine consensus conference: Definitions for sepsis and organ failure and guidelines for the use of innovative therapies in sepsis. *Chest, 101,* 1644–1655.

Boyce, J.M., & Pittet, D. (2002). Guidelines for hand hygiene in health-care settings: Recommendations of the healthcare infection control practices advisory committee and the HICPAC/SHEA/APIC/IDSA hand hygiene task force. *Morbidity and Mortality Weekly Report: Recommendations and Reports, 51*(RR-16), 1–45.

Cerra, F.B., Benitez, M.R., Blackburn, G.L., Irwin, R.S., Jeejeebhoy, K., Katz, D.P., et al. (1997). Applied nutrition in ICU patients: A consensus statement of the American College of Chest Physicians. *Chest, 111,* 769–778.

Chaiyakunapruk, N., Veenstra, D.L., Lipsky, B.A., & Saint, S. (2002). Chlorhexidine compared with povidone-iodine solution for vascular catheter-site care: A meta-analysis. *Annals of Internal Medicine, 136,* 792–801.

Chumillas, S., Ponce, J.L., Delgado, F., Viciano, V., & Mateu, M. (1998). Prevention of postoperative pulmonary complications through respiratory rehabilitation: A controlled clinical study. *Archives of Physical Medicine and Rehabilitation, 79,* 5–9.

Connors, A.F., Speroff, T., Dawson, N.V., Thomas, C., Harrell, F.E., Wagner, D., et al. (1996). The effectiveness of right heart catheterization in the initial care of critically ill patients: SUPPORT Investigators. *JAMA, 276,* 889–897.

Cook, D., Guyatt, G., Marshall, J., Leasa, D., Fuller, H., Hall, R., et al. (1998). A comparison of sucralfate and ranitidine for the prevention of upper gastrointestinal bleeding in patients requiring mechanical ventilation. Canadian Critical Care Trials Group. *New England Journal of Medicine, 338,* 791–797.

Dellinger, R.P., Carlet, J.M., Masur, H., Gerlach, H., Calandra, T., Cohen, J., et al. (2004). Surviving Sepsis Campaign guidelines for management of sepsis and septic shock. *Critical Care Medicine, 32,* 858–873.

ello, C.A. (1997). Proinflammatory and anti-inflammatory cytokines as mediators in pathogenesis of septic shock. *Chest, 112*(Suppl. 6), 321S–329S.

ic, M.B., Torres, A., Bauer, T.T., Nicolas, J.M., Nogue, S., & Ferrer, M. (1999). Study position as a risk factor for nosocomial pneumonia in mechanically ventilated A randomized trial. *Lancet, 354,* 1851–1858.

Harbarth, S., Constantin, M.N., Touveneau, S., Chevrolet, J.C., & Pittet, D. act of a prevention strategy targeting vascular-access care on incidence of uired in intensive care. *Lancet, 355,* 1864–1868.

04). Xigris (drotrecogin alfa [activated]) [Package insert]. Indianapolis,

00). Infection. In C.H. Yarbro, M.H. Frogge, & M. Goodman (Eds.), *Cannd practice* (5th ed., pp. 691–708). Sudbury, MA: Jones and Bartlett.

olin, R., Francis, J., May, L., Speroff, T., et al. (2001). The impact ive care unit on hospital length of stay. *Intensive Care Medicine,*

t., Gil, A., Gordo, F., Vallverdu, I., et al. (1999). Effect of ration on outcome of attempts to discontinue mechanical ventilation. Spanish Lung Failure Collaborative Group. *American Journal of Respiratory Critical Care Medicine, 159,* 512–518.

Filbin, M.R., & Stapczynski, J.S. (2002). *Septic shock.* Retrieved March 1, 2005, http://www.emedicine.com/emerg/topic533.htm

Finfer, S., Bellomo, R., Boyce, N., French, J., Myburgh, J., & Norton, R. (2004). A comparison of albumin and saline for fluid resuscitation in the intensive care unit. *New England Journal of Medicine, 350,* 2247–2256.

Fisher, C.J., Jr., & Yan, S.B. (2000). Protein C levels as a prognostic indicator of outcome in sepsis and related diseases. *Critical Care Medicine, 28*(Suppl. 9), S49–S56.

Friedman, G., Silva, E., & Vincent, J.L. (1998). Has the mortality rate of septic shock changed with time? *Critical Care Medicine, 26,* 2078–2086.

Gilbert, D.N., Moellering, R.C., Eliopoulos, G.M., & Sande, M.A. (2004). *The Sanford guide to antimicrobial therapy* (34th ed.). Hyde Park, VT: Antimicrobial Therapy, Inc.

Gobel, B.H. (2005). Metabolic emergencies. In J.K. Itano & K.N. Taoka (Eds.), *Core curriculum for oncology nurses* (4th ed., pp. 383–421). St. Louis, MO: Elsevier.

Grinnell, B.W., & Joyce, D. (2001). Recombinant human activated protein C: A system modulator of vascular function for treatment of severe sepsis. *Critical Care Medicine, 29*(Suppl. 7), S53–S61.

Hachem, R., & Raad, I. (2002). Prevention and management of long-term catheter related infections in cancer patients. *Cancer Investigation, 20,* 1105–1113.

Hollenberg, S.M., Ahrens, T.S., Annane, D., Astiz, M.E., Chalfin, D.B., Dasta, J.F., et al. (2004). Practice parameters for hemodynamic support of sepsis in adult patients. *Critical Care Medicine, 32,* 1928–1948.

Hotchkiss, R.S., & Karl, I.E. (2003). The pathophysiology and treatment of sepsis. *New England Journal of Medicine, 348,* 138–150.

Huber-Lang, M.S., Sarma, J.V., McGuire, S.R., Lu, K.T., Guo, R.F., Padgaonkar, V.A., et al. (2001). Protective effects of anti-C5a peptide antibodies in experimental sepsis. *Federation of American Societies for Experimental Biology Journal, 15,* 568–570.

Ibrahim, E.H., Sherman, G., Ward, S., Fraser, V.J., & Kollef, M.H. (2000). The influence of inadequate antimicrobial treatment of bloodstream infections on patient outcomes in the ICU setting. *Chest, 118,* 146–155.

Kress, J.P., Pohlman, A.S., O'Connor, M.F., & Hall, J.B. (2000). Daily interruption of sedative infusions in critically ill patients undergoing mechanical ventilation. *New England Journal of Medicine, 342,* 1471–1477.

Lefering, R., & Neugebauer, E.A. (1995). Steroid controversy in sepsis and septic shock: A meta-analysis. *Critical Care Medicine, 23,* 1294–1303.

Little, J.R., Murray, P.R., Traynor, P.S., & Spitznagel, E. (1999). A randomized trial of povidone-iodine compared with iodine tincture on venipuncture site disinfection: Effects on rates of blood culture contamination. *American Journal of Medicine, 107,* 119–125.

Luzzani, A., Polati, E., Dorizzi, R., Rungatscher, A., Pavan, R., & Merlini, A. (2003). Comparison of procalcitonin and C-reactive protein as markers of sepsis. *Critical Care Medicine, 31,* 1737–1741.

Mangram, A.J., Horan, T.C., Pearson, M.L., Silver, L.C., & Jarvis, W.R. (1999). Guideline prevention of surgical site infection, 1999. Hospital Infection Control Practices Advisory Committee. *Infection Control and Hospital Epidemiology, 20,* 250–278.

Marchetti, O., Cometta, A., & Calandra, T. (2001, December). *Fluoroquinolone prophyla granulocytopenic cancer patients: Pro's and con's.* 5th International Symposium on F Neutropenia. Retrieved March 1, 2005, from http://www.febrileneutropeni abstract/e_caland.htm

Martin, G.S., & Bernard, G.R. (2001). Airway and lung in sepsis. *Intensive Care* 27(Suppl. 1), S63–S79.

Martin, G.S., Mannino, D.M., Eaton, S., & Moss, M. (2003). The epidemiolog in the United States from 1979 through 2000. *New England Journal of Me* 1546–1554.

McClave, S.A., DeMeo, M.T., DeLegge, M.H., DiSario, J.A., Heyland, D.K., Maloney, J.P., et al. (2002). North American Summit on Aspiration in the Critically Ill Patient: Consensus statement. *Journal of Parenteral and Enteral Nutrition, 26*(Suppl. 6), S80–S85.

Meduri, G.U., & Chrousos, G.P. (1998). Duration of glucocorticoid treatment and outcome in sepsis: Is the right drug used the wrong way? *Chest, 114,* 355–360.

Metnitz, P.G., Krenn, C.G., Steltzer, H., Lang, T., Ploder, J., Lenz, K., et al. (2002). Effect of acute renal failure requiring renal replacement therapy on outcome in critically ill patients. *Critical Care Medicine, 30,* 2051–2058.

Meyer, M. (2000). Renal replacement therapies. *Critical Care Clinics, 16,* 29–58.

Moore, S. (2005). Septic shock. In C.H. Yarbro, M.H. Frogge, & M. Goodman (Eds.), *Cancer nursing: Principles and practice* (6th ed., pp. 895–909). Sudbury, MA: Jones and Bartlett.

Morrison, C. (2003). Identification and management of delirium in the critically ill patient with cancer. *AACN Clinical Issues, 14,* 92–111.

Muckart, D.J.J., & Bhagwanjee, S. (1997). American College of Chest Physicians/Society of Critical Care Medicine Consensus definitions of the systemic inflammatory response syndrome and allied disorders in relation to critically injured patients. *Critical Care Medicine, 25,* 1789–1795.

National Comprehensive Cancer Network. (2004). *NCCN clinical practice guidelines in oncology, version 1.2005.* Jenkintown, PA: Author.

Nimah, M., & Brilli, R.J. (2003). Coagulation dysfunction in sepsis and multiple organ system failure. *Critical Care Clinics, 19,* 441–458.

Oberhoffer, M., Karzani, W., Meier-Hellmann, A., Bogel, D., Fasssbinder, J., & Reinhart, K. (1999). Sensitivity and specificity of various markers of inflammation for the prediction of tumor necrosis factor-alpha and interleukin-6 in patients with sepsis. *Critical Care Medicine, 27,* 1814–1818.

Oberholzer, A., Oberholzer, C., & Moldawer, L.L. (2001). Sepsis syndromes: Understanding the role of innate and acquired immunity. *Shock, 16,* 83–96.

Ognibene, F.P. (1996). Hemodynamic support during sepsis. *Clinical Chest Medicine, 17,* 279–287.

O'Grady, N.P., Alexander, M., Dellinger, E.P., Gerberding, J.L., Heard, S.O., Maki, D.G., et al. (2002). Guidelines for the prevention of intravascular catheter-related infections. *Morbidity and Mortality Weekly Report: Recommendations and Reports, 51*(RR-10), 1–29.

Patel, B.M., Chittock, D.R., Russell, J.A., & Walley, K.R. (2002). Beneficial effects of short-term vasopressin infusion during severe septic shock. *Anesthesiology, 96,* 576–582.

lletier, L.L., Jr. (2003). Microbiology of the circulatory system. In S. Baron (Ed.), *Medical microbiology* (4th ed.). Retrieved March 1, 2005, from http://gsbs.utmb.edu/ crobook/ch094.htm

n, P.G. (1998). Sepsis and septic shock. In C.C. Chernecky & B.J. Berger (Eds.), ced and critical care oncology nursing (pp. 549–565). Philadelphia: Saunders.

Harbarth, S., Suter, P.M., Reinhart, K., Leighton, A., Barker, C., et al. (1999). Immunomodulating therapy on morbidity in patients with severe sepsis. *American espiratory and Critical Care Medicine, 160,* 852–857.

Clementi, G. (2004). Pulmonary artery catheterization in 9,071 cardiac ts: A review of complications [Abstract]. *Italian Heart Journal Supplement,*

& Wenzel, R.P. (1997). The epidemiology and natural history of sepsis. raham, & R.A. Balk (Eds.), *Sepsis and multiorgan failure* (pp. 27–34). Wilkins.

M.J. (2003). Sepsis and treatment-induced immunosuppres-cancer. *Critical Care Nursing Clinics of North America, 15,*

Li, J., Han, J., Wang, H., Yang, H., et al. (2003). IFN-gamma box 1 protein release partly through a TNF-dependent gy, 170,* 3890–3897.

Richard, C., Warszawski, J., Anguel, N., Deye, N., Combes, A., Barnoud, D., et al. (2003). Early use of the pulmonary artery catheter and outcomes in patients with shock and acute respiratory distress syndrome: A randomized controlled trial. *JAMA, 290,* 2713–2720.

Riedemann, N.C., Guo, R.F., Gao, H., Sun, L., Hoesel, M., Hollmann, T.J., et al. (2004). Regulatory role of C5a on macrophage migration inhibitory factor release from neutrophils. *Journal of Immunology, 173,* 1355–1359.

Rivers, E., Nguyen, B., Havstad, S., Ressler, J., Muzzin, A., Knoblich, B., et al. (2001). Early goal-directed therapy in the treatment of severe sepsis and septic shock. *New England Journal of Medicine, 345,* 1368–1377.

Rossiter, A., Souney, P.F., McGowan, S., & Carvajal, P. (1991). Pancuronium-induced prolonged neuromuscular blockade. *Critical Care Medicine, 19,* 1583–1587.

Sachdeva, K. (2002). *Granulocytopenia.* Retrieved March 15, 2005, from http://www.emedicine.com/med/topic927.htm

Safdar, A., & Armstrong, D. (2001). Infectious morbidity in critically ill patients with cancer. *Critical Care Clinics, 17,* 531–570.

Sama, A.E., D'Amore, J., Ward, M.F., Chen, G., & Wang, H. (2004). Bench to bedside: HMGB1-a novel proinflammatory cytokine and potential therapeutic target for septic patients in the emergency department. *Academic Emergency Medicine, 11,* 867–873.

Schleder, B., Stott, K., & Lloyd, R.C. (2002). The effect of a comprehensive oral care protocol on patients at risk for ventilator-associated pneumonia. *Journal of Advocate Health Care, 4,* 27–30.

Segal, B.H., Walsh, T.J., & Holland, S.T. (2001). Infections in the cancer patient. In V.T. DeVita, S. Hellman, & S.A. Rosenberg (Eds.), *Cancer: Principles and practice of oncology* (6th ed., pp. 2815–2868). Philadelphia: Lippincott Williams & Wilkins.

Shapiro, B.A., Warren, J., Egol, A.B., Greenbaum, D.M., Jacobi, J., Nasraway, S.A., et al. (1995). Practice parameters for systemic intravenous analgesia and sedation for adult patients in the ICU. An executive summary. *Society of Critical Care Medicine, 23,* 1596–1600.

Shelly, M.P. (1999). Sedation, where are we now? *Intensive Care Medicine, 25,* 137–139.

Shelton, B.K. (1999). Sepsis. *Seminars in Oncology Nursing, 15,* 209–221.

Stoll, E.H. (2001). Sepsis and septic shock. *Clinical Journal of Oncology Nursing, 5,* 71–72.

Tazbir, J. (2004). Sepsis and the role of activated protein C. *Critical Care Nurse, 24,* 40–45.

Turkoski, B.B., Lance, B.R., & Bonfiglio, M.F. (2004). *Lexi-Comp's drug information handbook for advanced practice nursing.* Hudson, OH: Lexi-Comp.

van den Berghe, G., Wouters, P., Weekers, F., Verwaest, C., Bruyninckx, F., Schetz, M., et al. (2001). Intensive insulin therapy in critically ill patients. *New England Journal of Medicine, 345,* 1359–1367.

Ware, L.B., & Matthay, M.A. (2000). The acute respiratory distress syndrome. *New England Journal of Medicine, 342,* 1334–1348.

Wheeler, A.P., & Bernard, G.R. (1999). Treating patients with severe sepsis. *New England Journal of Medicine, 340,* 207–214.

Williams, M.D., Braun, L.A., Cooper, L.M., Johnston, J., Weiss, R.V., Qualy, R.L., et al. (2004). Hospitalized cancer patients with sever sepsis: Analysis of incidence, mortality, and associated costs of care. *Critical Care, 8,* 291–298.

Jeanne K. Clancey, RN, MSN, CNRN

⊃ Chapter 7

Syndrome of Inappropriate Antidiuretic Hormone Secretion

Introduction

The syndrome of inappropriate antidiuretic hormone (SIADH) is a rare but serious endocrine disorder. The abnormal production and secretion of antidiuretic hormone (ADH) that is inappropriate for the feedback mechanisms regulating ADH release characterize this disorder. In SIADH, the excessive release of ADH causes disturbances in normal fluid and electrolyte balance. The kidney absorbs free water despite normal intravascular osmolality and blood volume, resulting in dilutionally low serum sodium levels (hyponatremia) and inappropriately concentrated urine (Fojo, 2005; Moore, 1998; Richerson, 2004).

Malignancy, particularly small cell lung cancer (SCLC), is the most common cause of SIADH, but a variety of nonmalignant conditions also are associated with this syndrome (Richerson, 2004). The signs and symptoms of SIADH can be mild and nonspecific or severe, manifested by neurologic changes such as seizures, coma, or death. The severity of the syndrome is related to the degree of hyponatremia and its rapidity of onset. Oncology nurses should be aware of the patient population at risk for SIADH and of the subtle signs and symptoms associated with this syndrome. Early recognition and intervention are essential to prevent symptoms from progressing to a life-threatening oncologic emergency (Keenan, 2005; Langfeldt & Cooley, 2003).

Incidence

SIADH is primarily associated with bronchogenic cancer, especially SCLC. This type of cancer constitutes approximately 20% of all lung cancers. About

10% of all patients with SCLC will develop SIADH (Keenan, 2005). Other malignancies, including carcinomas of the pancreas, duodenum, colon, bladder, and prostate, lymphomas, thymoma, and primary brain tumors, also produce SIADH (Richerson, 2004). These malignant cells synthesize, store, and release biologic ADH, known as arginine vasopressin (AVP), which is identical to native ADH. Nonmalignant conditions such as infections, pulmonary disease, CNS disorders, chronic illness, and increasing age account for the remaining causes of SIADH (Keenan; Moore, 1998; Richerson). Morbidity and mortality rates are higher in patients with severe hyponatremia that developed acutely. Hospitalized patients with hyponatremia have up to a 60% greater mortality rate than hospitalized patients with normal levels of serum sodium (Foster, 2005).

Normal Physiology of Water Regulation

A review of the normal physiology of water regulation and of key definitions (see Table 7-1) is essential to understanding the processes involved in SIADH. Approximately 60%–80% of body weight is water, which is distributed between two compartments, intracellular and extracellular. Intracellular fluid (within the cells) contains two-thirds of total body water; the other third is extracellular fluid, which includes interstitial fluid and intravascular fluid (plasma). Potassium and phosphate are the major intracellular electrolytes, whereas sodium and chloride are the primary extracellular electrolytes. The movement of water and dissolved particles (solutes) across semipermeable cell membranes—a process called *osmosis*—maintains equilibrium in the fluid and electrolyte balance of the intracellular and extracellular fluid compartments (Flounders, 2003). Figure 7-1 illustrates the effect of osmosis on the cell. The total concentration of solutes in the fluid compartments is called the *osmolality* of the solution.

Table 7-1. Definitions Related to Syndrome of Inappropriate Antidiuretic Hormone

Term	Definition
Osmosis	Movement of water and dissolved particles across semi-permeable cell membrane
Osmolality	The total concentration of solutes in the fluid compartments
Serum osmolality	Measures the number of dissolved particles per unit of water in serum. Reliable measure of hydration status.

Note. Based on information from Flounders, 2003; Grant & Kubo, 1975.

Figure 7-1. Effect of Osmosis Across a Cell Membrane

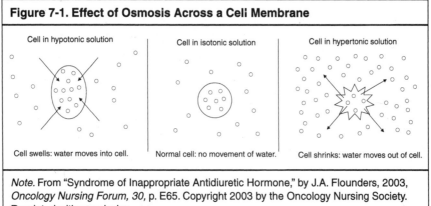

Note. From "Syndrome of Inappropriate Antidiuretic Hormone," by J.A. Flounders, 2003, *Oncology Nursing Forum, 30,* p. E65. Copyright 2003 by the Oncology Nursing Society. Reprinted with permission.

One of the most reliable measures of hydration status is *serum osmolality,* which measures the number of dissolved particles (solutes) per unit of water in serum (Grant & Kubo, 1975). Sodium serves as the principal determinant of serum osmolality and reflects the relative ratio of sodium to water in the blood. Changes in serum osmolality most often reflect changes in serum sodium concentration. The terms *osmolarity* and *osmolality* are interchangeable when discussing fluid and electrolyte balance (Grant & Kubo). Normal osmolality in serum is approximately 280–300 milliosmols per kilogram (mOsm/kg) (Craig, 2005; Keenan, 2005).

Homeostatic mechanisms involving thirst, ADH, and renal handling of sodium (reabsorption or excretion) normally maintain serum sodium concentration and serum osmolarity within a narrow range (Craig, 2005). ADH, known as a AVP in its biologically active form, is a peptide hormone that is produced by specialized neurosecretory cells in the hypothalamus and then stored and released by the posterior pituitary gland. The most important role of ADH is to conserve body water by reducing the output of urine (Foster, 2005). Dehydration causes increased serum osmolality; overhydration results in decreased serum osmolality. Neurons in the hypothalamus known as *osmoreceptors* sense increased serum osmolality and then, in turn, cause an increase in thirst and in the secretion of ADH (Craig).

ADH acts in the kidneys to conserve water by binding to receptors in the distal or collecting renal tubules, thus promoting reabsorption of water and excretion of a lesser amount of concentrated urine. The reabsorbed water dilutes the blood, reducing the serum osmolality toward normal, with a concomitant increase in urine osmolarity. In the opposite situation, when serum osmolality is low, as with fluid overload, the osmoreceptors are not stimulated, and ADH release is suppressed. In the absence of ADH, water is not reabsorbed in the renal tubules, and greater amounts of dilute urine are excreted, resulting in an increase in serum concentration (Agha, 2004).

Another mechanism involved in regulating ADH production takes place within the cardiovascular system. Changes in blood volume and pressure, which are sensed by stretch receptors in the heart and large arteries, stimulate or suppress secretion of ADH. Elevated blood volume and blood pressure increase the atrial stretch, causing the release of atrial natriuretic peptide (ANP). ANP is a hormone produced by cardiac atria tissue that responds to increased blood volume and atrial stretch by promoting excretion of sodium and water through the kidneys (Batcheller, 1994; Terpstra & Terpstra, 2000). ANP acts to reduce blood pressure by stimulating decreased water and sodium reabsorption in the renal tubules so that more water is lost in the urine. In contrast, when blood volume and pressure are low, the atrial stretch decreases, as does the stimulus for ANP release. Decreased ANP levels stimulate the release of ADH, which acts to conserve water by increasing water and sodium reabsorption in the kidneys. Changes in blood pressure and volume are not as sensitive a stimulator of ADH as increased osmolality but can be effective in conditions of severe fluid volume loss. Hemorrhage that results in 15%–20% loss of blood volume will stimulate massive ADH secretion (Colorado State University, 1998).

ADH secretion also increases in response to stimulation of the limbic system in the brain by psychological factors such as stress, pain, fear, and major trauma, such as surgery. The limbic system functions in behavior control but also participates in the control of body fluid osmolality by inducing ADH release (Langfeldt & Cooley, 2003).

Nausea is another potent stimulator of ADH release. Patients experiencing nausea and vomiting often develop hyponatremia because of ADH release in response to volume depletion. Water then is retained in excess of sodium, leading to mild hyponatremia (Terpstra & Terpstra, 2000).

Pathophysiology

SIADH is a disorder of water intoxication in which some of the excess free water in the body is distributed into the vascular space, where it dilutes the plasma, thus causing hyposmolality and dilutional hyponatremia. Signs of fluid volume overload are absent in SIADH because most of the free water diffuses across its osmotic gradient into the intracellular space, where the effects of intracellular edema are felt most strongly in the central nervous system (CNS) (Craig, 2005; Flounders, 2003; Keenan, 2005).

SIADH represents a failure of the negative feedback mechanisms that regulate the release and inhibition of ADH. The primary abnormality causing SIADH is the acquired ability of some malignant tissue (which is not responsive to regulatory feedback mechanisms) to inappropriately secrete ectopic ADH (Foster, 2005). Excessive secretion of ADH results in uncontrolled water reabsorption in the renal tubules despite decreasing serum sodium concentration and decreasing osmolality, indicating the presence of a nonosmotic stimulus for ADH release. The kidneys are unable to put out dilute urine because of the antidiuretic effects of ADH; they also increase sodium excretion in response to the increase in intravascular volume. The result is that the urine concentration (osmolality) becomes inappropriately high compared to serum osmolality, and urine sodium levels increase (Richerson, 2004; Terpstra & Terpstra, 2000).

Risk Factors

The risk factors for SIADH depend on its causes, which range from clinical disorders to medication side effects, as discussed in this section and outlined in Figure 7-2.

Central Nervous System Disorders

Central hypothalamic-pituitary SIADH may occur from several CNS disorders, including meningitis, brain tumors, brain abscess, subarachnoid hemorrhage, and head injuries. In these disorders, there is a sustained production of ADH from the posterior pituitary gland. As these conditions improve, the signs of SIADH will disappear, unlike with SIADH from an endocrine paraneoplastic syndrome (Batcheller, 1994). Patients with multiple sclerosis and Guillain-Barré syndrome may have increased ADH production as part of their disease process (Procyk, 2004).

Malignancy

SIADH most often occurs as an endocrine *paraneoplastic syndrome* that is the result of a malignant disease process. Tumor invasion or compression does not directly cause paraneoplastic syndromes. They result from the acquired ability of malignant cells to synthesize and release hormones (e.g., ectopic production of ADH) or other physiologically active substances, which can produce distant systemic effects that interfere with normal homeostasis (Santacroce, Gagliardi, & Balducci, 2005). In SIADH, malignant cells are able to inappropriately synthesize, store, and release AVP (Foster, 2005). The production and release of ectopic ADH by this process disrupts the normal fluid and electrolyte balance in the body (Flounders, 2003).

The most common type of malignancy associated with paraneoplastic SIADH is SCLC. Up to 80% of patients with SCLC have evidence of impaired water excretion (Miaskowski, 1999).

Several other malignancies also may stimulate SIADH, including non-small cell lung cancer, lymphomas, and carcinomas of the head and neck, prostate, pancreas, breast, ovary, duodenum, and esophagus (Batcheller, 1994; Flounders, 2003; Keenan, 2005; Procyk, 2004; Robinson, 2000). SIADH caused by ectopic ADH secretion is more difficult to treat than SIADH from central pituitary disease (Batcheller).

Figure 7-2. Risk Factors for Syndrome of Inappropriate Antidiuretic Hormone

Malignant Conditions

Cancers of the
- Bladder
- Brain
- Breast
- Cervix
- Colon
- Duodenum
- Esophagus
- Hypopharynx
- Lung (especially small cell lung cancer)
- Ovary
- Pancreas
- Prostate

Carcinoid
Leukemia
Lymphomas (Hodgkin and non-Hodgkin)
Mesothelioma
Neuroblastoma
Sarcoma
Thymoma

Nonmalignant Conditions

AIDS
Asthma
Chronic obstructive pulmonary disease
Hypothyroidism
Lung abscess
Older age
Pneumonia
Systemic lupus erythematosus
Tuberculosis

Neurologic Conditions

Stroke
Encephalitis
Guillain-Barré syndrome
Meningitis
Skull fracture
Subarachnoid hemorrhage
Subdural hematoma
Cerebral atrophy
Multiple sclerosis

Miscellaneous Conditions

Anxiety
Nausea
Positive end-expiratory pressure breathing devices
Severe pain
Stress
Trauma

Medications

Analgesics
- Aspirin
- Barbiturates
- General anesthetics
- Morphine
- Meperidine
- Nicotine
- Nonsteroidal anti-inflammatory drugs
- Acetaminophen

Antidepressants
- Imipramine
- Monoamine oxidase inhibitors
- Selective serotonin reuptake inhibitors

Chemotherapy
- Cisplatin
- Cyclophosphamide
- Docetaxel
- Ifosfamide
- Melphalan
- Vincristine

Other medications
- Bromocriptine
- Carbamazepine
- Chlorpropamide
- Haloperidol
- Thiazide diuretics

Note. Based on information from Keenan, 2005; Miaskowski, 1999; Terpstra & Terpstra, 2000.

Nonmalignant Conditions

Pulmonary Disease

Many pulmonary infections and inflammatory conditions can stimulate ectopic production of ADH. Pulmonary disorders such as pneumonia, fungal infections, tuberculosis, lung abscess, chronic obstructive pulmonary disease, and asthma are associated with SIADH occurrence (Flounders, 2003; Foster, 2005; Moore, 1998). Benign lung tissue also is thought to be able to produce and secrete ADH (Moore). Patients on mechanical ventilation or positive end-expiratory pressure breathing devices may develop SIADH. These treatments may reduce the venous return to the heart and decrease cardiac output and atrial stretch, thereby stimulating a decrease in the production of ANP. Decreased ANP production stimulates the release of ADH, which conserves water and sodium (Batcheller, 1994; Terpstra & Terpstra, 2000).

Medications and Hydration Factors

Many of the pharmacologic agents used in the daily management of patients with cancer may contribute to SIADH development (see Figure 7-2). Chemotherapy agents used in treating the patient's malignancy may increase SIADH occurrence by stimulating release of ADH from the posterior pituitary gland (Moore, 1998). The chemotherapeutic and biologic agents most commonly associated with SIADH include cyclophosphamide, cisplatin, ifosfamide, vincristine, vinblastine, melphalan, and interferon-alpha and interferon-gamma (Flounders, 2003; Langfeldt & Cooley, 2003). Administration of cyclophosphamide and cisplatin requires vigorous hydration to minimize toxicity to the bladder and kidneys and can lead to water overload and severe hyponatremia in those at risk. Aggressive hydration to prevent nephrotoxicity increases the risk of SIADH, as does hydration with hypotonic IV fluids (0.45% normal saline or less) (Flounders; Moore).

Conditions that increase water loss, such as dehydration, vomiting, diarrhea, and hyperthermia, may contribute to SIADH by stimulating ADH release (Miaskowski, 1999). Following surgery, patients are at increased risk for SIADH, related, in part, to the type and extent of fluid replacement. Fluids lost during surgery often are replaced with hypotonic IV solutions, such as 5% dextrose in water. These fluids dilute the concentration of plasma electrolytes and predispose patients to dilutional hyponatremia (Batcheller, 1994).

Many medications may contribute to SIADH development because they increase the levels of ADH or potentiate its actions, causing hyponatremia. This includes antidepressants (monoamine oxidase inhibitors, tricyclic antidepressants, selective serotonin reuptake inhibitors), nonsteroidal anti-inflammatory drugs, opioid analgesics, thiazide diuretics, barbiturates, angiotensin-converting enzyme inhibitors, oral hypoglycemic agents (chlorpropamide, tolbutamide), celecoxib, phenothiazines, gabapentin, haloperidol, proton pump inhibitors, and some anesthetic agents (Craig, 2005; Flounders, 2003; Foster, 2005; Langfeldt & Cooley, 2003; Miaskowski, 1999; Richerson, 2004). Nicotine in cigarettes stimulates ADH production and also may contribute to SIADH occurrence (Flounders).

Other Conditions

Many patients hospitalized with AIDS have hyponatremia, with more than 60% of the incidence related to SIADH. Patients with AIDS are at increased risk for developing SIADH because of the frequency of secondary malignancies and opportunistic infections, such as *Pneumocystis carinii* pneumonia, and the multitude of medications they take (Akalin, Chandrakantan, Keane, & Hamburger, 2001; Langfeldt & Cooley, 2003). Endocrine disorders, such as hypothyroidism and glucocorticoid deficiency (Addison disease), may be risk factors for developing SIADH (Foster, 2005). Postoperative patients are at increased risk for SIADH because of factors associated with increased secretion of ADH, trauma, stress, pain, general anesthesia, and use of opioid narcotics (Langfeldt & Cooley). Older adults, as well, have an increased incidence of SIADH from any disease state. With the aging process, total body fluid decreases and changes occur in renal function, which cause ineffective regulation of sodium and diminished ability to concentrate urine. Results of a study of older adult patients in long-term care revealed that 18%–22% had serum sodium levels < 135 mEq/L, and the incidence of hyponatremia was 50% (Larson & Martin, 1994). Many older adults also take multiple medications, some of which may be associated with increased risk for SIADH (Terpstra & Terpstra, 2000).

Clinical Manifestations

With SIADH, most of the excess free water in the body is distributed within the intracellular compartment rather than the intravascular space. Most tissues tolerate intracellular edema well, but not the brain, which is confined within the skull and has little room for expansion. Therefore, clinical manifestations of hyponatremia are related primarily to cerebral edema (Craig, 2005). The rate of onset and the degree of hyponatremia are critical to the extent of the clinical manifestations seen in SIADH (Craig; Keenan, 2005; Richerson, 2004) (see Table 7-2). When serum sodium concentrations fall gradually, over several days to weeks, symptoms may be minimal even with sodium levels as low as 110 mEq/L. This is because the brain possesses compensatory mechanisms that allow it to handle slowly developing hyponatremia by extruding solutes and fluid to the extracellular space. The flow of free water into the intracellular space within the brain is reduced, and the symptoms are milder than would be expected for a given degree of hyponatremia (Craig). However, a rapid decline in serum sodium to less than

Table 7-2. Clinical Manifestations of Syndrome of Inappropriate Antidiuretic Hormone*

Type	Laboratory Test	Signs/Symptoms
Mild hyponatremia	Sodium 125–134 mEq/L	Nonspecific or none; may present with thirst, anorexia, nausea, fatigue, weakness, muscle cramps, headache
Moderate hyponatremia	Sodium 115–124 mEq/L	Weight gain, oliguria, progressive neurologic symptoms
Severe hyponatremia	Sodium < 115 mEq/L	Signs/symptoms related to cerebral edema: papilledema, delirium, hypoactive reflexes, ataxia, gait disturbance, seizures, coma, death

* Varies depending on the rate of onset of hyponatremia; signs of fluid volume depletion or overload are absent.

Note. Based on information from Flounders, 2003; Foster, 2005; Keenan, 2005.

120 mEq/L over 24–48 hours overwhelms this compensatory mechanism in the brain, and severe cerebral edema, along with seizures, coma, brain stem herniation with respiratory arrest, and death, may occur (Craig; Terpstra & Terpstra, 2000). Mortality rates from acute, severe hyponatremia may reach 50% and, if accompanied by alcoholism or cachexia, can be as high as 70% (Terpstra & Terpstra).

Symptom severity depends on the absolute concentration of sodium in the serum (Foster, 2005). Patients with mild hyponatremia (125–134 mEq/L) may present with thirst, anorexia, nausea, fatigue, weakness, muscle cramps, and headache (Keenan, 2005). These are nonspecific symptoms that also may be related to side effects of malignancy or treatment; therefore, the hyponatremia often is undiagnosed. Significant symptoms usually do not become apparent until the serum sodium level decreases to moderate hyponatremia (115–124 mEq/L). Weight gain and oliguria may appear along with progressive neurologic symptoms.

The fluid and electrolyte imbalances related to SIADH affect the CNS the most. Changes in the level of consciousness and in cognitive function, including confusion, lethargy, irritability, disorientation, combativeness, or psychotic behavior, are manifestations of increasing cerebral edema (Craig, 2005; Foster, 2005; Keenan, 2005; Richerson, 2004). Severe hyponatremia (< 115 mEq/L) is a medical emergency and may be associated with papilledema, delirium, psychosis, hypoactive reflexes, ataxia or gait disturbance, seizures, coma, and death (Foster). The intravascular volume minimally increases in SIADH, so signs associated with fluid overload, such as peripheral edema, ascites, and heart failure, usually are absent (Flounders, 2003; Foster).

Patient Assessment

History

A variety of conditions can cause hyponatremia, but without the intracellular water excess indicative of SIADH. A thorough patient history is essential because disorders other than ectopic production of ADH must be excluded as the cause of SIADH in patients with cancer. Nurses should obtain information about patients' history of the CHART diseases (cardiac failure, hepatic dysfunction, adrenal insufficiency [Addison disease], renal disorders, and hypothyroidism), which may be associated with increased ADH secretion (Foster, 2005; Moore, 1998). Healthcare providers also should obtain patients' history of pulmonary and mediastinal diseases, CNS infections or conditions, and medication use (numerous drugs are associated with decreased serum sodium), plus recent dietary and fluid intake and gastrointestinal losses (Craig, 2005). All of these factors may cause hyponatremia or affect its severity (Foster). Questioning related to patients' history of cancer and cytotoxic treatments is essential. Often, the development of SIADH may be the first indication of malignancy, particularly with lung cancer (Terpstra & Terpstra, 2000).

Physical Examination

Physical examination of patients with hyponatremia focuses on assessing their neurologic and hydration status. Physical findings are highly variable depending on the severity and chronicity of hyponatremia, but most abnormal findings are neurologic, as described in "Clinical Manifestations." The patient's hydration status is important to assess because appropriate treatment interventions depend on an accurate diagnosis of the underlying cause of the hyponatremia. Initial patient assessment includes observing for signs of volume depletion or fluid overload; either condition would rule out SIADH as the cause of hyponatremia (Flounders, 2003). Signs of volume depletion (e.g., dry mucous membranes, poor skin turgor, tachycardia, orthostatic hypotension) would suggest hypovolemic hyponatremia resulting from excessive loss of body fluids followed by replacement with inappropriately dilute fluids. Signs of volume overload (e.g., pulmonary rales, S3 gallop, peripheral edema, jugular distension, ascites) would suggest hypervolemic hyponatremia caused by excess retention of sodium and free water. This type of dilutional hyponatremia can occur with liver disease, nephrotic syndrome, or congestive heart failure (Foster, 2005; Moore, 1998). SIADH usually is not associated with either fluid overload or depletion. Physical signs expected in SIADH would support a normal extracellular fluid volume (euvolemia) and would include normal blood pressure and pulse (without orthostatic changes), moist mucous membranes, normal skin turgor, and absence of peripheral edema (Craig, 2005).

Diagnostic Evaluation

Multiple laboratory tests are necessary to arrive at a confident diagnosis of SIADH. Healthcare professionals make the diagnosis of SIADH based upon the biochemistry parameters included in Table 7-3. Specific diagnostic criteria that define SIADH include the following: hyponatremia (serum sodium level < 135 mEq/L); hypotonicity (decreased plasma osmolality level < 280 mOsm/kg); increased urine osmolality (> 1,200 mOsm/kg water); increased urine sodium concentration (> 220 mEq/L in 24 hours); absence of clinical hypovolemia (euvolemia); and normal renal, adrenal, and thyroid function (Foster, 2005; Moore, 1998; Terpstra & Terpstra, 2000).

Measures of urine osmolarity may be helpful in establishing the diagnosis of SIADH. Patients with SIADH typically have inappropriately concentrated urine with urine osmolalities greater than 100 mOsm/L, whereas patients with other forms of hyponatremia have urine osmolalities below 100 mOsm/L (Foster, 2005). Serum concentrations of blood urea nitrogen (BUN), creatinine, uric acid, and albumin tend to be low because the small increase in intravascular volume seen with SIADH dilutes the plasma (Foster; Keenan, 2005).

Both hypothyroidism and adrenal insufficiency can increase ADH secretion and should be ruled out as a cause of hyponatremia. To rule out hypothyroidism, healthcare providers should check serum thyroid-stimulating hormone and free thyroxine levels. Adrenal insufficiency can be ruled out via random serum cortisol levels or an adrenocorticotropic hormone stimulation test in

---

Table 7-3. Biochemistry Parameters in Syndrome of Inappropriate Antidiuretic Hormone (SIADH)

Laboratory Test	Normal Value	Value in SIADH
Serum sodium	135–145 mEq/L	< 135 mEq/L
Serum osmolality	275–295 mOsm/kg	< 275 mOsm/kg
Urine sodium	50–220 mEq/L in 24 hours	> 220 mEq/L in 24 hours
Urine osmolality*	400–1,200 mOsm/kg water	> 1,200 mOsm/kg water
Urine specific gravity	1.025–1.032	> 1.032
Blood urea nitrogen (BUN)	6–22 mg/dl	Low BUN
Water loading test	80% of water load excreted in 5 hours	< 40% of water load excreted in 5 hours; Absence of diuresis

* Normal ratio of urine osmolality to serum osmolality is 4:1; this varies with diet.

Note. Based on information from Foster, 2005; Grant & Kubo, 1975; Langfeldt & Cooley, 2003; Moore, 1998.

patients who have recently taken oral steroids or in any patients suspected of having Addison disease (Foster, 2005; Moore, 1998).

Clinicians may perform a water loading test to diagnosis SIADH, but this usually is not necessary to obtain the diagnosis. Patients must have a serum sodium level greater than 125 mEq/L and be asymptomatic to undergo this test. Patients drink an oral water load of 20 cc per kg of body weight over 15–20 minutes. Urine then is collected hourly for five hours and tested for specific gravity and osmolality. Normally, patients excrete 80% of the water by the end of five hours, and the urine osmolality is < 100 mOsm/kg. In the presence of SIADH, however, the specific gravity is normal or increased, and less than 40% of the water is excreted by five hours (Langfeldt & Cooley, 2003; Moore, 1998). The water loading test can be very dangerous if the serum sodium is not corrected upward to at least 125 mEq/L before starting (Moore). Physicians may order a chest x-ray to rule out a pulmonary cause for the hyponatremia. They also may obtain a computed tomography (CT) scan of the head to assess for cerebral edema or to rule out other CNS conditions, such as a brain tumor, that may be responsible for the patient's hyponatremia and neurologic changes (Foster, 2005).

Treatment Modalities

After confirming the diagnosis of SIADH, healthcare professionals must identify and treat the precipitating etiology. If SIADH is medication induced, discontinuing the offending medications should be sufficient to correct the problem. If a disease process (i.e., pulmonary, CNS, renal, thyroid, adrenal) is causing SIADH, it will require appropriate treatment. If SIADH is malignancy induced, prompt initiation of antineoplastic treatment to eradicate or reduce the tumor burden will help to correct the sodium-water imbalance (Keenan, 2005; Langfeldt & Cooley, 2003). Several modalities may successfully treat the underlying malignancy. Surgery, radiation therapy, or the administration of antineoplastic agents, either alone or in combination, may be used. The urgency with which the patient's hyponatremia needs to be resolved depends on the degree of the condition and the rapidity with which it occurred (Fojo, 2005). SIADH is a medical emergency only when the hyponatremia is symptomatic or severe (Richerson, 2004). The treatment modalities used to correct the sodium-fluid imbalance are based on the degree of hyponatremia.

Severe Hyponatremia

Severe symptoms (e.g., seizures, coma) and severe hyponatremia (serum sodium level between 110–115 mEq/L) require immediate attention and are considered to be an oncologic emergency. The ultimate danger for patients with sodium levels below 120 mEq/L is brain stem herniation (Craig, 2005). Patients should receive treatment in an intensive care unit because they require frequent monitoring (every one to two hours) of their serum sodium and electrolyte levels and their neurologic status. Treatment measures include restricting patients' fluids to 500 ml per day and withholding any drugs that may contribute to fluid retention (Langfeldt & Cooley, 2003; Moore, 1998). Immediate sodium-fluid correction techniques may include administering IV hypertonic saline (3%) slowly via infusion pump at a rate of 0.05 ml/kg/minute over two to three hours (Keenan, 2005). During the infusion, healthcare professionals watch patients closely for manifestations of hypernatremia. Patients with severe neurologic dysfunction may receive concurrent treatment with furosemide, a loop diuretic that promotes diuresis and spares sodium from excretion. The dose of furosemide is individualized for each patient at 1 mg/kg of body weight. Serum electrolyte levels, especially potassium, require close monitoring during furosemide therapy (Foster, 2005; Langfeldt & Cooley; Terpstra & Terpstra, 2000).

The goal of treatment is to quickly correct the low serum sodium level toward normal, but only enough to stop the progression of symptoms (Craig, 2005). The serum sodium should increase no more than 1–2 mEq/L per hour. Hypertonic saline infusions are restricted to two to three hours; at that point, the serum sodium should have increased by 4–6 mEq/L, to the range of mild hyponatremia. The initial treatment with hypertonic saline infusion then is discontinued, and more conservative measures are instituted. The total increase in serum sodium should be limited to 12 mEq/L in the first 24 hours (Craig; Foster, 2005; Keenan, 2005; Richerson, 2004).

Too rapid correction of serum sodium may dehydrate brain cells too quickly, resulting in brain damage and a permanent neurologic condition called *central pontine myelinolysis* (CPM) (Foster, 2005; Keenan, 2005). CPM results from osmotic injury to the endothelial cells in the brain and a breakdown in the blood-brain barrier leading to nerve demyelination with cavitation in the pons. The condition destroys myelin sheaths but spares neurons and axons. Clinical examination indicates a subacute or acute pontine lesion, which typically occurs two to six days after the hyponatremia is corrected. Characteristic symptoms of CPM include progressive muscle weakness, dysarthria, dysphagia, and/or flaccid quadriplegia (locked-in syndrome). The mental status changes may progress to permanent brain damage or death. A CT scan or magnetic resonance imaging will reveal severe edema and damage to the pontine area (Foster; Keenan; Langfeldt & Cooley, 2003; Lindsay & Bone, 2004; Procyk, 2004).

Mild to Moderate Hyponatremia

Fluid restrictions and oral medications that inhibit the actions of ADH may adequately manage mild to moderate hyponatremia. Successful treatment for mild hyponatremia (serum sodium level between 125–134 mEq/L) may only require restricting fluids to 800–1,000 ml/day. The fluid restriction allows the plasma osmolality and the sodium level to gradually return to normal as the loss of free water occurs, usually over a period of three to five days. Response is measured by increases in the serum sodium concentration and osmolality and by weight loss (Keenan, 2005; Moore, 1998; Richerson, 2004).

The fluid restriction may continue in the outpatient setting if patients are compliant and if the serum sodium level does not continue to decline. Fluid restriction may be difficult for patients to maintain because a normal diet contains 750–1,000 ml of water, exclusive of voluntary fluid intake. Patients must restrict voluntary fluid intake to 250–500 ml/day (Foster, 2005; Lindsay & Bone, 2004; Procyk, 2004).

If patients are being treated for malignancy-induced SIADH with chemotherapy agents that require increased hydration, fluid management may be a challenge. The use of aggressive hydration to prevent nephrotoxicity with the administration of drugs such as cyclophosphamide and cisplatin increases the risk of SIADH. Hydrating patients with normal saline, giving furosemide as ordered, and closely monitoring intake and output and electrolyte balance, with replacement as needed, often can manage this situation (Richerson, 2004).

Moderate hyponatremia (serum sodium level between 120–125 mEq/L) may be treated with a daily dose of demeclocycline, a tetracycline derivative antibiotic that inhibits the action of ADH on the renal tubules, thereby promoting water excretion. The drug may take more than a week to improve diuresis and hyponatremia, so it is not indicated for emergency management of symptomatic hyponatremia. A normal intake of fluid is allowed with demeclocycline, so the drug is useful for patients who cannot comply with fluid restrictions or for those with chronic hyponatremia. The usual oral dose of demeclocycline is 150 mg four times daily or 300 mg twice a day (Foster, 2005). Patients should not take the drug with food (take at least one hour prior to meals and at least two hours after meals) or with antacids containing aluminum, magnesium, calcium, or iron, which may delay its absorption. Common side effects of demeclocycline include nausea, photosensitivity, and azotemia. Renal function should be monitored because the drug may cause nephrotoxity (Terpstra & Terpstra, 2000). Superinfections and hematologic changes may occur with demeclocycline, and it may diminish the effectiveness of oral contraceptives, causing breakthrough bleeding and increasing pregnancy risk (Foster; Keenan, 2005; Lindsay & Bone, 2004; Procyk, 2004; Richerson, 2004). Patients may receive furosemide at a daily oral maintenance dose of 20–80 mg to maintain urine output and block secretion of ADH (Foster; Langfeldt & Cooley, 2003). This therapy entails monitoring of serum electrolytes, especially potassium, and replacing dietary salt (Batcheller, 1994; Keenan; Moore, 1998).

Urea, an osmotic diuretic, may be administered to induce diuresis. It acts by increasing the osmolality of the glomerular filtrate, which hinders tubular reabsorption of water. Urea is not used unless SIADH is refractory to treatment or if patients have been noncompliant with other therapies (Foster, 2005; Richerson, 2004). For treating chronic SIADH, the use of lithium has achieved some success because it inhibits ADH action. However, it rarely is used because of its toxic side effects on the CNS, cardiac, thyroid, gastrointestinal, and renal systems. Serum levels of lithium must be monitored to detect lithium toxicity levels (Moore, 1998; Richerson). In addition, 35%–70% of patients taking urea develop diabetes insipidus (Richerson).

Nursing Management

Early Detection

Although prevention of SIADH may not be possible, early detection may keep the complication from progressing to an oncologic emergency. Nurses need to be aware of the population at risk for SIADH and the factors that contribute to its development. Early signs and symptoms of SIADH often are nonspecific and may be attributed to effects of malignancy or its treatment or to neurologic disorders. Nurses need to understand the early signs and symptoms of hyponatremia so that they can recognize the subtle changes in patient status and the presenting symptoms that may indicate SIADH. Ongoing monitoring of fluid and electrolyte status and physical assessment to detect changes in neurologic status are essential to early recognition of SIADH, especially in high-risk patients, such as those with SCLC. Nursing assessment of hydration status includes measuring intake and output and daily weights, and checking skin turgor and mucous membranes. Pertinent laboratory results that should be reviewed include serum electrolyte levels and osmolality, and urine osmolality and specific gravity. Nurses should follow BUN and creatinine levels to monitor renal function. The presence of signs of fluid overload (e.g., fluid intake greater than output, weight gain), hyponatremia, and mental status changes (especially lethargy and drowsiness) should raise the level of suspicion for SIADH in high-risk patients (Langfeldt & Cooley, 2003; Moore, 1998). Table 7-4 provides an overview of nursing interventions in the care of patients with SIADH.

Supportive Care

With a diagnosis of SIADH, nursing interventions focus on managing the signs and symptoms of SIADH and instituting measures to correct the underlying cause. Initial interventions aim to increase free water loss through the kidneys. Evaluating patients' fluid status includes strict intake and output measurements and daily weight monitoring. Initially, an hourly assessment of intake and output data as well as urine specific gravity may be necessary (Terpstra & Terpstra, 2000). For accuracy, the nursing staff should obtain daily weights on the same scale, at the same time of day, with the patient wearing the same amount of clothing. Patients with SIADH are at risk for congestive heart failure caused by fluid overload, so auscultation of the lungs is important to detect overhydration. The use of a urinary catheter can measure output in patients with an altered level of consciousness who are incontinent (Terpstra & Terpstra).

Table 7-4. Nursing Management of Syndrome of Inappropriate Antidiuretic Hormone (SIADH)

Nursing Management	Nursing Interventions
Initial nursing assessment for early detection	Identify patients with risk factors for development of SIADH: Small cell lung cancer; carcinoma of the pancreas, duodenum, prostate, lymphoid tissue; pulmonary infections, chemotherapy treatment regimens. Review all medications to identify drugs that increase the risk of SIADH. Closely monitor serum and urine electrolytes and osmolality. Assess for early signs of hyponatremia: headache, nausea, anorexia, generalized weakness, muscle cramps.
Severe hyponatremia	Hospitalize patients for medication administration, and closely monitor serum and urine electrolytes and osmolality, intake and output, vital signs, and neurologic status. Administer IV hypertonic saline as ordered, and possibly admit patients to intensive care for monitoring serum sodium every one to two hours. Administer furosemide as ordered to increase diuresis. Monitor potassium level. Institute safety measures and seizure precautions as indicated. Assess for adequate symptom management related to pain, anxiety, depression, nausea, and vomiting. Assess coping abilities.
Moderate hyponatremia	Administer demeclocycline as ordered. May be given alone or in conjunction with fluid restriction. Avoid giving with food (at least one hour prior to and at least two hours after meals). Avoid use of aluminum or magnesium antacids. Observe for side effects: decreased urine output, azotemia, infection. Monitor electrolytes, urine output, renal function. Document response to treatment: fluid weight loss, increased serum sodium and osmolality. Relieve pain, anxiety, and stress with relaxation techniques. Opioids, barbiturates, and tricyclic antidepressants increase antidiuretic hormone release and should be minimized.
Mild hyponatremia	Restrict fluids to 800–1,000 ml/day. Monitor electrolyte levels frequently, especially sodium and potassium. Educate patients and caregivers about the importance of fluid restriction. Provide an easy method to measure and record oral fluid intake.
Neurologic changes	Monitor for changes in level of consciousness and behavior. Institute seizure precautions for sodium level > 120 mEq/L. Provide safety measures, and assist with daily care: walking, eating, self-care, administration of medications. Generalized weakness: Provide means of safety with ambulation (e.g., walker, cane).

(Continued on next page)

Table 7-4. Nursing Management of Syndrome of Inappropriate Antidiuretic Hormone (SIADH) (Continued)

Nursing Management	Nursing Interventions
Pain management	Assess for adequate pain control and evidence of side effects with discontinuation of medications associated with SIADH risk.
Fluid and electrolyte balance	Restrict fluids as ordered. Closely monitor electrolytes and daily weights; encourage a diet high in sodium. If loop diuretics are ordered, monitor serum sodium and potassium levels; provide a diet high in potassium. Administer hypertonic saline as ordered, using caution with the rate of administration—0.05 ml/kg/minute. Watch for signs of central pontine myelinolysis, which often are delayed two to six days after correction of hyponatremia.
Seizure precautions	Monitor closely for seizures; institute seizure precautions for serum sodium level < 120 mEq/L. Administer anticonvulsants for seizure activity as ordered. Institute safety precautions and fall-prevention measures.
Patient and caregiver education	Restrict fluids, and record and measure intake. Control thirst and dry mouth. Use ice, hard candy, and artificial saliva, and avoid alcohol-based mouthwashes. Recognize nonspecific signs of mild hyponatremia that should be promptly reported: nausea, headache, anorexia, muscle cramps. Provide medication instructions about the schedule and side effects of demeclocycline and furosemide. Maintain a diet high in sodium. Reinforce coping strategies related to fluid restrictions, muscle weakness, mental changes, cancer diagnosis.

Note. Based on information from Foster, 2005; Keenan, 2005; Miaskowski, 1999; Moore, 1998; Richerson, 2004.

Interventions for SIADH include fluid restriction, usually to a total of 800–1,000 ml fluid per day, which includes ordered oral and IV medications. Fluid restriction presents a challenge for both nurses and patients. To help patients to stay within the restriction, nurses should administer IV medications in the least amount of fluid possible and should avoid solutions of 5% dextrose in water and hypotonic solutions. Patients with cancer who are receiving nephrotoxic agents as part of their cytotoxic therapy require careful assessment of the effects of fluid restriction. The risks of hemorrhagic cystitis and nephropathy secondary to the administration of cyclophosphamide and cisplatin, respectively, may increase with reduced IV hydration (Richerson, 2004). If not contraindicated, patients should receive oral medications with meals. Furthermore, they should not receive enemas of tap water or saline because the fluid may be absorbed from the intestines. Nasogastric and other enteral tubes should be irrigated with normal saline solution rather than water (Batcheller, 1994). The nursing staff should work with patients in planning how to divide the daily fluid intake. Patients also must increase the amount of sodium in their daily diet, which will increase the thirst sensation. Nursing care should encourage fluids that are high in sodium, such as tomato and orange juice and beef and chicken broth. Supportive nursing care to relieve dry mouth may include providing frequent mouth care, oral rinses without swallowing, or artifical saliva (Richerson). Sucking on hard, sugarless candy, chewing sugarless gum, and drinking chilled beverages may help patients to tolerate the fluid restriction. Commercial mouthwashes containing alcohol and mouth swabs of lemon and glycerin are very drying and should be avoided (Langfeldt & Cooley, 2003).

Assessment of patients for effective control of SIADH, resolution of symptoms, and presence of treatment side effects is ongoing. Nurses frequently monitor the laboratory results for sodium concentration and osmolality in the plasma and the urine to assess the effectiveness of treatment interventions in correcting hyponatremia. Care involves following serum potassium levels as well. Hypernatremia may result from overcorrection by hypertonic saline, and as the serum sodium increases, a risk develops for potassium loss and hypokalemia (Moore, 1998). Assessing patients for changes in neurologic status and maintaining safety for patients who are weak or confused are essential parts of nursing care. With decreasing sodium levels, a patient's mental status can range from fully alert, to confused and disoriented, to comatose. When caring for older adult patients with neurologic symptoms, nurses can obtain information about their previous level of functioning and awareness from family members or caregivers to use as a baseline for comparison (Terpstra & Terpstra, 2000). Seizure precautions are indicated when the serum sodium level falls below 120 mEq/L and include placing the bed in the lowest position, padding the side rails, and having suction and airway equipment at the bedside for emergency use (Richerson, 2004). Nurses also should provide skin care and monitor skin integrity in patients on bed rest.

Another challenge for nurses is relieving the patient's pain and minimizing stress, which are factors that stimulate ADH release, while at the same time limiting the use of barbiturates, narcotics, or tricyclic antidepressants, which also are associated with SIADH development (Moore, 1998; Richerson, 2004). Medications for pain or anxiety should be changed to those without the side effect of SIADH (Batcheller, 1994). Treatment may involve instituting complementary methods for pain relief, including distraction, massage, or heat or cold therapy. Relaxation techniques, guided imagery, and self-hypnosis may help patients to reduce stress (Richerson). The nursing staff should monitor patients for adequate pain relief and control of symptoms of stress and depression. Nurses should offer reassurance and emotional support to patients and caregivers and assess their ability to cope with the treatment regimens and fluid restrictions, as well as with the diagnosis of cancer, if SIADH was the initial presenting sign.

Patient and Caregiver Education

Involving patients and their caregivers in the management of SIADH is essential to early detection and reversal of symptoms. Management of SIADH may continue at home, and the condition possibly may recur or become chronic. Nurses should discuss the rationale for fluid restriction and the importance of compliance and should include patients and caregivers in planning the fluid allocation schedule. Education should emphasize the importance of monitoring daily weights in assessing fluid status. Nurses should provide written instructions and a form on which to record accurate daily weights and intake and output data. Patients need to report rapid weight gains or losses of more than 1 kg (2.2 pounds) (Terpstra & Terpstra, 2000). Giving patients and caregivers a sense of control over the situation may increase their adherence to the fluid regimen. Patients should increase the amount of sodium in their diet, if not contraindicated by other health conditions. Patient education also focuses on the potential side effects of and proper schedule for taking prescribed medications, such as demeclocycline, which should not be taken with food or near mealtime or with certain antacids. Patients and caregivers also must understand that certain signs and symptoms such as generalized weakness, nausea and vomiting, muscle cramps, difficulty concentrating, decreased urine output, and weight gain without swelling in the extremities may be early manifestations of SIADH that they need to report promptly. Additionally, they should receive information regarding stress reduction techniques, relaxation exercises, and pain management strategies that minimize the use of drugs associated with SIADH risk. Referral to home care may be necessary to monitor patients' clinical status and facilitate the collection of frequent serum electrolyte specimens. Nurses should provide emotional support and referral to social services, if necessary, to help patients and caregivers to learn coping strategies for dealing with a distressing situation.

Conclusion

A number of factors, ranging from disease states to various medications, can precipitate the development of SIADH, but most commonly the condition arises as a paraneoplastic syndrome associated with SCLC. Oncology nurses should have a high index of suspicion for this complication while caring for these patients. Knowledge of the physiologic mechanisms regulating normal fluid and electrolyte balance will help nurses to understand and recognize the pathologic processes involved in SIADH development. SIADH may have a vague, insidious onset, but it can progress to severe neurologic dysfunction, coma, and death. Early detection, prompt diagnosis, and effective treatment can prevent SIADH from becoming a life-threatening oncologic emergency.

References

Agha, I.A. (2004, February 23). *Osmolality.* Retrieved August 7, 2005, from http://www.nlm .nih.gov/medlineplus/ency/article/003463.htm

Akalin, E., Chandrakantan, A., Keane, J., & Hamburger, R.J. (2001). Normouricemia in the syndrome of inappropriate antidiuretic hormone secretion. *American Journal of Kidney Diseases, 37,* 1–3.

Batcheller, J. (1994). Syndrome of inappropriate antidiuretic hormone secretion. *Critical Care Nursing Clinics of North America, 6,* 687–692.

Colorado State University. (1998, October 11). *Antidiuretic hormone (vasopressin).* Retrieved August 10, 2005, from http://arbl.cvmbs.colostate.edu/hbooks/pathphys/endocrine/ hypopit/adh.html

Craig, S. (2005, January 20). *Hyponatremia.* Retrieved August 2, 2005, from http://www .emedicine.com/emerg/topic275.htm

Flounders, J.A. (2003). Syndrome of inappropriate antidiuretic hormone [Online exclusive]. *Oncology Nursing Forum, 30,* E63–E68.

Fojo, A.T. (2005). Metabolic emergencies. In V.T. DeVita, S. Hellman, & S.A. Rosenberg (Eds.), *Cancer: Principles and practice of oncology* (7th ed., pp. 2292–2300). Philadelphia: Lippincott Williams & Wilkins.

Foster, J. (2005, June 7). *Syndrome of inappropriate antidiuretic hormone secretion.* Retrieved August 2, 2005, from http://www.emedicine.com/emerg/topic784.htm

Grant, M.M., & Kubo, W.M. (1975). Assessing a patient's hydration status. *American Journal of Nursing, 75,* 1306–1311.

Keenan, A.K. (2005). Syndrome of inappropriate antidiuretic hormone. In C.H. Yarbro, M.H. Frogge, & M. Goodman (Eds.), *Cancer nursing: Principles and practice* (6th ed., pp. 940–945). Sudbury, MA: Jones and Bartlett.

Langfeldt, L.A., & Cooley, M.E. (2003). Syndrome of inappropriate antidiuretic hormone secretion in malignancy: Review and implications for nursing management. *Clinical Journal of Oncology Nursing, 7,* 425–430.

Larson, P., & Martin, J. (1994). Renal system changes in the elderly. *AORN Journal, 60,* 298–301.

Lindsay, K.W., & Bone, I. (2004). *Neurology and neurosurgery illustrated* (4th ed.). London: Churchill Livingstone.

Miaskowski, C. (1999). Syndrome of inappropriate antidiuretic hormone secretion. In C. Miaskowski & P.C. Buchsel (Eds.), *Oncology nursing: Assessment and clinical care* (pp. 221–243). St. Louis, MO: Mosby.

Moore, J.M. (1998). Syndrome of inappropriate antidiuretic hormone secretion. In B.L. Johnson & J. Gross (Eds.), *Handbook of oncology nursing* (3rd ed., pp. 711–721). Sudbury, MA: Jones and Bartlett.

Procyk, L.F. (2004). Hyponatremia. In M.K. Bader & L.R. Littlejohns (Eds.), *AANN core curriculum for neuroscience nursing* (4th ed., pp. 109–111). St. Louis, MO: Saunders.

Richerson, M.T. (2004). Electrolyte imbalances. In C.H. Yarbro, M.H. Frogge, & M. Goodman (Eds.), *Cancer symptom management* (3rd ed., pp. 440–453). Sudbury, MA: Jones and Bartlett.

Robinson, A.G. (2000). Syndrome of inappropriate secretion of antidiuretic hormone—hypersecretion of vasopressin. In H.D. Humes (Ed.), *Kelley's textbook of internal medicine* (4th ed., pp. 2689–2691). Philadelphia: Lippincott Williams & Wilkins.

Santacroce, L., Gagliardi, S., & Balducci, L. (2005, July 21). *Paraneoplastic syndromes.* Retrieved August 7, 2005, from http://www.emedicine.com/med/topic1747.htm

Terpstra, T.L., & Terpstra, T.L. (2000). Syndrome of inappropriate antidiuretic hormone secretion: Recognition and management. *MEDSURG Nursing, 9,* 61–68.

Marcelle Kaplan, RN, MS, OCN®, AOCN®

→ **Chapter 8**

Spinal Cord Compression

Introduction

Spinal cord compression is one of the most dreaded complications of cancer and is a true clinical emergency. It affects 5%–10% of the adult population with cancer (more than 25,000 people) every year in the United States (Schiff, 2003) and is the second most frequent neurologic complication of cancer, following brain metastases (Myers, 2001). The most common cause of cord compression is metastatic disease that extends into or invades the epidural space; henceforth, this chapter will refer to *metastatic spinal cord compression* (MSCC). MSCC occurs when malignant disease or a pathologically collapsed vertebra either compresses or displaces the thecal sac containing the spinal cord and its extension, the cauda equina (Osowski, 2002; Prasad & Schiff, 2005). Clinicians use specific radiographic and clinical criteria to further refine the diagnosis of MSCC. Radiologic evidence must demonstrate indentation of the thecal sac at the level of key clinical features, which include any of the following: pain (local or radicular), weakness, sensory disturbance, and/or sphincter dysfunction (Loblaw & Laperriere, 1998). Although MSCC usually is a late manifestation of metastatic bone involvement, it can occur at any time during the course of malignant disease. In approximately one-third of cases, the appearance of spinal cord compression is the first evidence that cancer is present (Eakin, 2002).

Back pain is an early and sensitive indicator of MSCC, but it is such a nonspecific symptom and common acute problem that its significance often is missed. The relationship between back pain and previous cancer history, or back pain as the initial manifestation of cancer, may not be appreciated until it is too late (Wilkes, 2004). As time passes without appropriate treatment, the likelihood of neurologic recovery diminishes. The natural course of untreated MSCC is one of relentless neurologic injury and permanent loss that typically follows a progressive sequence of pain, motor weakness, sensory loss, sphincter dysfunction, and ultimately paralysis (Loblaw, Perry, Chambers, & Laperriere, 2005). As the length of cancer survival increases, the importance of early recognition and prompt intervention cannot be overemphasized in limiting devastating losses. Nurses must be able to recognize which patients are at increased risk for MSCC and should raise their level of suspicion at the appearance of the often subtle and nonspecific signs and symptoms of MSCC.

Incidence

Solid tumors that preferentially metastasize to vertebral bone are associated with the highest incidence of MSCC (see Table 8-1). This is especially true for cancers of the breast, lung, and prostate, which together account for more than 60% of all cases of MSCC (Manzullo, Rhines, & Forman, 2002;

Table 8-1. Cancers Associated With Risk for Metastatic Spinal Cord Compression

Tumor Type	Incidence
Most common	
Breast	15%–20%
Lung	15%–20%
Prostate	15%–20%
Multiple myeloma	10%–15%
Unknown primary	10%
Renal cell carcinoma	5%–10%
Non-Hodgkin lymphoma	5%–10%
Hodgkin disease	5%
Less common	
Gastrointestinal malignancies	
Soft tissue sarcoma	
Thyroid cancer	
Neuroblastoma	
Uncommon	
Melanoma (intradural and leptomeningeal involvement more common than vertebral involvement)	
Uterine and cervical cancers	
Bladder cancer	
Leukemia (tumor cells circulating in cerebrospinal fluid form metastatic deposits in epidural space)	
Rare	
Head and neck cancers	
Brain, pancreatic, liver, and ovarian cancers	
Testicular cancer (direct extension from retroperitoneal space)	
Esophageal cancer (direct extension to thoracic spine)	

Note. Based on information from Abrahm, 2004; Eakin, 2002; Gabriel & Schiff, 2004; Kazierad, 1998; Osowski, 2002; Prasad & Schiff, 2005; Schuster & Grady, 2001; Weinstein, 2002.

Maranzano, Trippa, Chirico, Basagni, & Rossi, 2003; Yalamanchili & Lesser, 2003). These cancers are followed in incidence by renal cell carcinoma, non-Hodgkin lymphoma, and multiple myeloma. Multiple myeloma, the most common primary tumor of bone, contributes 10%–15% to the total incidence of MSCC (Weinstein, 2002). Colorectal cancer, cancers of unknown origin, sarcoma, melanoma, thyroid, and head and neck cancers also contribute to the incidence of MSCC (Gabriel & Schiff, 2004; Grandt, 2000; Wilkes, 2004). Cancers of unknown origin account for 10% of cases; they most likely represent unrecognized lung or gastrointestinal primary malignancies (Posner, 1995).

Although cord compression usually occurs in patients with a known history of cancer, MSCC may be the first indication of malignant disease in up to a third of cases (Prasad & Schiff, 2005; Wilkes, 2004). This type of disease presentation may be seen with lung cancer, cancer of unknown origin, multiple myeloma, and non-Hodgkin lymphoma, but it is extremely unlikely with breast cancer (Gabriel & Schiff, 2004; Posner, 1995). MSCC associated with breast cancer can develop as late as 20 years after initial diagnosis (Wilkes). Compression of the spinal cord occurs at more than one site in 10%–38% of patients and reappears at a new site after a median interval of four months in approximately 10% of patients (Abrahm, 2004; Tharpar & Laws, 1995). The average age of MSCC occurrence is 58 years (Waller & Caroline, 2000).

Risk Factors

Eighty-five percent to 90% of cases of MSCC result from the effects of metastatic disease involving the vertebral bodies (Weinstein, 2002; Wilkes, 2004). Regardless of the origin of the primary tumor, the most common site of bone metastasis is the spine. An estimated one of every five patients who have vertebral metastases will develop MSCC at some time over the course of his or her disease (Eakin, 2002). Autopsy studies have demonstrated the incidence of vertebral metastasis in several common cancers associated with increased risk for MSCC: prostate, 90%; breast, 74%; lung, 45%; and gastrointestinal, 25% (Prasad & Schiff, 2005). However, only a small percentage of vertebral metastases will cause compression of the spinal cord or cauda equina (Posner, 1995).

A retrospective review of data has led investigators to identify six independent risk factors predictive for the development of MSCC in patients with cancer. These are neurologic factors (loss of ambulation and increased deep tendon reflexes), radiologic factors (recent vertebral compression fractures and presence of bone metastases), and clinical factors not commonly assessed (duration of bone metastases for longer than one year and age younger than 60 years). Patients with all six risk factors demonstrated the highest risk for MSCC (87%), whereas those with none of the predicted risk factors had a 4% risk of developing MSCC (Loblaw et al., 2005; Talcott et al., 1999).

Another group of researchers analyzed potential risk factors for MSCC based on the results of spinal magnetic resonance imaging (MRI) demonstrating compression of the thecal sac. They identified four independent predictors of risk: (a) abnormal neurologic examination, (b) pain in the middle or upper back, (c) known vertebral metastases, and (d) metastatic disease at initial presentation. Clinicians can readily obtain this type of clinical data and use it to stratify risk in the initial evaluation of patients with a history of cancer suspected of having MSCC (Lu, Gonzalez, Jolesz, Wen, & Talcott, 2005).

Pathophysiology

Spinal Anatomy

Prior to a discussion of the pathophysiology of MSCC, the anatomy of the spinal column and spinal cord is briefly reviewed to provide insight into the pathologic processes associated with MSCC.

The spinal column consists of 33 vertebrae joined in series. From head to tail, 7 cervical, 12 thoracic, 5 lumbar, 5 sacral (fused to form the sacrum), and 4 coccygeal (fused into the coccyx) vertebrae comprise the spinal column. Except for the fused sacrum and coccyx, intervertebral discs separate each vertebra and cushion shocks. Spaces formed between adjacent vertebrae are called *intervertebral foramina* and serve as openings through which the spinal nerves emerge. The vertebrae form the spinal canal, which encloses and protects the spinal cord, which "floats" in cerebrospinal fluid (CSF) within a membrane called the *thecal (or dural) sac* (Sunderland, 1994).

The spinal cord essentially is a long column of nervous tissue that mediates the transmission of messages between the brain and the body. It extends from the medulla at the base of the brain only to the level of the first or second lumbar vertebra and is divided into 31 segments. Each spinal segment has a pair of anterior (motor) and posterior (sensory) spinal nerve roots, which merge to form a mixed spinal nerve as they exit the vertebral column through the intervertebral foramina (see Figure 8-1). In the cervical region, the spinal nerves exit the vertebral canal immediately above their corresponding vertebra; in the thoracic, lumbar, and sacral regions, they exit immediately below their corresponding vertebra (Schreiber, 2004).

The spinal cord serves as a central switching and processing station. Motor (efferent) impulses are relayed along descending pathways from the brain to the cord. The appropriate cord segment transmits the motor impulse via the anterior (ventral) nerve root to segments of the body formed by groups of muscles. The individual body segments are called *myotomes.* Posterior (dorsal) nerve roots transmit sensory (afferent) information related to temperature, pain, touch, body position, pressure, vibration, and other sensory stimuli from the body to the spinal cord. Sensory information reaches awareness when ascending pathways relay it to the brain. The skin segment that sends sensory signals into a given spinal cord segment is called a *dermatome.* Dermatomes vary in size and shape and are mapped on the surface of the skin, loosely corresponding with

Figure 8-1. Location of Metastases to the Spine

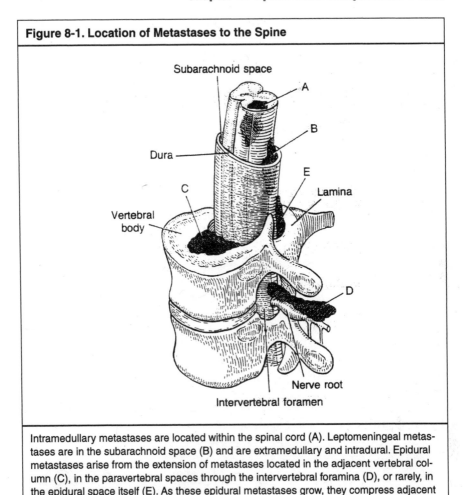

Intramedullary metastases are located within the spinal cord (A). Leptomeningeal metastases are in the subarachnoid space (B) and are extramedullary and intradural. Epidural metastases arise from the extension of metastases located in the adjacent vertebral column (C), in the paravertebral spaces through the intervertebral foramina (D), or rarely, in the epidural space itself (E). As these epidural metastases grow, they compress adjacent blood vessels, nerve roots, and spinal cord, resulting in local and referred pain, radiculopathy, and myelopathy.

Note. From "Spinal Cord Compression From Epidural Metastases," by T.N. Byrne, 1992, *New England Journal of Medicine, 327,* p. 615. Copyright 1992 by the Massachusetts Medical Society. Reprinted with permission.

the spinal cord segments. Only a general relationship exists between the sensory segments and the muscles innervated by the same segment of the cord. Some overlapping of the spinal nerves also occurs, so that one muscle or one area of skin usually is supplied by more than one nerve (Sunderland, 1994).

The spinal cord is composed of a butterfly-shaped inner core of gray matter, composed of nerve cell bodies and synapses, which is completely surrounded by an outer band of white matter. The white matter contains myelinated axons that ascend or descend within the spinal cord (Ballenger, 1991). Damage to ascending nerve tracts, which carry sensory messages toward the brain, may result in both pain and sensory changes. Damage to descending nerve tracts, which carry motor messages from the brain, may cause deficits in motor function and impair bowel, bladder, and sexual function (Myers, 2001).

At the level of the first or second lumbar vertebra, the spinal cord terminates in a cone-like structure called the *conus medullaris*. Distal to the conus is a bundle of lumbar and sacral spinal nerve roots called the *cauda equina* (Latin for *horse's tail*, which it resembles). The nerve roots of the cauda equina fill the lower part of the spinal canal to the level of the second sacral vertebra and are arranged according to the spinal segments from which they originate. They exit the spinal canal through their respective intervertebral foramina to supply the legs, bowel, bladder, and genitalia and are the anatomic connection between the central and peripheral nervous systems (Dawodu & Lorenzo, 2005).

The brain and spinal cord are covered with three layers of protective membranes, or meninges: the dura mater, the arachnoid membrane, and the pia mater. The innermost membrane, the pia mater (Latin for *gentle mother*), is a delicate, lacelike membrane that adheres directly to the brain and spinal cord. The middle layer, the arachnoid membrane, has a spongy, web-like structure and is separated from the pia mater by the subarachnoid space, which contains CSF. Between the arachnoid membrane and the outermost layer, the dura mater, is the subdural space, which is traversed by small bridging veins. The dura mater (Latin for *hard mother*) is a tough, thick, nonelastic membrane to which the spinal nerves are attached. The space formed between the dura mater and the inner surface of the spinal canal is the *epidural space*. It contains blood vessels and connective and adipose tissue (Myers, 2001).

Mechanisms Promoting Metastatic Spinal Cord Compression

The most common pathologic mechanism responsible for MSCC is direct pressure on the cord. The metastatic tumor mass within the vertebral body expands into the epidural space and impinges on the anterior aspect of the thecal sac, directly compressing the spinal cord and the surrounding epidural venous plexus. The second mechanism is mechanical cord destruction. Metastatic tumor erodes and collapses the vertebral body, displacing bone fragments into the epidural space. The fragments further compress the spinal cord and epidural venous plexus or cause spinal instability. These two mechanisms are associated with 85% of MSCC cases. The third and least common mechanism of MSCC is direct invasion of tumor into the epidural space without destruction of bone (10%–15% of cases). This may occur when lung cancer, lymphoma, or retroperitoneal sarcoma grows along nerve roots and penetrates into the epidural space through the intervertebral foramina (Abrahm, 2004; Klimo, Kestle, & Schmidt, 2003; Manzullo et al., 2002; Maranzano et al., 2003; Tharpar & Laws, 1995). Direct extension of tumor into vertebral structures and the epidural space also may occur with Pancoast tumor of the lung apex and with cancers of the colon, kidney, prostate, and head and neck (Baehring, 2005). Tumors rarely metastasize directly to the epidural space or to the spinal cord itself (Byrne, 1992; DeAngelis & Posner, 2003). Figure 8-1 depicts locations of spinal metastases.

The propensity for MSCC to occur in a specific area of the spine correlates with several factors: the potential for a tumor to metastasize to vertebral bone, the number of vertebrae in the region, the size of the epidural space in each spinal segment, and the properties of the venous blood supply to the vertebral column. The thoracic spine is the most common site of epidural compression because of its unique properties. With 12 vertebrae, the thoracic spine contains the largest volume of bone and active bone marrow (supporting the growth of metastatic deposits) in the spinal column and has the greatest incidence of vertebral bone metastases (70%). A poor blood supply and a narrow epidural space that allows little room for expansion further contribute to risk of compression. The thoracic spine is followed by the lumbosacral spine and cervical spine in incidence of epidural compression in a ratio of 4:2:1 (DeAngelis & Posner, 2003; Manzullo et al., 2002; Posner, 1995). Metastases from breast and lung cancers typically involve the thoracic vertebrae but also may be distributed fairly equally throughout the spinal regions. Cancers of the prostate, kidney, and colon are associated mostly with lesions of the lower thoracic or lumbosacral spine (Abrahm, 2004; Gabriel & Schiff, 2004; Weinstein, 2002) (see Table 8-2).

A small percentage (5%) of cases of cord compression develop because of primary tumors arising within the spinal cord or associated structures (see Figure 8-2). Because these tumors grow slowly and are located within the dural membrane (intradurally), the spinal cord can tolerate the presence of primary tumors for quite some time without loss of function (Tharpar & Laws, 1995). Primary cancers arising within the spinal cord (intramedullary) include ependymomas, astrocytomas, and gliomas (Myers, 2001). Common primary tumors arising in the dura (meningioma) or nerve roots (schwannoma) are called *extramedullary intradural tumors*; they compress and displace, rather than invade, the spinal cord (Batzdorf & Haskell, 2001). However, the vast majority of cord compression is extradural, resulting from the encroachment of metastatic tumor into the epidural space. Invasion of the epidural space in the cervical and thoracic regions produces compression of the cord itself; invasion in the lumbosacral region produces either conus medullaris syndrome or cauda equina syndrome (Heary & Bono, 2001).

Mechanisms Promoting Vertebral Metastases

Knowledge of how metastatic disease reaches the vertebrae has increased in recent years. The major mechanism of vertebral bone involvement currently is understood to be through direct arterial transport of tumor microemboli from the primary tumor to the vertebral body. Studies with mice have dem-

Table 8-2. Etiology and Clinical Manifestations of Spinal Cord Compression by Spinal Level

Spinal Level and Incidence	Malignancy	Pain Characteristics	Potential Clinical Manifestations
Cervical spine (10%)	Head and neck* Melanoma Lung (Pancoast tumor) Lymphoma	Occipital headache Radicular pain in neck, shoulder, arm May be exacerbated by neck flexion Neck stiffness	• Lesion at or above C4: diaphragmatic weakness/paralysis (unilateral or bilateral) and respiratory insufficiency • Weakness, spasticity and wasting of neck, shoulder, arm muscles; in time progressing to opposite arm and leg(s) • Neurogenic shock: hypotension, bradycardia, peripheral vasodilation • Quadriplegia • Paresthesias and sensory loss for position, vibration, temperature in areas of weakness • Lhermitte sign: electric tingling sensation down the back and upper/lower extremities on neck flexion/extension • Horner syndrome: constricted pupil, upper eyelid droop, loss of sweating on affected side of face (with C8 involvement) • Reflexes: hyperactive deep tendon reflexes, extensor plantar response (positive Babinski sign) • Autonomic effects: Late onset. Bladder, bowel, and sexual dysfunction. Risk of autonomic hyperreflexia: hypertension, bradycardia, pounding headache, profuse sweating; autoregulation mechanisms interrupted by spinal lesion.
Thoracic spine (70%)	Breast* Lung* Lymphoma Multiple myeloma Pancreatic Esophageal	Pain is local, radicular, or both, in chest and back.	• Weakness of abdominal muscles; arm muscles spared • Lower extremity weakness or paralysis (low T-spine lesion) • Band-like paresthesias around waist • Decreased sensation below level of lesion, increased above • Reflexes: increased deep tendon reflexes distal to lesion, extensor plantar response, Beevor sign • Autonomic effects: Late onset. Bladder, bowel, and sexual dysfunction. Risk of autonomic hyperreflexia with lesion at or above T6.
Lower levels	Prostate Colon Renal		

(Continued on next page)

Table 8-2. Etiology and Clinical Manifestations of Spinal Cord Compression by Spinal Level *(Continued)*

Spinal Level and Incidence	Malignancy	Pain Characteristics	Potential Clinical Manifestations
Lumbosacral spine (20%)	Prostate Renal cell Ovarian	Pain is local, radicular, or both, in groin region or sciatic distribution in leg(s). Pain on straight leg raising	• Weakness in pelvic muscles • Weakness to paralysis in lower extremities, with muscle atrophy; ataxic gait • Numbness, paresthesias, sensory loss in lower extremities • Reflexes: Decreased to absent knee and ankle reflexes; extensor plantar response • Autonomic effects: Bladder, bowel, and sexual dysfunction
Lower levels	Colon Uterine Cervix		Conus medullaris syndrome • Muscle weakness; fasciculations in lower extremities; spasticity possible • Saddle anesthesia: numbness in buttocks, thighs, perineum • Reflexes: knee jerk preserved; decreased to absent ankle and plantar reflexes; bulbocavernosus and anal reflexes may be preserved. • Autonomic effects: Early onset. Urinary retention and overflow incontinence, bowel incontinence, impotence
Cauda equina	Prostate Bladder Renal Colorectal Uterine Cervical	Pain is local, radicular, or referred, in back and leg(s).	Cauda equina syndrome • Muscle weakness, flaccidity (foot drop)/paralysis in lower extremities • Saddle anesthesia: numbness in buttocks, thighs, perineum • Reflexes: decreased to absent knee, ankle, plantar, bulbocavernosus, and anal reflexes • Autonomic effects: Early onset. Urinary retention, overflow incontinence, constipation, impotence

* May be distributed throughout the spine.

Note. Based on information from Behin & Delattre, 2004; Bucholtz, 1999; Dawodu & Lorenzo, 2005; Kazierad, 1998; Labovich, 1994; Miaskowski, 1999; Osowski, 2002; Schuster & Grady, 2001; Weinstein, 2002.

Figure 8-2. Classification of Primary Spinal Tumors

Location in the spinal canal:
Extramedullary—71%
- Extradural
  - Metastatic solid tumors (most commonly breast, lung, prostate)
  - Lymphoma
  - Myeloma
  - Sarcoma
- Intradural tumors
  - Schwannoma
  - Meningioma

Intramedullary—29%
- Ependymoma
- Astrocytoma (grades 1, 2)
- Glioblastomas
- Oligodendroglioma
- Hemangioblastoma

Note. Based on information from Batzdorf & Haskell, 2001; Myers, 2001.

---

onstrated that tumor cells injected into the arterial circulation disseminate to the marrow of the vertebrae rather than to vertebral bone itself (Gabriel & Schiff, 2004; Manoso & Healey, 2005; Prasad & Schiff, 2005). The bone marrow provides a hospitable environment for cell proliferation; growth factors and cytokines within bone promote the growth of metastatic deposits. Formerly, the Batson plexus was considered the predominant route for metastatic spread to the spinal column. It is a large, low-pressure, venous plexus system of small valveless veins that connects the visceral organs to the spine and pelvis. The unique circulation pattern in the Batson plexus system allows changes in direction of blood flow within the vertebral canal, depending on pressure gradients (Baehring, 2005; Manoso & Healey; Weinstein, 2002). Activities that increase the intra-abdominal or intrathoracic pressures, such as sneezing, coughing, or performing the Valsalva maneuver, may cause malignant cells to circulate from the viscera to the spinal column. This pattern of spread is common for prostate cancer (Heary & Bono, 2001; Manoso & Healey).

Mechanisms Promoting Spinal Cord Damage

The pathophysiology of MSCC is vascular in nature. When metastatic tumor invades the epidural space and exerts direct pressure on the spinal cord, normal venous blood flow from the cord into the vertebral venous plexus is obstructed, and venous stasis ensues (Abrahm, 2004; Maranzano et al., 2003; Prasad & Schiff, 2005). Initially, congestion of blood in the venous plexus system causes vasogenic edema of white matter, swelling of the nerve axons, loss of myelin, and ischemia in the area of compression (Byrne, 1992). Progressive cord compression, venous stasis, and demyelination of the axons in the white matter result in symptomatic neurologic dysfunction. Blood flow to the spinal cord may decrease to such an extent that circulation in the arterioles in deep white matter almost totally ceases, thus creating the potential for spinal cord infarction. Once the cord infarcts, the neurologic injury is irreversible (Abrahm, 2004; Prasad & Schiff).

In addition, evidence suggests that compressed neural tissue releases potentially neurotoxic substances, including cytokines (interleukin [IL]-1, IL-6), inflammatory mediators (prostaglandin E_2), and excitatory neurotransmitters (serotonin), that may contribute to further injury and neurologic impairment (Bucholtz, 1999; DeAngelis & Posner, 2003; Wilkes, 2004). Inflammation increases vascular permeability and may disrupt the blood-spinal barrier at the tumor site (Gabriel & Schiff, 2004). Spinal cord hypoxia stimulates the production of vascular endothelial growth factor (VEGF), which acts to increase vascular permeability and vasogenic edema (Wilkes). In the later stages of MSCC, vasogenic edema is replaced by ischemic-hypoxic neuronal injury and by the onset of cytotoxic edema, resulting in progressive neuronal injury and disintegration and neurologic loss (Prasad & Schiff, 2005). Without correction of the pathologic mechanisms damaging the spinal cord in MSCC, neurologic damage and functional losses become increasingly extensive and ultimately irreversible.

Clinical Manifestations

The clinical presentation of MSCC is similar in all patients regardless of the origin of the malignancy. The earliest symptom of MSCC is typically pain, which, if not promptly recognized and treated, will progress sequentially to motor weakness, sensory loss, autonomic dysfunction (i.e., sphincter disturbance and loss of bladder and bowel control), and, finally, paralysis, which treatment will not reverse (Ruckdeschel, 2004; Tharpar & Laws, 1995). The premium on early diagnosis cannot be too strongly emphasized if healthcare providers are to prevent devastating consequences. See Table 8-2 for an overview of the types of pain and clinical manifestations associated with different levels of spinal involvement.

Back Pain

The hallmark manifestation of MSCC is back pain, which presents as the first symptom in approximately 95% of cases. It may be the first evidence of malignancy in a small percentage of patients, but back pain typically represents recurrent cancer or metastatic disease to the spine (Posner, 1995; Wilkes, 2004). Although back pain is not a specific symptom of MSCC, healthcare professionals should assume that patients with a known or suspected history of cancer who present with new-onset back pain have spinal cord compression until proved otherwise, and they should urgently proceed with a neurologic examination (Gabriel & Schiff, 2004; Maranzano et al., 2003; Ruckdeschel, 2004). The location of back pain also is clinically relevant. Sixty percent to 90% of the U.S. population will experience pain in the lower back at some time; pain in the middle or upper back is less common and is an independent predictive risk factor for MSCC (Lu et al., 2005). However, because back pain usually is treated initially with rest and non-narcotic analgesics, the evaluation and diagnosis of MSCC frequently is delayed. Recognition of MSCC also may be delayed by the presence of painful lesions of herpes zoster, which sometimes erupts at the dermatomal level of the cord compression (DeAngelis & Posner, 2003). Furthermore, most cases of MSCC seem to present on Fridays, when it is more difficult to arrange for prompt diagnostic evaluations and initiate treatment (Baehring, 2005; Manzullo et al., 2002).

Malignant cells in the vertebral bone marrow do not stimulate pain because no pain receptors are present in bone marrow (Waller & Caroline, 2000). Patients experience the pain of MSCC when the expanding vertebral mass stretches the periosteum (nociceptive pain), erodes or fractures the vertebral body (mechanical pain), or involves spinal nerve roots (neuropathic pain) (Osowski, 2002; Tharpar & Laws, 1995; Waller & Caroline; Weinstein, 2002). Pain associated with MSCC can occur at any level of the spine and can be *local* (near the site of compression), *radicular* (distributed along dermatomes), or *referred* (in a nonradicular distribution) or can have combined features (Abrahm, 1999; Myers, 2001; Weinstein; Wilkes, 2004).

Local Pain

At the outset, back pain generally is localized near the midline within one to two spinal segments of the cord compression (Quinn & DeAngelis, 2000). It presents as a constant, dull ache that worsens in the supine position and improves with sitting or standing. Many patients experience the greatest pain intensity on awakening in the morning, because of the increased venous stasis and cord edema related to overnight recumbency. They report that sleeping in a sitting position provides relief (Baehring, 2005; Flaherty, 2005). This characteristic may help to distinguish the pain of MSCC from the pain of degenerative joint disease or herniated disc, which generally is alleviated by lying down and mostly is confined to the lower cervical or lower lumbar spine. The local pain of MSCC increases in intensity over time, and actions that increase intra-abdominal or intrathoracic pressures, such as coughing, sneezing, straining at stool, and performing the Valsalva maneuver, may exacerbate pain (DeAngelis & Posner, 2003; Flounders & Ott, 2003; Grandt, 2000; Kazierad, 1998). Local pain that increases with movement implies spinal instability and is particularly immobilizing (Coyle & Foley, 1991).

Radicular Pain

Radicular pain is less common than local back pain and is triggered by compression of spinal nerve roots or the cauda equina. The pain radiates along dermatomes innervated by the affected nerve roots. Radicular pain can vary from a constant, dull ache that is difficult to localize to intermittent, burning, shooting pain that is easy to localize and is provoked by movement of the spine. The pain intensifies with coughing, sneezing, performing the Valsalva maneuver, and being in the supine position and is relieved by sitting or standing (Grandt, 2000; Osowski, 2002; Quinn & DeAngelis, 2000). Nerve root involvement in the cervical or lumbosacral spine usually produces unilateral pain that radiates down the involved extremity, but it may progress to the other extremity over time. A lesion in the thoracic spine generally produces pain that radiates bilaterally across the chest or abdomen from back to front and is experienced as a tight, squeezing band of pain (Coyle & Foley, 1991; Gabriel & Schiff, 2004; Osowski; Quinn & DeAngelis). The greatest reported incidence of radicular pain is with lesions involving the lumbosacral spine (90%), the cervical spine (79%), and the thoracic spine (55%) (Waller & Caroline, 2000; Weinstein, 2002).

Referred Pain

Patients with MSCC also may experience nonradicular referred pain that may be mistaken for a lesion at the perceived site. A lesion confined to the vertebral body may produce referred pain, which is poorly localized because of the involvement of multiple dermatomes. For example, disease at the seventh vertebra of the cervical spine (C7) may refer pain to the intrascapular region, whereas disease at the first lumbar vertebra (L1) may refer pain to the iliac crests, hips, or sacroiliac region. Sacral involvement often causes midline pain that radiates to the buttocks and intensifies with sitting (Quinn & DeAngelis, 2000; Weinstein, 2002). Compression in the cervical region rarely produces funicular pain, experienced as a band of paresthesias, which is referred to the lower extremities, thorax, or abdomen (Weinstein). The site of pain and the sensory levels frequently do not correspond with the site of cord compression. In a prospective study of patients diagnosed with MSCC, 54% with cord compression located in the thoracic vertebrae (between T1–T6) experienced pain in the lumbosacral area. A similar number of patients with lumbosacral compression reported thoracic pain. In 16% of patients, the sensory level correlated with the level of cord compression seen on MRI scans (Abrahm, 2004).

Motor Weakness

Weakness is the second most common feature of MSCC, presenting in up to 85% of patients at the time of diagnosis. Motor weakness usually follows pain by weeks to months and precedes sensory findings (Kazierad, 1998; Quinn & DeAngelis, 2000). The correlation between weakness and cord compression may be missed because weakness is one of the most common symptoms in advanced cancer (Waller & Caroline, 2000). Delayed diagnosis of MSCC can have devastating consequences on the patient's ability to walk; within one week of presentation of motor weakness, approximately 30% of patients will develop irreversible paraplegia (Maranzano et al., 2003). A survey of primary care physicians, conducted in 2002, indicated that an average of two months elapsed between patients' reports of pain and a diagnosis of MSCC. The delay to diagnosis following reports of motor deficits averaged 20 days, with the result that 82% of the surveyed patients were unable to walk or required assistance to walk at the time of diagnosis (Gabriel & Schiff, 2004).

Regardless of the level of cord compression, motor weakness typically begins in the legs. Early on, the weakness primarily affects the proximal muscles in the lower extremities, manifested by difficulty in rising from a low chair or toilet seat or in climbing stairs. Patient reports of heaviness, spasticity, or stiffness in the legs indicate increased muscle tone (Glick & Glover, 1995; Maranzano et al., 2003; Posner, 1995). In general, weakness related to upper motor neuron dysfunction is associated with increased muscle tone and hyperreflexia, and weakness caused by lower motor neuron involvement is accompanied by muscle flaccidity, atrophy, and hyporeflexia (Manzullo et al., 2002). Disease involving the conus medullaris (the termination of the spinal cord) often produces a combination of upper motor neuron and lower motor neuron signs and symptoms in the dermatomes and myotomes of the affected segments because of the proximity of the conus to the spinal nerve roots. In contrast, a lesion of the cauda equina is considered to be a lower motor neuron lesion because those nerve roots are part of the peripheral nervous system (Dawodu & Lorenzo, 2005).

As MSCC progresses, motor weakness becomes more profound, leading to difficulty in walking and finally to paralysis (Gabriel & Schiff, 2004; Posner, 1995). Occasionally, paralysis develops abruptly, without prior clinical signs (Quinn & DeAngelis, 2000). Involvement of the high cervical spine (at or above C4) may cause weakness or paralysis of the diaphragm and respiratory insufficiency (Baehring, 2005). An ataxic gait sometimes may be the only neurologic finding and reflects spinocerebellar tract dysfunction (Yalamanchili & Lesser, 2003). Ataxia may be the most confusing sign of MSCC. Although back pain usually precedes ataxia, healthcare providers often overlook the reports of pain and mistake ataxia for alcoholism or cerebellar metastases (Baehring; Gabriel & Schiff; Maranzano et al., 2003).

Sensory Loss

Sensory changes occur less frequently than weakness but still are common, presenting in approximately 50% of patients at diagnosis of MSCC. Sensory changes may develop in conjunction with signs of motor weakness or shortly thereafter (Quinn & DeAngelis, 2000; Yalamanchili & Lesser, 2003). The type of sensory disturbance depends on the level and degree of cord compression, but it usually begins as numbness in the toes (usually without paresthesias) and ascends in a stocking-like distribution, eventually reaching one to two spinal segments below the level of cord compression (Waller & Caroline, 2000). Sensory loss gradually progresses to diminished vibration and position sense and ultimately to loss of sensation for touch, pain, and temperature (DeAngelis & Posner, 2003; Gabriel & Schiff, 2004). Lesions of the conus medullaris or the cauda equina may produce conus medullaris syndrome or cauda equina syndrome, characterized by sensory loss in the area of the body that would come into contact with a saddle (saddle anesthesia), including the buttocks, thighs, and perineal region (Glick & Glover, 1995; Maranzano et al., 2003; Quinn & DeAngelis).

Autonomic Dysfunction

Autonomic dysfunction is a common late finding in patients with MSCC. It often indicates bilateral cord damage and portends a poor prognosis (Manglani, Marco, Picciolo, & Healey, 2000; Yalamanchili & Lesser, 2003). The most common autonomic abnormality is bladder dysfunction, followed by impaired bowel function. Weakness of the bladder sphincters or paralysis of the muscles controlling bladder emptying causes early symptoms of urinary hesitancy and urgency, progressing to urinary retention and overflow incontinence (Flaherty, 2005; Waller & Caroline, 2000). Patients frequently present with painless urinary retention, which correlates with severe weakness and sensory loss in the lower extremities, and may not be aware of retained urine because bladder sensation is lost (Gabriel & Schiff, 2004; Glick & Glover, 1995). At diagnosis, almost half of the patients with MSCC are incontinent or require urinary catheterization (Manzullo et al., 2002). The presence of paralysis and urinary retention are the two most significant factors associated with a poor outcome for MSCC (DeAngelis & Posner, 2003), especially if the urinary retention has been present for more than 30 hours (Weinstein, 2002). Urinary retention is defined as a postvoid residual of more than 150 ml and is determined by catheterizing the bladder after micturition (Flaherty). Disturbance of bowel function occurs related to the loss of both voluntary and reflex constriction of the anal sphincter and loss of perineal sensation. Difficulty expelling stool progresses to constipation and fecal incontinence. Impotence develops in males (Maranzano et al., 2003; Quinn & DeAngelis, 2000).

Autonomic dysfunction typically appears late in the course of MSCC; however, it may occur early when compression involves the upper lumbar spine at the level of the conus medullaris or the level of the cauda equina. Decreased sphincter tone and loss of bulbocavernosus (perineal muscles in males and females) and anal reflexes result in disturbances of the bladder, rectum, and genitalia (Abrahm, 2004; Baehring, 2005; Manglani et al., 2000). The appearance of Horner syndrome, a combination of drooping eyelid, constricted pupil, and decreased sweating on the affected side of the face, represents autonomic dysfunction of the sympathetic nerves of the face, which is caused by tumor involvement around the junction of the cervical and thoracic spines (Baehring; Gabriel & Schiff, 2004). Injury to the spinal cord at or above the level of the sixth or seventh thoracic vertebra may trigger autonomic hyperreflexia. The classic symptoms of autonomic hyperreflexia include a pounding headache, hypertension, bradycardia, nasal congestion, profuse sweating, and pilomotor erection (goose bumps) above the level of the lesion (Myers, 2001).

Prognostic Factors

Early recognition, diagnosis, and initiation of treatment for MSCC are powerful predictors of functional outcome and survival. The most important prognostic factor for functional outcome is ambulatory status at the time of presentation (Abrahm, 2004; Weinstein, 2002). Once neurologic symptoms progress beyond back pain, the progression to complete paralysis of the lower extremities (i.e., paraplegia) can occur in a matter of hours to days (Coyle & Foley, 1991; Maranzano et al., 2003). Studies have shown that 67%–100% of patients who were ambulatory at diagnosis remain so following treatment. In contrast, only approximately 10% of patients who present with paraplegia will ever walk again, despite intervention (Gabriel & Schiff, 2004; Weinstein). The presence of urinary retention for a period of more than 30 hours predicts a poor outcome, regardless of treatment (Weinstein). A major factor influencing length of survival is the patient's ability to ambulate on presentation of MSCC. In one study, 40% of patients who were able to walk before and after radiation therapy (RT) were alive one year later. Patients who did not regain ambulation after RT had a particularly poor survival prognosis—only 7% were alive at one year (Bucholtz, 1999; Weinstein).

The type of histology and extent of the underlying malignancy also are important factors influencing response to treatment, functional outcome, and length of survival. Patients with tumors sensitive to antineoplastic therapy have the potential for long-term survival after diagnosis of MSCC (Baehring, 2005). Tumors with favorable histologies related to their high degree of radiosensitivity include breast and prostate cancers, myeloma, and lymphoma. These cancers are significantly associated with a better functional outcome than unfavorable radioresistant cancers, such as lung, bladder, and renal cell carcinomas (Maranzano et al., 2003; Talcott et al., 1999). Long-term survival is common for patients with myeloma; 100% survival at one year has been reported. Most lymphomas demonstrate a good response to chemotherapy and RT, and up to 75% of patients with melanoma and MSCC respond to radiation. Patients with prostate cancer have a median survival of six months following diagnosis of MSCC, although those with a prior good response to hormonal manipulation of their cancer may live longer (Weinstein, 2002). Renal cell carcinoma is poorly radioresponsive and is associated with a median survival of less than four months after diagnosis of MSCC. Overall survival prognosis for all patients diagnosed with MSCC is less than 50% at two months (Baehring). Figure 8-3 lists prognostic factors predictive for functional outcome and length of survival after diagnosis of MSCC.

Figure 8-3. Prognostic Factors for Functional Recovery and Survival Following Metastatic Spinal Cord Compression

Favorable prognostic factors
- Early recognition and diagnosis of metastatic spinal cord compression (MSCC)
- Prompt initiation of therapy
- Able to ambulate at presentation
- Slow onset of motor weakness
- Radiosensitive tumors—myeloma, lymphoma, breast, prostate
- Good performance status
- Responsive to steroid treatment
- Female gender
- Long interval between diagnosis of primary tumor and appearance of MSCC

Poor prognostic factors
- Paraplegia prior to treatment
- Urinary retention
- Sphincter incontinence
- Rapidly deteriorating neurologic function (in less than 72 hours)
- Radioresistant tumors—lung, renal, gastrointestinal, sarcoma, bladder
- Extensive disease
- Poor performance status

Note. Based on information from Abrahm, 2004; Baehring, 2005; DeAngelis & Posner, 2003; Klimo et al., 2003; Maranzano et al., 2003; Talcott et al., 1999; Waller & Caroline, 2000; Weinstein, 2002.

Patient Assessment

History

A thorough, detailed history and physical exam are essential for prompt identification of the classic signs and symptoms of MSCC. Nurses should question patients carefully about the history and duration of the presenting symptoms and the use of relief measures. A pain history consists of collecting information regarding pain onset, location, intensity and quality, exacerbating and relieving factors, prior pain treatment methods, and actual use of medications prescribed for pain (Paice, 1999). Cancer risk factors in patients without a known history of cancer are assessed by questioning them regarding smoking status, recent breast, prostate, or colorectal screening tests, suspicious skin lesions, unplanned weight loss, and changes in bladder and bowel habits

(Heary & Bono, 2001). Assessment of patients with a known history of cancer includes gathering information regarding the initial date, type of malignancy, and disease stage at diagnosis, treatment history, history of metastatic disease and location, and dates of imaging and biomarker studies (Bucholtz, 1999). The patient's use of medications is reviewed, including prescribed and over-the-counter drugs and herbal and nutritional supplements (Wilkes, 2004). Older patients require careful questioning and examination to prevent delays in diagnosing MSCC. Older patients may have other preexisting health conditions, such as diabetes and osteoarthritis, as well as a history of constipation or urinary incontinence that can produce overlapping symptoms and confound the diagnosis of MSCC (Guberski & Belcher, 2005).

Laboratory Tests

No laboratory test is diagnostic for MSCC. Laboratory tests that may be ordered include a complete blood count, erythrocyte sedimentation rate (indicates inflammation), basic blood chemistries, clotting parameters, prostate-specific antigen (to assess for prostate cancer), urinalysis (presence of hematuria may indicate renal or bladder cancer), and serum and urine electrophoresis (to rule out myeloma). Healthcare professionals also should review serum albumin levels in conjunction with ionized calcium, because patients with bone metastases may be hypercalcemic. Patients with MSCC caused by spinal metastases often have multiple areas of bone involvement, and whole body bone scanning may be useful to detect other lesions (Heary & Bono, 2001).

Physical Examination

A thorough, systematic neurologic examination is essential to determine the presence, location, and type of pain, manifestations of motor, sensory, and autonomic dysfunction, and functional losses affecting activities of daily living. A performance scoring system such as the Karnofsky Performance Scale (see Table 5-4) or the Eastern Cooperative Oncology Group scale can grade functional assessment, reflecting patients' general performance and ambulation abilities (Bilsky, Lis, Raizer, Lee, & Boland, 1999).

Back Pain

Pain elicited by gentle vertebral palpation and percussion, neck flexion, or straight leg raises can indicate the level of cord compression (Glick & Glover, 1995). The use of a visual analog scale can assess pain intensity. Gentle palpation and percussion over the vertebrae can locate tenderness or radicular pain at the level of compression. Pain caused by neck flexion indicates compression in the cervical spine (Wilkes, 2004), but extreme care must be taken when performing range-of-motion maneuvers on the neck. Instability of the cervical vertebrae may trigger muscle spasms, and forced neck movements may dislodge vertebral bone fragments, causing acute spinal cord or brain stem injury (Weinstein, 2002). Straight leg raising, which provokes radicular pain that radiates from the back into the leg and increases on foot dorsiflexion, is indicative of nerve root compression in the lumbar or thoracic spine (Baehring, 2005; Flounders & Ott, 2003). Lateral flexion and rotation of the trunk may provoke thoracic and abdominal radicular pain, indicating nerve root involvement in those areas (Weinstein).

Musculoskeletal Assessment

Musculoskeletal assessment begins with observation of the patient's posture, spinal curvature, symmetry of the paraspinal muscles, and gait and coordination (Weinstein, 2002). The natural curve of the spine may straighten in the cervical or lumbar regions from spasm of the paravertebral muscles caused by irritation of involved nerve roots (Baehring, 2005). Healthcare professionals should observe patients for fluidity of movement and arm swinging while walking and turning and for ability to walk heel-to-toe in a straight line. Loss of balance indicates ataxia (Mueller, 2002). Motor weakness begins in the proximal muscles of the leg and may be indicated by patient reports of leg stiffness or heaviness and difficulty arising from a seated position or climbing stairs (Baehring). Leg strength may be tested by asking patients to do heel walking, toe walking, and deep knee bends (DeAngelis & Posner, 2003; Kazierad, 1998) or by having patients perform active movements against the examiner's resistance, depending on the patients' abilities (Bucholtz, 1999). If pain is present, patients may receive analgesics prior to strength testing to permit adequate evaluation (Manzullo et al., 2002). Ideally, a standardized strength scale should be used at baseline as a guide to following the clinical course of MSCC. Clinicians should test each muscle group individually and compare the results from each side of the body for muscle strength and symmetry of movement (Manzullo et al.). The American Spinal Injury Association (ASIA, 2001) uses grading categories ranging from 0 (total paralysis) to 5 (active movement against full resistance) to score muscle strength in the presence of spinal cord injury. ASIA has created standardized forms that can be used at baseline and at follow-up to classify existing motor and sensory function and impairment (Bilsky et al., 1999; Klimo et al., 2003). See Figure 8-4, the ASIA Impairment Scale, and Figure 8-5, the Standard Neurologic Classification of Spinal Cord Injury.

Sensory Assessment

Sensory assessment is an essential part of the neurologic exam and includes evaluation of patients' ability to sense pain, temperature, light touch, vibration, and position sense (proprioception). Sensory testing should be done when patients are as relaxed and comfortable as possible, because

---

Figure 8-4. American Spinal Injury Association Impairment Scale

❏ A = Complete: No motor or sensory function is preserved at the sacral segments S4–S5.
❏ B = Incomplete: Sensory but not motor function is preserved below the neurologic level and includes the sacral segments S4–S5.
❏ C = Incomplete: Motor function is preserved below the neurologic level, and more than half of key muscles below the neurologic level have a muscle grade less than 3.
❏ D = Incomplete: Motor function is preserved below the neurologic level, and at least half of key muscles below the neurologic level have a muscle grade of 3 or more.
❏ E = Normal: Motor and sensory functions are normal.

Note. Figure courtesy of the American Spinal Injury Association, Chicago, IL. Used with permission.

---

results may be unreliable when patients are in pain (Manzullo et al., 2002). Careful dermatomal mapping may help to locate the areas of sensory loss and indicate the level of cord damage (Bucholtz, 1999) (see Figure 8-5 for key sensory points). Reduced sensation may be detected up to five segmental levels below or one to two segments above the level of neural damage (Weinstein, 2002). Pinprick testing for pain localization involves alternately tapping a sharp and dull object against the skin along the lines of the dermatomes, applying equal pressure throughout. The sharp and blunt ends of a safety pin can be used to test relative sharpness. The safety pin is then discarded. The patient's eyes remain closed during this testing (Bucholtz; Mueller, 2002). Healthcare providers can test patients' sensitivity to warm and cold temperatures using warmed and chilled metal tuning forks. They also can use a tuning fork over bony prominences to test vibration sense. Testing patients' sense of light touch entails brushing a fingertip or a fine wisp of cotton against the skin along a dermatome (Bucholtz; Manzullo et al.). To test proprioception, patients stand with their feet together and eyes closed. If they cannot maintain this posture and they begin to sway or fall, this is considered a positive Romberg test (Mueller). Loss of sensation for light touch, pain, or temperature and diminished or absent vibration or proprioception sense indicate progressive neurologic dysfunction (Maranzano et al., 2003).

Autonomic Function Assessment

A detailed micturition history is essential to determine the presence of autonomic dysfunction. Patients frequently may overlook or rationalize symptoms of neurogenic bladder because they believe that increased fluid intake is causing new-onset nocturia or greatly increased urinary frequency during the day. Reports of frequent, small voids may indicate urinary reten-

Figure 8-5. Standard Neurologic Classification of Spinal Cord Injury

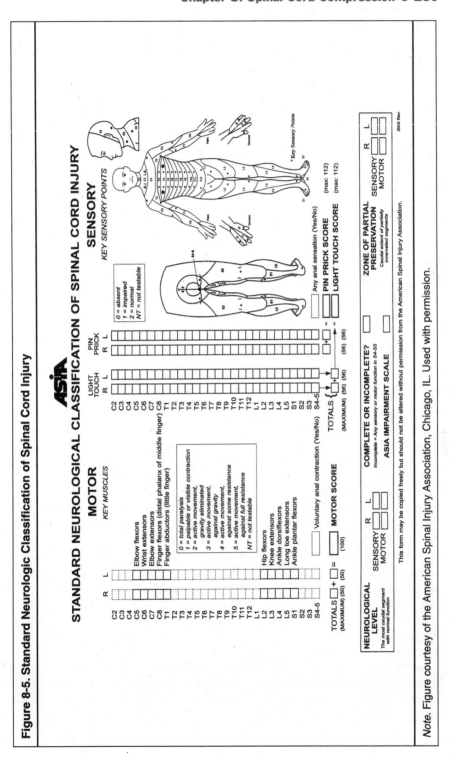

Note. Figure courtesy of the American Spinal Injury Association, Chicago, IL. Used with permission.

tion, and abdominal palpation may reveal distension of the bladder and colon (DeAngelis & Posner, 2003; Weinstein, 2002). Healthcare professionals ask patients to urinate and then catheterize the bladder to measure residual urine volume. Volumes exceeding 150 ml suggest neurogenic bladder (Huff, 2005). Patients should be questioned about changes in bowel habits or difficulty passing stool. Digital rectal examination is performed to check the tone or laxity of the anal sphincter. If patients are immunosuppressed or have a bleeding risk, clinicians can place a cotton-padded examining finger next to the anal opening and have the patients gently squeeze on the finger (Manzullo et al., 2002). Additionally, assessment includes eliciting information about sexual function and new onset of impotence.

Reflex Assessment

Assessment of reflexes is an important indicator of patients' neurologic status. Normal reflex response is brisk; changes in reaction time and intensity may indicate the level of neural damage (Flounders & Ott, 2003). Deep tendon reflexes generally decrease at the level of compression and become hyperactive below (Wilkes, 2004). Hyperactive deep tendon reflexes in the lower extremities and extensor plantar responses (positive *Babinski sign*) indicate cord compression in the thoracic region (Glick & Glover, 1995; Maranzano et al., 2003; Posner, 1995). The presence of a positive Babinski sign is always an abnormal finding in adults and is evidence of corticospinal tract dysfunction. To elicit the Babinski sign, clinicians stroke a tool across the sole of the foot, from the heel to the small toe, and then draw an arc across to under the big toe. Dorsiflexion of the great toe with fanning of the other toes indicates a positive response, which reflects upper motor neuron disease. Checking the Babinski sign can be unpleasant and can be put off until the end of a neurologic exam (Manzullo et al., 2002). Observation of the *Beevor sign* (vertical movement of the umbilicus with neck flexion) may determine the level of lower thoracic nerve root dysfunction. To elicit the Beevor sign, the examiner flexes the supine patient's head forward against resistance while observing the movement of the umbilicus. Movement in a caudal direction (toward the foot) indicates that nerve root involvement is above T10; cephalad movement (toward the head) indicates the dysfunction is below T10 (Manzullo et al.). In contrast to the hyperreflexia seen with higher lesions, compression at the level of the cauda equina produces hyporeflexia or areflexia in the legs (DeAngelis & Posner, 2003). Weakness of the hip flexor muscles and loss of the knee jerk reflex reflect nerve root involvement of the upper lumbar plexus. Foot drop and a diminished ankle jerk reflex indicate lesions of the nerve roots of the lower lumbar plexus (Weinstein, 2002). Lesions of the conus medullaris present a mixed picture. The knee jerk, bulbocavernosus, and anal reflexes may be preserved, whereas the ankle and plantar reflexes are decreased to absent (Dawodu & Lorenzo, 2005).

Diagnostic Evaluation

After a thorough history and physical examination, diagnostic evaluation should proceed urgently. The patient's clinical presentation and neurologic status guide the selection of imaging tests to detect MSCC. Although clinicians now consider MRI to be the imaging procedure of choice, this section will begin with a review of the various imaging modalities used to detect MSCC.

Plain Films

Plain films (x-rays) of the spine may be appropriate for patients who present solely with pain and no other neurologic dysfunction. Plain films are a readily available initial test but are associated with a high false-negative rate (Schiff, 2003). Researchers estimate that 50% of vertebral bone must be destroyed before plain films become abnormal (Gabriel & Schiff, 2004; Tharpar & Laws, 1995). Plain films can image bony changes, such as vertebral erosion, vertebral collapse, and bone fragment dislocation, but cannot show the extent of soft tissue lesions and impingement on the spinal cord (Rude, 2000; Schiff). One study found that extensive vertebral destruction seen on spinal x-rays of patients presenting with back pain was indicative of MSCC in approximately 75% of cases. However, plain films do not have adequate predictive value to warrant routine use (Schiff).

Bone Scans

Radionuclide bone scintigrams (bone scans) may be ordered following normal plain films of the spine for patients who have back pain but no other neurologic impairment. Bone scans are more sensitive than x-ray and can detect tumor growth up to six months before it becomes visible on x-ray (Yalamanchili & Lesser, 2003). However, bone scans have several limitations. They are not as specific as x-ray for diagnosing metastatic lesions, do not provide structural detail, and produce false-positive results related to nonmalignant skeletal conditions. In addition, bone scans depend on blood flow and new bone growth to demonstrate metastases; they may produce false-negative results with tumors that do not stimulate new bone formation, such as myeloma, lung carcinoma, and melanoma (Manoso & Healey, 2005; Schiff, 2003).

Myelography

Before MRI became widely available, myelography was the gold standard for assessing MSCC. Myelography is an uncomfortable and invasive procedure. It requires manipulation of the spine for lumbar punctures to inject contrast dye into the spinal canal and is used in conjunction with computed tomography (CT) imaging (Yalamanchili & Lesser, 2003). Clinicians can collect CSF simultaneously with CT myelography for diagnostic purposes, but they must do so with caution. Removal of CSF in the presence of a tumor may worsen cord compression and exacerbate existing neurologic deficits (Huff, 2005). Myelography is contraindicated in patients with coagulation disorders and thrombocytopenia (Weinstein, 2002). CT myelography now usually is reserved for situations in which MRI is contraindicated, including patients with pacemakers, mechanical heart valves, or other metal implants and those who cannot lie in one position for an extended period of time or cannot tolerate the claustrophobia of an MRI machine (Hatchett & Kripas, 2002; Ruckdeschel, 2004).

Magnetic Resonance Imaging

Symptomatic patients with neurologic findings, severe or progressive pain, or suspected pathology found on plain film require emergent evaluation with MRI scans. MRI is currently the most sensitive, specific, and accurate test for detecting MSCC and has many advantages over other imaging tests. It is non-invasive, requires minimal patient manipulation, and has the ability to show the extent of the lesion and soft tissue anatomy in detail to distinguish between benign and malignant lesions, to diagnose other unsuspected sites of MSCC, and to image multiple levels of cord involvement in a single examination. Consequently, MRI also is of great value to radiation oncologists in defining a target treatment volume that encompasses the full scope of the spinal lesions (DeAngelis & Posner, 2003; Gabriel & Schiff, 2004; Maranzano et al., 2003). Contrast enhancement with gadolinium is not necessary to detect MSCC but is needed to help to identify intramedullary and intradural tumors, radiation myelopathy, or leptomeningeal disease (Hatchett & Kripas, 2002).

Ruckdeschel (2004) described a detailed diagnostic algorithm to guide the workup and treatment of MSCC. A patient with any sign of myelopathy receives an emergent MRI of the entire spine so that discontiguous or skip lesions are not missed. An IV bolus of high-dose corticosteroids also is administered without waiting for the MRI results. The expectation is that the benefits of steroid therapy outweigh the possible risks of a single bolus of drug, even if MSCC is not confirmed. If MRI cannot be done on an emergent basis, as in the middle of the night, treatment involves corticosteroid administration until MRI can be performed. Using MRI as the initial imaging method is a faster, more efficient, and more cost-effective approach to early diagnosis of MSCC than first obtaining plain films or performing bone scans (Ruckdeschel).

Treatment Modalities

The goal of treatment is to optimize patients' quality of life by relieving pain, palliating symptoms, preventing permanent disability, preserving or recovering motor and sphincter function, and extending the active portion of the patients' remaining life. Healthcare providers tailor the intensity of intervention to patients' prognosis and life expectancy. Therapy for MSCC is divided into temporizing therapy with corticosteroids and definitive therapy using RT and surgery, either alone or in combination (Lamont, Rudin, & Hoffman, 2003). A multidisciplinary approach is necessary to achieve effective implementation of the various treatment modalities (Klimo et al., 2003). Pain relief is always a priority regardless of the prognosis, and healthcare professionals consider the therapeutic and rehabilitation goals for each patient on an individual basis (Abrahm, 2004).

Corticosteroids

The initial treatment for all patients with MSCC is corticosteroids. Corticosteroids can reduce vasogenic edema in the spinal cord and downregulate expression of VEGF, thereby improving neurologic function in some patients (Lamont et al., 2003; Prasad & Schiff, 2005) and diminishing pain in the short term (Rude, 2000). Corticosteroids also may relieve cord compression by shrinking tumors, particularly lymphoma but also breast cancer (DeAngelis & Posner, 2003). Corticosteroids should be held if lymphoma is suspected as the cause of MSCC, except in emergent situations, because they are so effective in minimizing lymphoma that diagnosis could be difficult (Weinstein, 2002).

The most widely used steroid for MSCC is dexamethasone, but no consensus exists among clinicians about the optimal dose, which remains controversial. A systematic review of the literature by Klimo et al. (2003) revealed loading doses ranging between 10–100 mg followed by a range of maintenance doses of 4–24 mg four times daily, tapering over several weeks. In general, high doses were initiated for patients who presented with severe symptoms or worsening neurologic status. Results of clinical studies vary in demonstrating that high-dose dexamethasone followed by standard maintenance therapy (with or without the addition of RT) makes a difference in outcomes related to pain relief, ambulation, or bladder function. In addition, higher doses of steroids are associated with more severe complications. The authors' recommendation, based on their extensive literature review, is that the appropriate regimen for dexamethasone is an initial bolus of 10 mg followed by 16 mg per day, with doses tapering over several weeks while the patients receive definitive treatment with either RT or surgery (Klimo et al.).

Although disagreement exists, other clinicians recommend that patients who present with moderate pain but no other neurologic symptoms or those with evidence of spinal cord compression on MRI should be started on a standard dose of 6 mg of dexamethasone given four times a day, with dose escalations if pain persists or new symptoms develop. Patients experiencing severe pain or those with evidence of neurologic deficits on presentation would receive an IV loading dose of 100 mg dexamethasone, followed by 96–100 mg every 24 hours in divided doses, despite the potential for serious side effects. The drug is tapered once more definitive treatment has begun (DeAngelis & Posner, 2003; Yalamanchili & Lesser, 2003). No studies have

yet determined the efficacy of other forms of steroids, such as methylprednisolone or hydrocortisone, as adjuncts to RT in treating patients with MSCC
(Yalamanchili & Lesser).

Infusion of dexamethasone should be done slowly over a period of 5–10
minutes; rapid administration can cause severe genital burning (DeAngelis &
Posner, 2003). Side effects of corticosteroids depend on the duration of drug
administration, the cumulative dose, and the regimen. Review studies have
demonstrated that patients receiving high-dose maintenance dexamethasone
experienced a significant increase in serious adverse effects, including severe
psychoses, gastric ulcers, and bowel perforations requiring surgery (Loblaw
et al., 2005). Other side effects of maintenance steroid therapy include increased risk of postoperative infections, adrenal insufficiency, hyperglycemia,
fluid retention, osteoporosis, depression, and emotional lability (Rude, 2000).
Prolonged administration of corticosteroids can cause immunosuppression
and the appearance of opportunistic infections, such as *Pneumocystis carinii*.
Also, corticosteroids are metabolized through the cytochrome P450 system,
thus creating a potential for drug interactions with other medications, such as
anticonvulsants, that are metabolized in the same way (Weinstein, 2002).

Radiation Therapy

The best therapy for MSCC has not yet been established. Where no specific
indication for surgery exists, RT generally is accepted as first-line treatment
for patients with mostly asymptomatic MSCC (Manoso & Healey, 2005; Maranzano et al., 2003; Yalamanchili & Lesser, 2003). Based on the results of
retrospective analyses, both surgery followed by RT and RT alone provided
similar outcomes if performed early, before significant neurologic symptoms
developed (DeAngelis & Posner, 2003; Maranzano et al.). An evidence-based
review of the literature arrived at several indications for using RT to treat
MSCC (Klimo et al., 2003). These were the presence of radiosensitive tumors
(lymphoma, multiple myeloma, small cell lung cancer, testicular seminoma,
neuroblastoma, and Ewing sarcoma), expected survival of less than three to
four months, inability to tolerate surgery, duration longer than 24–48 hours
of total neurologic deficit below the level of cord compression, and multilevel
or diffuse spinal involvement (Klimo et al.).

RT should start soon after administration of corticosteroids, usually within
24 hours of the diagnosis of MSCC (Manglani et al., 2000). The optimal dose
and fractionation schedule for RT has not been established because of lack
of comparison studies (Yalamanchili & Lesser, 2003). Most centers use a total
of 3,000 cGy divided into 10 fractions. RT is delivered to a single posterior
portal centered on the spine that usually is 8–10 cm wide and extends two
vertebral bodies above and below the compression site (DeAngelis & Posner,
2003; Yalamanchili & Lesser).

Radiation to the spinal cord does not cause acute clinical symptoms, but
early-delayed radiation myelopathy may develop 12–20 weeks following treat-

ment (Posner, 1995). This is related to transient demyelination of spinal posterior columns and white matter necrosis caused by radiation injury. MRI of the spinal cord usually is normal, and clinical signs usually are limited to paresthesias or Lhermitte sign, a sudden, mild, electric shock–like sensation triggered by neck flexion that radiates down the spine into the extremities. No specific treatment exists for this condition, and in most cases, the symptoms usually resolve spontaneously within one year (Behin & Delattre, 2004; Yalamanchili & Lesser, 2003).

A late-delayed complication that may arise 6 months to 10 years following spinal radiation is chronic progressive myelitis. It is caused by axon demyelination and loss and vascular derangements related to the dose of radiation received by the spinal cord. Clinical signs begin with weakness and paresthesias, which in the worst case may progress to complete loss of motor, sensory, and autonomic function below the level of the treated lesion (Behin & Delattre, 2004; Posner, 1995; Yalamanchili & Lesser, 2003).

RT does not cure spinal instability and may cause further bone weakening (Heary & Bono, 2001). Bracing the spine may be necessary until bone healing occurs. Patients usually wear spinal braces for 6–10 weeks, which ideally are custom-made with a moldable synthetic material. The spinal segments that are most important to immobilize are junctional areas—where two regions of the spine join together, such as the cervicothoracic, thoracolumbar, and lumbosacral junctions (Manglani et al., 2000).

Surgery

The superiority of surgery over RT is not statistically significant, and the decision to undertake surgery is made on an individual basis (Maranzano et al., 2003). Traditional indications for surgery as the first-line treatment of choice in patients with MSCC include rapidly progressing paraplegia, spinal instability, pathologic fracture with dislocation of bone fragments, circumferential epidural tumor, biopsy for unknown histologic diagnosis, intractable pain, recurrence after prior RT, and radioresistant tumors (Jacobs & Perrin, 2001; Klimo et al., 2003; Manoso & Healey, 2005; McClain & Bell, 1998). Researchers who conducted an evidence-based review of surgical management of MSCC concluded that the evidence is not sufficient to support a surgical treatment standard. They found that surgery can improve quality of life by alleviating pain, producing spinal stability, and improving neurologic function in patients who did not present with complete paraplegia (Ryken et al., 2003). Surgical decompression cannot reverse a complete paralysis of more than 24 hours' duration and should not be attempted (Jacobs & Perrin).

Several factors determine the selection of the surgical approach: tumor location and extent, integrity of adjacent segments, type of reconstruction planned, and general condition of the patient (DeAngelis & Posner, 2003; Weinstein, 2002). In general, candidates for palliative surgery should have a life expectancy of at least 12 weeks. A minimum of three weeks should be allowed between completion of RT and surgery in the same area (Manoso & Healey, 2005).

Laminectomy

Laminectomy, the traditional surgical procedure to decompress MSCC, has fallen out of favor because it does not allow for complete tumor resection and increases spinal instability, therefore worsening neurologic symptoms (Abrahm, 2004; McClain & Bell, 1998; Rude, 2000). Laminectomy provides direct access to tumors located posteriorly; however, most metastatic disease involves the vertebral body, which is anterior to the spinal cord. Vertebral bone fragments and tumor cannot be removed from the anterior cord surface without manipulating the spinal cord and risking further neurologic injury (McClain & Bell). Decompressive laminectomy still may be indicated for patients whose neurologic status continues to worsen following irradiation, for those with posteriorly located radioresistant tumors, in the absence of vertebral involvement, or possibly to obtain a tissue diagnosis (Gabriel & Schiff, 2004).

More aggressive operative choices to decompress the spinal cord include anterior, posterior, or combined approaches, all with advantages and disadvantages. Newer percutaneous procedures, such as vertebroplasty, can be effective in a selected group of patients who do not have neurologic deficits (Heary & Bono, 2001).

Anterior Vertebral Body Resection With Stabilization

In 85% of MSCC cases, the location of metastatic disease is anterior to the spinal cord, so an anterior surgical approach is an important advance. The anterior approach to the spine is a more aggressive technique than laminectomy and is known as *vertebral corpectomy*. It involves accessing the affected vertebral body and the epidural space via thoracotomy or laparotomy to completely debulk the tumor and relieve pressure on the spinal cord (Gabriel & Schiff, 2004; McClain & Bell, 1998). Vertebral body resection (VBR) leaves a defect in the anterior spinal column, which must be reconstructed using a stabilizing device. Surgeons usually use polymethyl methacrylate (PMMA), a bone cement filler, in conjunction with a variety of internal fixation devices to reconstruct the spine and provide stability for the remainder of the patient's life. Metallic fixation devices, such as pins, rods, plates, or titanium cages, are attached to intact vertebral bodies above and below the involved area. The primary objective is immediate spinal stability that is durable enough to last for one year (Heary & Bono, 2001; Manglani et al., 2000). Bone grafts also can be used to fill the defect but require six weeks to fuse before RT can begin, whereas RT can start one week after PMMA insertion (Gabriel & Schiff).

Renal cell carcinoma and thyroid metastases are highly vascular tumors, and blood loss during VBR can be life threatening. To minimize bleeding, these tumors usually are embolized prior to surgery (Abrahm, 2004; Jacobs &

Perrin, 2001). Particularly in cases of renal cell carcinoma, clinicians should obtain a preoperative arteriogram to help to avoid embolizing major spinal feeding arteries located in the lower thoracic spine, which would create further neurologic compromise (Heary & Bono, 2001).

The risk-benefit ratio for VBR must be assessed on an individual basis. Most patient series show a high morbidity (48%) and mortality (6%–10%) rate for VBR (Yalamanchili & Lesser, 2003). Morbidity is related to the occurrence of deep venous thrombosis, pulmonary embolism, wound infection and breakdown, hemorrhage, stabilization failure, hematoma, pneumonia, and cardiac infarct (Gabriel & Schiff, 2004; Yalamanchili & Lesser). Significant predisposing factors for complications related to this procedure include age older than 65, history of prior spinal RT, and the presence of paraparesis (Abrahm, 2004; Gabriel & Schiff). Patients who have had prior RT for MSCC may have a complication rate as high as 30% for spinal surgery (Weinstein, 2002). Patients who have not had prior irradiation to the spine usually receive postoperative RT beginning 7–10 days after surgery (Quinn & DeAngelis, 2000; Weinstein).

Vertebroplasty

Vertebroplasty is a minimally invasive percutaneous technique of stabilizing the vertebrae in patients with MSCC who are experiencing pain but do not have neurologic manifestations. The procedure initially was developed for treatment of osteoporotic compression fractures (Manglani et al., 2000). It involves injecting PMMA into the vertebral body with a hollow-bore needle. The posterior wall of the vertebral body must be intact to prevent extravasation of PMMA into the spinal canal. The primary goal of vertebroplasty is to increase the stability of the anterior column of the spine; however, 50%–80% of carefully selected patients also have experienced dramatic pain relief (Heary & Bono, 2001).

Kyphoplasty

Kyphoplasty is a procedure that has evolved from vertebroplasty. During kyphoplasty, a balloon is introduced into the fractured vertebral body under x-ray guidance and is expanded and removed. The space created by the expanded balloon is filled with PMMA, which hardens quickly, thereby producing stability and restoring height to the fractured vertebral body, reducing kyphosis deformity, and relieving pain (Flaherty, 2005).

Posterolateral Approach

A posterolateral approach is an alternative route for lesions of the upper thoracic spine (above T6), which are technically difficult to reach via an anterior approach. Posterolateral surgery involves removing part of a rib to approach and remove anterior disease from the side, without the need for a thoracotomy. With this approach, access to MSCC always is limited, and neurologic recovery is less reliable (McClain & Bell, 1998). Spine stabilization generally follows this surgery to prevent kyphosis (Abrahm, 2004). Surgeons are developing new posterolateral approaches for specific MSCC syndromes in patients with advanced cancer. Several authors have suggested reserving a limited posterolateral approach to tumor resection for patients whose expected survival is less than six months (Weinstein, 2002).

Chemotherapy

The epidural space is on the systemic side of the blood-brain barrier, so chemotherapy may serve as an adjunct in treating MSCC caused by chemosensitive tumors, such as Hodgkin disease, non-Hodgkin lymphoma, neuroblastoma, germ cell tumors, and breast cancer (Abrahm, 2004; Gabriel & Schiff, 2004). Chemotherapy can be especially helpful in patients with recurrent MSCC and in nonoperable patients who have not responded to RT. Hormone therapy with tamoxifen, aromatase inhibitors, or androgen blockade may be of benefit in metastatic breast and prostate cancers not previously exposed to hormones. Patients generally receive chemotherapy and hormonal treatments in conjunction with more rapidly effective modalities such as RT or surgery (Gabriel & Schiff); however, chemotherapy may be effective as the sole treatment for MSCC caused by highly chemosensitive tumors, such as non-Hodgkin lymphoma (Baehring, 2005).

Bisphosphonates

Bisphosphonates now are widely used to inhibit tumor-induced bone resorption, especially in the treatment of breast cancer and multiple myeloma. Bisphosphonates can effectively reduce pain and other skeletal complications of vertebral metastases; however, their benefit may not become apparent before three to six months, so they should be started early in the treatment process. Pamidronate has been shown to be effective for lytic metastases, and zoledronate for lytic and blastic metastases. For metastatic bone disease, the approved dosing regimens are 4 mg zoledronate and 90 mg pamidronate every three to four weeks via IV infusion (Manoso & Healey, 2005). Although bisphosphonates can improve the quality of life for patients with bone metastases, they have not been shown to prolong survival with or reduce the incidence of MSCC (Flaherty, 2005). For a more complete description of bisphosphonates, see Chapter 3.

Nursing Management

The role of nurses caring for patients with MSCC changes as patients progress along a continuum from early detection and diagnosis, to emergent and definitive treatment, to rehabilitation or supportive palliative care. Early on, nurses play a key role in recognizing the subtle signs and symptoms of spinal cord compression and prompting rapid diagnostic evaluation. Once the diagnosis of MSCC is confirmed, nurses provide individualized care based on the patient's neurologic condition and spinal stability while the patient receives appropriate therapies. Nursing care centers on issues of pain relief, motor and sensory loss, bladder and bowel dysfunction, treatment preparation and side-effect management, safety, skin integrity, and nutrition (see Figure 8-6). Nurses incorporate rehabilitation principles in the care of patients to maximize and restore function where feasible and to prevent injuries and

---

Figure 8-6. Nursing Interventions in the Care of Patients With Metastatic Spinal Cord Compression

- Institute pain relief measures, and evaluate effectiveness.
- Conduct ongoing assessment of sensory and motor functions.
- Measure vital signs, with attention to respiration, and fluid intake and output.
- Provide education and reassurance related to treatment modalities.
- Evaluate objective and subjective responses to therapy.
- Institute safety measures to prevent injury and further neurologic damage.
- Mobilize patients, and assist them with weight-bearing activities and proper body mechanics as appropriate.
- Manage preventive skincare regimen.
- Monitor nutritional and fluid status.
- Assess for bladder distension and need for urinary catheter.
- Assess bowel function, and establish an elimination program.
- Coordinate activity regimen and rehabilitation program.
- Assess coping mechanisms related to cancer diagnosis, altered body image, and changes in sexual function.
- Facilitate adaptation to neurologic deficits and advancing disease.
- Support patients and caregivers in accepting functional limitations and addressing end-of-life issues.

Note. Based on information from Bucholtz, 1999; Camp-Sorrell, 1998; Forster, 1998; Kazierad, 1998; Miaskowski, 1999; Myers, 2001; Osowski, 2002; Rude, 2000.

---

further neurologic damage, coordinate care with the rehabilitation team, and prepare patients for discharge to home or hospice. They provide patient and caregiver teaching at an appropriate level, assess coping mechanisms, and offer encouragement and emotional support throughout the entire continuum (Flaherty, 2005; Myers, 2001; Osowski, 2002; Rude, 2000; Wilkes, 2004).

Pain Management

Pain management is a priority in patients with MSCC. The only reliable way to assess pain is to ask the patients. Conducting a baseline pain assessment is essential, noting the pain quality and intensity, location, pattern (local/radiating), actions that increase pain or provide relief, and treatments that have been effective in the past (Miaskowski, 1999; Paice, 1999). The analgesia regimen begins immediately upon presentation of MSCC. The administration of corticosteroids immediately after diagnosis provides pain relief, but the pain-reducing effect of RT typically does not occur before five fractions of RT have been delivered and may not be fully appreciated for up to two weeks after completion of treatment (Bucholtz, 1999). Inadequate pain relief has a significant negative effect on patients' functional capacity and quality of life, so ongoing pain assessment is necessary throughout treatment. Management of cancer-related pain should involve pain specialists (if they are available) early in the course of treatment (Schuster & Grady, 2001).

The appropriate combination of therapeutic agents and nonpharmacologic techniques can control pain in 85%–95% of patients with MSCC (Abrahm, 1999). Nurses need to be familiar with the principles of pharmacologic analgesia and equianalgesic dosing, the risks, benefits, and costs of different drug regimens, and nonpharmacologic behavioral approaches to managing pain, such as relaxation techniques and hypnosis (Abrahm, 1999; Flaherty, 2005). The World Health Organization has developed a well-validated three-step analgesic ladder for providing pain relief based on escalating pain severity (Abrahm, 1999). With this approach, standard nonsteroidal anti-inflammatory drugs (NSAIDs) are used for mild pain, and other agents, including opioids and adjuvant drugs, are added as needed for moderate and severe pain. NSAIDs are effective in managing bone pain but are associated with gastrointestinal toxicity in the older adult population and should be taken with antiulcer drugs. Bleeding and renal problems also may occur when NSAIDs are used on a prolonged basis, so patients taking these drugs should be closely monitored (Abrahm, 1999; Flaherty).

Nurses should question patients about existing pain levels and their response to analgesics, as corticosteroids or definitive treatments relieve pain, so that doses can be modified or adjuvant drugs added if necessary (Wilkes, 2004). Chronic opioid therapy often is required for persistent pain and should be used on an around-the-clock or fixed schedule rather than as necessary. Stool softeners and laxatives may be ordered to prevent constipation, with dose elevations as the opioid dose increases (Paice, 1999). Adjuvant agents, such as anticonvulsants, antidepressants, and antianxiety drugs, also may be helpful in pain management (Flaherty, 2005). Neuropathic pain related to tumor involvement of spinal nerve roots or peripheral nerves typically does not respond to opioids. Anticonvulsants (e.g., phenytoin) and tricyclic antidepressants (e.g., amitriptyline) may be effective in treating this type of pain (Rude, 2000). Patients may require benzodiazepines if spastic reactions occur below the level of cord compression (Flaherty). When systemic analgesics are no longer effective, epidural blocks, with local anesthetic or opioids, or intrathecal administration of opioids may become necessary (Camp-Sorrell,

1998). Cordotomy, cutting through spinal nerve tracts that transmit pain, can be considered as an extreme measure in cases of intractable pain (Schuster & Grady, 2001).

Mobility and Safety Issues

Care of patients with MSCC is individualized, but in all situations, the patients' comfort and safety are the primary goals. Nursing actions center on preventing further damage to the spine and the vertebral column, which should be considered unstable until diagnostic evaluation proves otherwise (Kazierad, 1998). Providing safe and comfortable patient transfers, assisting with ambulation, implementing prescribed safety measures, such as padded and raised side rails, maintaining proper body alignment and support, and moving bedbound patients with great caution are essential nursing measures (Myers, 2001). Prevention and detection of deep venous thromboses are critical in immobilized patients (Schuster & Grady, 2001). Nurses apply antiembolic stockings as ordered and measure the patient's calves daily, noting any redness, warmth, or swelling (Myers).

If vertebral fractures are present, patients may be fitted with a brace to provide external stabilization until surgery can be performed. Treatment in the postoperative period also includes using braces until internal stabilization devices or bone grafts heal and strengthen the spine (Flaherty, 2005; Kazierad, 1998). Following surgical intervention, the principles of postoperative nursing care include serial neurologic assessment, pain management, wound care, body alignment, and spinal stability (Flaherty). Before initiating a mobility program, clinicians may consider prophylactic fixation of impending osteoporotic or pathologic fractures in the extremities to aid in mobility and weight bearing (Weinstein, 2002). A hard or soft cervical collar or a halo fixator may be used for patients with lesions of the cervical spine to provide nonsurgical stabilization (Heary & Bono, 2001).

Patients who have lesions of the cervical or high thoracic spine are at risk for acute respiratory insufficiency and for autonomic hyperreflexia. Nurses should institute pulmonary hygiene measures as ordered to prevent hypoventilation, atelectasis, and pneumonia and should be prepared to place patients on mechanical ventilation if necessary. They also should be familiar with and alert for signs indicating autonomic hyperreflexia, such as elevated blood pressure, bradycardia, pounding headache, chest pain, vasodilation, flushing, and profuse sweating above the level of the spinal block (Myers, 2001).

Skin Care

Skin care and skin protection are essential components of nursing care and begin upon admission (Kazierad, 1998). Patients with advanced cancer frequently are malnourished; therefore, their skin is at increased risk for breakdown and infection. Meticulous skin care is essential, especially if patients are not mobile or are wearing supportive spinal braces (Weinstein, 2002). Nurses should assess patients' nutritional status by monitoring their serum protein and albumin levels. If necessary, nutritional supplementation may aid post-surgical wound healing (Schuster & Grady, 2001). Patients receiving RT for MSCC require routine skin assessments. During radiation, the potential for skin reactions is related to the size of the treatment portals and the sensitivity of the patient's skin. Radiation oncology nurses should instruct patients about care of the skin and the use of water-soluble lotions in the irradiated area during treatment (Flaherty, 2005).

Bowel and Bladder Function

Loss of the ability to fully empty the bladder results in urinary retention, bladder distension, and chronic urinary tract infections (UTIs). Nursing activities include monitoring fluid intake and output, assessing for bladder distension, and catheterizing for residual urine after voiding. If retained urine is present, a schedule of intermittent catheterization may be instituted during the acute phase of MSCC. Nurses check for signs of UTI, such as cloudy urine with a foul odor, frequency, urgency, or burning on urination, and monitor the results of the urinalysis and cultures (Bucholtz, 1999; Labovich, 1994). Fluoroquinolones or sulfa-containing antibiotics usually are ordered to treat most UTIs (Flaherty, 2005).

Nurses provide instruction to patients who will be discharged home and/or their caregivers regarding intermittent catheterization (if indicated) and recognizing signs of UTI. Intermittent catheterization may be necessary at home to help in establishing urinary continence, emptying the bladder more fully, and reducing the risk of UTI. Patients with progressive disease may require a permanent indwelling urinary catheter. Maintaining fluid intake greater than 2 L per day, including cranberry juice to acidify the urine, may reduce the risk of UTI secondary to an indwelling urinary catheter. Daily catheter care and perineal hygiene and regular catheter changes are important measures to decrease UTI risk (Flaherty, 2005).

Constipation, impaction, and loss of sphincter control can result from bowel dysfunction, which may progress to paralytic ileus and abdominal distension. Opioids used to control pain, inactivity, and immobility also contribute to constipation (Kazierad, 1998). Nurses should palpate the patient's abdomen for signs of distension, listen for bowel sounds, and check for stool impaction on a daily basis. A bowel maintenance program will help to reduce the incidence of constipation and stool incontinence. The use of stool softeners, laxatives, bulk-producing products, lubricants, and rectal suppositories, as ordered, can help to establish regular bowel evacuation. In addition, nurses should encourage patients to increase their intake of fluids and dietary bulk and fiber (Flaherty, 2005; Myers, 2001). Table 8-3 outlines supportive measures in the care of patients with MSCC.

Table 8-3. Supportive Measures in the Care of Patients With Metastatic Spinal Cord Compression

Problems	Patient Goals	Interventions
Pain caused by irritation and compression of nerve roots and neural tissue and/or vertebral collapse as evidenced by localized or radicular pain	Achieving maximum comfort as reported on a pain scale during rest and activity by appropriately using various types of analgesics and nonpharmacologic interventions	• Opioids—time release, immediate, transdermal release • Dexamethasone • NSAIDs • Anticonvulsants/antidepressants • Complementary medicine; capsicum cream, hydrotherapy, massage, acupressure • Vertebroplasty, kyphoplasty
Immobility caused by compression of neural tissue and motor neurons as evidenced by proximal muscle weakness that progresses to motor loss	Maintaining optimal level of mobility, range of motion, and strength through an activity and exercise program	• Refer to physical therapy. • Obtain equipment and devices to preserve alignment, enhance mobility, and stabilize spine. • Assist homecare agency in organizing environment to be conducive to mobility.
Risk of injury related to sensory loss, which includes paresthesia, loss of temperature, position and vibratory senses, and light touch	Preserving safety at all times	• Assess degree of sensory changes: touch, temperature, paresthesia. • Assess environment for physical, thermal, and chemical hazards, and organize environment to minimize hazards. • Assist patient with ADLs as needed.
Bladder dysfunction caused by disruption of lower motor neurons (autonomic function) as evidenced by incontinence, frequency, and/or retention	Maintaining adequate urinary elimination with early identification and treatment of urinary tract infections	• Ensure fluid intake greater than 2 quarts/day. • Encourage adequate intake of juices to maintain acidity (e.g., cranberry). • Use straight catheterization/indwelling catheter to maintain continence and empty bladder. • Change indwelling catheter each week. • Perform urinalysis/urine culture for pain, burning, foul-smelling/cloudy urine, fever, and increased WBC count. • Promptly treat urinary tract infection with antibiotic sensitive to the organism identified. • Maintain daily perineal hygiene.

(Continued on next page)

Table 8-3. Supportive Measures in the Care of Patients With Metastatic Spinal Cord Compression *(Continued)*

Problems	Patient Goals	Interventions
Bowel disturbances caused by opioid use and disruption of lower motor neurons (autonomic function) as evidenced by constipation, incontinence, and/or difficulty expelling stool	Maintaining adequate bowel elimination and preventing ileus from constipation	• Establish bowel regimen including stool softener (i.e., docusate sodium), intestinal lubricants, mineral oil, laxatives; senna products, magnesium-based products (i.e., milk of magnesia, magnesium citrate). • Follow dietary recommendations to include fresh fruits, vegetables, and high-fiber cereals. • Ensure adequate fluid intake greater than 2 quarts/day. • Provide periodic perineal hygiene.

ADLs—activities of daily living; NSAIDs—nonsteroidal anti-inflammatory drugs; WBC—white blood cell
Data from Wilkes (1999).

Note. From "Spinal Cord Compression" (p. 921), by A.M. Flaherty in C.H. Yarbro, M.H. Frogge, and M. Goodman (Eds.), *Cancer Nursing: Principles and Practice* (6th ed.), 2005, Sudbury, MA: Jones and Bartlett. Copyright 2005 by Jones and Bartlett. Adapted with permission.

Rehabilitation and Palliative Care

Rehabilitation is individualized and modified for each patient to provide optimum care. General rehabilitation goals are to improve ambulation, achieve weight-bearing and transfer ability, and restore bladder and bowel function, where possible (Weinstein, 2002). Achieving these goals is a multidisciplinary process, with nurses playing a key role in conjunction with physical and occupational therapy, social services, home health agencies, and patients and caregivers. After discharge home, healthcare professionals continue to monitor patients on a regular basis for pain control and functional status and assess them for signs of progressive disease or recurrent MSCC. Home visits from nurses and the pain team and physical or occupational therapy are necessary to assess patient and caregiver needs. During these visits, instruction is provided regarding pain management, mobility and weight bearing, safety measures and fall prevention, and regulation of bladder and bowel elimination. The physical and occupational therapists evaluate patients' functional abilities and need for assistive devices, such as a specialized hospital bed, wheelchair, or ramps in the home, and provide instruction in range-of-motion exercises, transfer methods, and use of assistive devices (Bucholtz, 1999; Osowski, 2002).

Following treatment for MSCC, patients' potential for regaining sexual function depends on the level and duration of the cord compression and whether sacral reflex pathways remain intact (Kazierad, 1998). Loss of bladder and bowel control, the presence of pain, and altered body image can greatly diminish libido. Nurses can help to promote dialogue between the affected partners and can discuss other methods of sharing physical intimacy, such as holding hands, cuddling, or giving gentle massages.

Nurses assist patients and caregivers in coping with patients' increasing dependence by encouraging them to express their feelings, fears, and concerns and support them in establishing realistic rehabilitation goals and accepting functional limitations. The appearance of MSCC is often an emblem of the cancer's progression and patients' approaching mortality. The nurse, who most likely has established a unique bond with the patients and caregivers, is the ideal healthcare provider to offer emotional support and referrals for professional assistance as they experience issues of loss and anticipatory grieving. Patients with irreversible or progressive neurologic deficits or those with end-stage disease may require more intensive nursing care and referral to hospice or comprehensive palliative homecare services to maintain their quality of life. Palliative care goals focus on relieving pain, making patients comfortable, preventing further injury, and managing bladder and bowel elimination. Caregivers coping with patients' neurologic decline are supported emotionally as they deal with losses and end-of-life issues (Bucholtz, 1999; Myers, 2001; Weinstein, 2002).

Patient and Caregiver Education

Educating patients and caregivers regarding recognition of the early signs and symptoms of MSCC is essential. Nurses should teach patients at high risk for cord compression—particularly those with known bone metastases, cancers of the lung, breast, or prostate, or lymphoma—the importance of promptly reporting all back pain, whether of new onset or changes in chronic back pain. Education emphasizes the need for reporting pain that is accompanied by sensory changes, especially if occurring in the lower extremities (Guberski & Belcher, 2005). Once the diagnosis of MSCC is made, teaching relating to treatment modalities, pain management, and safety and mobility issues is essential in helping patients and caregivers to adapt. Patients being discharged home and their caregivers must learn how to maintain the rehabilitation and strength-training regimen, and how to do urinary self-catheterization, if required. Pressure ulcer prevention measures, such as regular skin inspection, proper positioning, turning and transfer methods, and the use of skin-protecting products and pressure-reducing support surfaces are taught as indicated (Dawodu & Lorenzo, 2005). Patients and caregivers also receive instructions on medication schedules and side effects and the importance of keeping scheduled follow-up visits.

Conclusion

MSCC is a true oncologic emergency. Few conditions are as amenable to clinical improvement if managed promptly and appropriately or, conversely, have the potential for such dire consequences. Nurses caring for patients with cancer, especially those with known bone metastases, must maintain a high index of suspicion for this complication. Healthcare providers should regard the occurrence of new-onset back pain in patients with a known cancer history as a sign of possible spinal cord compression, even if the patient has had a long tumor-free interval since diagnosis. Prompt diagnosis and treatment may mean the difference between patients maintaining their functional independence and a reasonable quality of life or spending the remainder of their lives incapacitated and dependent on others.

References

Abrahm, J.L. (1999). Management of pain and spinal cord compression in patients with advanced cancer. ACP-ASIM End-of-Life Care Consensus Panel. American College of Physicians-American Society of Internal Medicine. *Annals of Internal Medicine, 131,* 37–46.

Abrahm, J.L. (2004). Assessment and treatment of patients with malignant spinal cord compression. *Journal of Supportive Oncology, 2,* 377–391.

American Spinal Injury Association. (2001). *ASIA impairment scale.* Retrieved July 29, 2005, from http://www.asia-spinalinjury.org/publications/2001_Classif_worksheet.pdf

Baehring, J.M. (2005). Spinal cord compression. In V.T. DeVita, S. Hellman, & S.A. Rosenberg (Eds.), *Cancer: Principles and practice of oncology* (7th ed., pp. 2287–2292). Philadelphia: Lippincott Williams & Wilkins.

Ballenger, S. (1991). Assessment of the nervous system. In D.D. Ignatavicius & M.V. Bayne (Eds.), *Medical-surgical nursing: A nursing process approach* (p. 835). Philadelphia: Saunders.

Batzdorf, U., & Haskell, C.M. (2001). Spinal cord: Natural history, diagnosis, and staging. In C.H. Haskell (Ed.), *Cancer treatment* (5th ed., pp. 1142–1145). Philadelphia: Saunders.

Behin, A., & Delattre, J.Y. (2004). Complications of radiation therapy on the brain and spinal cord. *Seminars in Neurology, 24,* 405–417.

Bilsky, M.H., Lis, E., Raizer, J., Lee, H., & Boland, P. (1999). The diagnosis and treatment of metastatic spinal tumor. *Oncologist, 4,* 459–469.

Bucholtz, J.D. (1999). Metastatic epidural cord compression. *Seminars in Oncology Nursing, 15,* 150–159.

Byrne, T.N. (1992). Spinal cord compression from epidural metastases. *New England Journal of Medicine, 327,* 614–619.

Camp-Sorrell, D. (1998). Clinical focus: Spinal cord compression. *Clinical Journal of Oncology Nursing, 2,* 112–113.

Coyle, N., & Foley, K.M. (1991). Alterations in comfort: Pain. In S.B. Baird, R. McCorkle, & M. Grant (Eds.), *Cancer nursing: A comprehensive textbook* (pp. 782–805). Philadelphia: Saunders.

Dawodu, S.T., & Lorenzo, N. (2005, August 9). *Cauda equina and conus medullaris syndromes.* Retrieved September 13, 2005, from http://www.emedicine.com/neuro/topic667.htm

DeAngelis, L.M., & Posner, J.B. (2003). Neurologic complications. In D.W. Kufe, R.E. Pollock, R.R. Weichselbaum, R.C. Bast, T. Gansler, J.F. Holland, et al. (Eds.), *Holland-Frei cancer medicine* (6th ed., pp. 2451–2467). Hamilton, Ontario, Canada: BC Decker.

Eakin, R. (2002). Bone emergencies. In P.G. Johnston & R.A.J. Spence (Eds.), *Oncologic emergencies* (pp. 175–198). Oxford, England: Oxford University Press.

Flaherty, A.M. (2005). Spinal cord compression. In C.H. Yarbro, M.H. Frogge, & M. Goodman (Eds.), *Cancer nursing: Principles and practice* (6th ed., pp. 910–924). Sudbury, MA: Jones and Bartlett.

Flounders, J.A., & Ott, B.B. (2003). Oncology emergency modules: Spinal cord compression [Online exclusive]. *Oncology Nursing Forum, 30,* E17–E21.

Forster, D.A. (1998). Spinal cord compression. In C.C. Chernecky & B.J. Berger (Eds.), *Advanced and critical care oncology nursing: Managing primary complications* (pp. 566–579). Philadelphia: Saunders.

Gabriel, K., & Schiff, D. (2004). Metastatic spinal cord compression by solid tumors. *Seminars in Neurology, 24,* 375–383.

Glick, J.H., & Glover, D. (1995). Oncologic emergencies. In G.P. Murphy, W. Lawrence, & E.L. Raymond (Eds.), *Clinical oncology* (2nd ed., pp. 597–618). Atlanta, GA: American Cancer Society.

Grandt, N.C. (2000). Spinal cord compression. In D. Camp-Sorrell & R.A. Hawkins (Eds.), *Clinical manual for the oncology advanced practice nurse* (pp. 799–804). Pittsburgh, PA: Oncology Nursing Society.

Guberski, T.D., & Belcher, A.E. (2005). Spinal cord compression. In P.G. Morton, D.K. Fontaine, C.M. Hudak, & B.M. Gallo (Eds.), *Critical care nursing: A holistic approach* (8th ed., pp. 1165–1167; 1171–1173). Philadelphia: Lippincott Williams & Wilkins.

Hatchett, R.J., & Kripas, C.J. (2002). Diagnostic imaging in oncologic emergencies. In S.C.J. Yeung & C.P. Escalante (Eds.), *Holland-Frei oncologic emergencies* (pp. 484–522). Hamilton, Ontario, Canada: BC Decker.

Heary, R.F., & Bono, C.M. (2001). Metastatic spinal tumors. *Neurosurgical Focus, 11*(6), Article 1. Retrieved June 20, 2005, from http://www.aans.org/education/journal/neurosurgical/dec01/11-6-1.pdf

Huff, S.J. (2005, March 24). *Neoplasms, spinal cord.* Retrieved April 5, 2005, from http://www.emedicine.com/med/topic337.htm

Jacobs, W.B., & Perrin, R.G. (2001). Evaluation and treatment of spinal metastases: An overview. *Neurosurgical Focus, 11*(6), Article 10. Retrieved June 20, 2005, from http://www.aans.org/education/journal/neurosurgical/dec01/11-6-10.pdf

Kazierad, D. (1998). Obstructive emergencies: Spinal cord compression. In B.L. Johnson & J. Gross (Eds.), *Handbook of oncology nursing* (3rd ed., pp. 631–644). Sudbury, MA: Jones and Bartlett.

Klimo, P., Jr., Kestle, J.R., & Schmidt, M.H. (2003). Treatment of metastatic spinal epidural disease: A review of the literature. *Neurosurgical Focus, 15*(5), Article 1. Retrieved June 20, 2005, from http://www.aans.org/education/journal/neurosurgical/nov03/15-5-1.pdf

Labovich, T.M. (1994). Selected complications in the patient with cancer: Spinal cord compression, malignant bowel obstruction, malignant ascites, and gastrointestinal bleeding. *Seminars in Oncology Nursing, 10,* 189–197.

Lamont, E.B., Rudin, C.M., & Hoffman, P.C. (2003). Diagnosis and management of oncologic emergencies. In E.E. Vokes & H.M. Golomb (Eds.), *Oncologic therapies* (2nd ed., pp. 108–114). New York: Springer.

Loblaw, D.A., & Laperriere, N.J. (1998). Emergency treatment of malignant extradural spinal cord compression: An evidence-based guideline. *Journal of Clinical Oncology, 16,* 1613–1633.

Loblaw, D.A., Perry, J., Chambers, A., & Laperriere, N.J. (2005). Systematic review of the diagnosis and management of malignant extradural spinal cord compression: The Cancer Care Ontario Practice Guidelines Initiative's Neuro-Oncology Disease Site Group. *Journal of Clinical Oncology, 23,* 2028–2037.

Lu, C., Gonzalez, R.G., Jolesz, F.A., Wen, P.Y., & Talcott, J. (2005). Suspected spinal cord compression in cancer patients: A multidisciplinary risk assessment. *Journal of Supportive Oncology, 3,* 305–312.

Manglani, H.H., Marco, R.A., Picciolo, A., & Healey, J.H. (2000). Orthopedic emergencies in cancer patients. *Seminars in Oncology, 27,* 299–310.

Manoso, M.W., & Healey, J.H. (2005). Metastatic cancer to bone. In V.T. DeVita, S. Hellman, & S.A. Rosenberg (Eds.), *Cancer: Principles and practice of oncology* (7th ed., pp. 2368–2381). Philadelphia: Lippincott Williams & Wilkins.

Manzullo, E.F., Rhines, L.D., & Forman, A.D. (2002). Neurologic emergencies. In S.C.J. Yeung & C.P. Escalante (Eds.), *Holland-Frei oncologic emergencies* (pp. 270–279). Hamilton, Ontario, Canada: BC Decker.

Maranzano, E., Trippa, F., Chirico, L., Basagni, M.L., & Rossi, R. (2003). Management of metastatic spinal cord compression. *Tumori, 89,* 469–475.

McClain, R.F., & Bell, G.B. (1998). Newer management options in patients with spinal metastasis. *Cleveland Clinic Journal of Medicine, 65,* 359–367.

Miaskowski, C. (1999). Spinal cord compression. In C. Miaskowski & P. Buchsel (Eds.), *Oncology nursing: Assessment and clinical care* (pp. 231–243). St. Louis, MO: Mosby.

Mueller, D.M. (2002, March 21). *Cervical conundrum: Neurologic examination.* Virtual Health Care Team. Retrieved June 20, 2005, from http://www.vhct.org/case1799/neurologic_examination.shtml

Myers, J.S. (2001). Oncologic complications. In S.E. Otto (Ed.), *Oncology nursing* (4th ed., pp. 498–581). St. Louis, MO: Mosby.

Osowski, M. (2002, October 14). Spinal cord compression: An obstructive oncologic emergency. *Topics in Advanced Practice Nursing eJournal, 2*(4). Retrieved April 14, 2005, from http://www.medscape.com/viewarticle/442735

Paice, J.A. (1999). Symptom management. In C. Miaskowski & P. Buchsel (Eds.), *Oncology nursing: Assessment and clinical care* (pp. 275–303). St. Louis, MO: Mosby.

Posner, J.B. (1995). *Neurologic complications of cancer.* Philadelphia: F.A. Davis.

Prasad, D., & Schiff, D. (2005). Malignant spinal cord compression. *Lancet Oncology, 6,* 15–24.

Quinn, J.A., & DeAngelis, L.M. (2000). Neurologic emergencies in the cancer patient. *Seminars in Oncology, 27,* 311–321.

Ruckdeschel, J.C. (2004). Spinal cord compression. In M.D. Abeloff, J.O. Armitage, J.E. Niederhuber, M.B. Kasten, & W.G. McKenna (Eds.), *Clinical oncology* (3rd ed., pp. 1063–1071). Philadelphia: Elsevier Churchill Livingstone.

Rude, M. (2000). Brain metastases and spinal cord compression. *Critical Care Nursing Clinics of North America, 12,* 269–279.

Ryken, T.C., Eichholz, K.M., Gerszten, P.C., Welch, W.C., Gokaslan, Z.L., & Resnick, D.K. (2003). Evidence-based review of the surgical management of vertebral column metastatic disease. *Neurosurgical Focus, 15*(5), Article 11. Retrieved June 20, 2005, from http://www.aans.org/education/journal/neurosurgical/nov03/15-5-11.pdf

Schiff, D. (2003). Spinal cord compression. *Neurology Clinics of North America, 21,* 67–86.

Schreiber, D. (2004, August 27). *Spinal cord injuries.* Retrieved April 5, 2005, from http://www.emedicine.com/emerg/topic553.htm

Schuster, J.M., & Grady, M.S. (2001). Medical management and adjuvant therapies in spinal metastatic disease. *Neurosurgical Focus, 11*(6), Article 3. Retrieved June 20, 2005, from http://www.aans.org/education/journal/neurosurgical/dec01/11-6-3.pdf

Sunderland, P.M. (1994). Structure and function of the nervous system. In K.L. McCance & S.E. Huether (Eds.), *Pathophysiology: The biologic basis for disease in adults and children* (2nd ed., pp. 397–436). St. Louis, MO: Mosby.

Talcott, J.A., Stomper, P.C., Drislane, F.W., Wen, P.Y., Block, C.C., Humphrey, C.C., et al. (1999). Assessing suspected spinal cord compression: A multidisciplinary outcomes analysis of 342 episodes. *Supportive Care in Cancer, 7,* 31–38.

Tharpar, K., & Laws, E.R. (1995). Tumors of the central nervous system. In G.P. Murphy, W. Lawrence, Jr., & R.E. Lenhard, Jr. (Eds.), *Clinical oncology* (2nd ed., pp. 406–410). Atlanta, GA: American Cancer Society.

Waller, A., & Caroline, N.L. (2000). *Handbook of palliative care in cancer* (2nd ed.). Boston: Butterworth-Heinemann.

Weinstein, S.H. (2002). Management of spinal cord and cauda equine compression. In A.M. Berger, R.K. Portenoy, & D.E. Weissman (Eds.), *Principles and practice of palliative care and supportive oncology* (2nd ed., pp. 532–543). Philadelphia: Lippincott Williams & Wilkins.

Wilkes, G.M. (1999). Neurological disturbances. In C.H. Yarbro, M.H. Frogge, & M. Goodman (Eds.), *Cancer symptom management* (2nd ed., pp. 344–381). Sudbury, MA: Jones and Bartlett.

Yalamanchili, M., & Lesser, G.J. (2003). Malignant spinal cord compression. *Current Treatment Options in Oncology, 4,* 509–516.

Elena Kuzin, RN, MSN, APRN,BC, AOCN®

⊃ Chapter 9

Superior Vena Cava Syndrome

Introduction

Superior vena cava syndrome (SVCS) is an uncommon problem, occurring in approximately 3%–4% of patients with cancer (Hemann, 2001). The superior vena cava (SVC), the major vein returning blood from the head, neck, upper extremities, and upper thorax to the right side of the heart, gradually may become obstructed or compressed by a variety of space-occupying lesions in the mediastinum. The presence of malignancy, especially locally advanced bronchogenic cancer, is the most common cause of obstruction, but thrombosis or tumor occurring within the lumen also may block the vessel (Flounders, 2003). Obstruction of the SVC causes venous congestion and increased venous pressure in the head, neck, upper extremities, and upper thorax and may restrict cardiac output. The resulting complex of symptoms and physical findings that develops is SVCS (DeMichele & Glick, 2001; Moore, 2005). Manifestations of the syndrome generally develop gradually but also may occur quickly. Although SVCS usually is not life threatening, it may become an oncologic emergency when SVC obstruction is severe and causes decreased cardiac filling, cerebral edema, respiratory distress, or upper airway tracheal obstruction (Aurora, Milite, & Vander Els, 2000; Moore; Pinover & Coia, 1998). Oncology nurses need to be aware of which patients are at risk for SVCS and be familiar with the early signs and symptoms. Prompt intervention may prevent SVCS from progressing to a life-threatening oncologic emergency.

Incidence

Annually, approximately 15,000 people in the United States develop SVC obstruction from a variety of causes (Wudel & Nesbitt, 2001). SVCS was first recognized in 1757 in a patient with a syphilitic aneurysm (Hunter, 1757) and has been associated over the centuries with cases of lung cancer (Rosenblatt, 1964). Before the mid-20th century, malignancy accounted for only about one-third of all cases of SVCS. Infectious conditions such as granulomatous infections secondary to tuberculosis, goiter, aortic aneurysms, or histoplasmo-sis-related mediastinal fibrosis caused by tuberculosis were responsible for the majority of cases (Aurora et al., 2000; Haapoja & Blendowski, 1999; Yahalom, 1997). Currently, with the development of successful treatments for these infections, mediastinal malignancies account for 70%–95% of the incidence of SVCS (Camp-Sorrell & Mayo, 1998; Markman, 1999). Figure 9-1 lists the etiologies associated with SVCS.

Figure 9-1. Causes of Superior Vena Cava Syndrome

Malignant (95%)	Nonmalignant (5%)
Small cell lung cancer	Indwelling central venous catheters
Non-small cell lung cancer	Benign tumor
Non-Hodgkin lymphoma (diffuse large cell, lymphoblastic)	Mediastinal fibrosis (tuberculosis, prior radiation therapy)
Esophageal carcinoma	Histoplasmosis
Thyroid carcinoma	Cardiac (aneurysm, arteriovenous fistula, pericarditis)
Breast carcinoma	
Thymoma	Sarcoidosis
Mesothelioma	Infection
Leukemia	Trauma

Note. Based on information from Camp-Sorrell & Mayo, 1998; Hunter, 1998.

The majority of cases arise from bronchogenic carcinoma (82%), particularly small cell lung cancer (SCLC) (65%–80%) and, less frequently, non-small cell lung cancer (NSCLC) (squamous cell carcinoma, adenocarcinoma). Lung cancers arising in the right lung carry the greatest risk for SVCS because of their proximity to the SVC, and these are associated with a fourfold greater incidence of SVCS than lesions on the left side of the chest (Escalante, 1993). SVCS occurs as the presenting feature of malignancy in 10% of patients who have SCLC and in approximately 2% of patients with NSCLC (Rowell & Gleeson, 2002). Lymphoma, primarily non-Hodgkin lymphoma (NHL), is the second most common malignancy associated with SVCS and accounts for 5%–15% of cases (Kreamer, 1998; Mack, 1997). SVCS is more likely to occur with the high-grade subtypes of NHL, such as diffuse large cell and lymphoblastic lymphoma, and rarely is seen with Hodgkin lymphoma, in spite of the high incidence of mediastinal involvement (Moore, 2005; Sitton, 2000).

The incidence of SVCS not directly related to cancer appears to be increasing (Mack, 1997). Nonmalignant conditions, such as intraluminal thrombus formation and external compression, may cause as many as

15%–22% of cases of SVCS (Kee et al., 1998; Yahalom, 1997). Thrombus formation related to vascular access devices, central venous monitoring catheters, and cardiac pacemaker electrodes account for 3%–5% of the incidence of SVCS.

Risk Factors

The major cause of SVCS is obstruction of upper central venous return to the heart by a mediastinal malignancy. The most common cause is SCLC, followed by squamous cell carcinoma and adenocarcinoma of the lung, NHL, and large cell lung cancer (Yellin, Rosen, Reichert, & Lieberman, 1990). In a significant number of cases (perhaps as many as 60%), SVCS is the presenting condition that leads to a diagnosis of cancer (Kreamer, 1998). Men between 50–70 years old who have mediastinal malignancies are at greater risk for SVCS (Flounders, 2003). Breast cancer metastatic to the mediastinum may be associated with SVCS, and, rarely, germ cell tumors, thymoma, and Kaposi sarcoma may cause the syndrome (Flounders; Mack, 1997). Less common causes include obstruction by a benign process, thrombosis of the SVC as a consequence of the placement of central venous catheters or pacemaker catheters (Yahalom, 1997), and mediastinal fibrosis, histoplasmosis, and thoracic aortic aneurysm (Kreamer).

Pathophysiology

Anatomy

The SVC is the major conduit for venous drainage from the head, neck, upper extremities, and upper thorax to the right atrium of the heart. It is located in the middle third of the right anterior superior mediastinum behind the sternum and is surrounded by such relatively rigid structures as the trachea, esophagus, right main bronchus, aorta, pulmonary artery, and vertebral bodies, as well as perihilar and paratracheal lymph nodes (see Figures 9-2 and 9-3). The SVC is a thin-walled, low-pressure (less than 5 mm Hg) vessel that is approximately 7 cm long and 1.5–2 cm wide and is formed by the junction of the left and right brachiocephalic veins in the middle third of the mediastinum and terminates in the right atrium. The SVC lies posterior to and to the right of the ascending aorta and is joined posteriorly by the azygos vein as it loops over the right mainstem bronchus. The mediastinal parietal pleura is lateral to the SVC, creating a confined space. The SVC is adjacent to several lymph node groups on the right, including the paratracheal, azygos, right hilar, and subcarinal lymph nodes. Blood flow through the SVC is at low pressure, a factor that may contribute to extrinsic compression and intraluminal thrombus formation (Abner, 1993).

Figure 9-2. Superior Vena Cava With Collateral Circulation

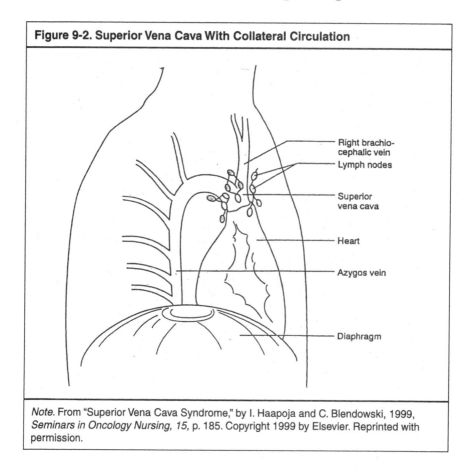

- Right brachio-cephalic vein
- Lymph nodes
- Superior vena cava
- Heart
- Azygos vein
- Diaphragm

Note. From "Superior Vena Cava Syndrome," by I. Haapoja and C. Blendowski, 1999, *Seminars in Oncology Nursing, 15,* p. 185. Copyright 1999 by Elsevier. Reprinted with permission.

Mechanisms of Superior Vena Cava Syndrome

Several features of the anatomy and location of the SVC render it particularly vulnerable to obstruction by any local space-occupying process. It has thin walls and low-pressure hemodynamics, so it collapses readily, and it is enclosed within a rigid anatomic compartment in the thorax, encircled by multiple lymph node chains. Its location in the right side of the superior mediastinum directly behind the sternum and adjacent to the right mainstem bronchus does not permit great flexibility when a space-occupying mediastinal lesion is present, such as expanding bronchogenic tumors, growing tumors within the mediastinal parietal pleura, and/or lymph nodes enlarged with disease (Yahalom, 1997). Metastasis to regional lymph nodes can obstruct the SVC through direct extension or extrinsic compression, resulting in congestion of the collateral veins of the neck, anterior chest wall, face, and right arm (Miaskowski, 1991).

Four mechanisms may cause SVCS: (a) occlusion by an extrinsic mass, (b) occlusion by direct tumor invasion through the vessel wall, (c) occlusion by a thrombus around a central venous catheter, and (d) occlusion by a thrombus occurring within the SVC (Miaskowski, 1991). Risk factors for thrombus formation include a hypercoagulable state induced by malignancy, intimal damage to the vein from central venous catheters, or venous stasis resulting from external compression to the SVC (Haapoja & Blendowski, 1999). Thrombosis is more likely to cause acute and complete obstruction of the SVC than tumor infiltration (Markman, 1999).

Partial or complete occlusion of the SVC (see Figure 9-3) results in an increase in venous pressure (venous hypertension) causing venous stasis and vein engorgement in the areas normally drained by the SVC. The rising venous pressure leads to third-spacing of fluid into adjacent tissue. *Third-spacing* refers to the accumulation of fluid that is unavailable to support the circulation but remains inside the body (Berkow & Fletcher, 1992). Fluid accumulation adds to the vena caval compression and may cause compression of other vital structures in the mediastinum, as well as pleural or pericardial effusion (Sitton, 2000). When the SVC is obstructed above the azygos vein, SVCS is less pronounced.

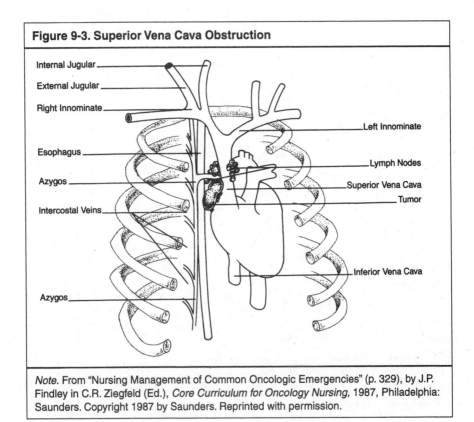

Figure 9-3. Superior Vena Cava Obstruction

Internal Jugular
External Jugular
Right Innominate
Esophagus
Azygos
Intercostal Veins
Azygos

Left Innominate
Lymph Nodes
Superior Vena Cava
Tumor
Inferior Vena Cava

Note. From "Nursing Management of Common Oncologic Emergencies" (p. 329), by J.P. Findley in C.R. Ziegfeld (Ed.), *Core Curriculum for Oncology Nursing,* 1987, Philadelphia: Saunders. Copyright 1987 by Saunders. Reprinted with permission.

The azygos vein is a major auxiliary vessel of the SVC and returns venous blood to the heart from the compensatory collateral circulation system that develops in the upper body. The azygos system can distend easily and accommodate the shunted blood so that the venous pressure does not increase greatly in the head, arms, and upper thorax (Markman, 1999). If SVC obstruction occurs below the azygos vein, more severe manifestations of SVCS develop.

Venous pressure is higher below the azygos arch, and blood flow back to the heart is more circuitous and complex. With lower SVC obstruction, the collateral circulation returns blood to the heart via the upper abdominal veins and inferior vena cava, requiring higher venous pressure. The resulting venous congestion may lead to laryngeal and cerebral edema, progressing to stupor, convulsions, and coma (Markman, 1999).

The degree of obstruction of the SVC may vary greatly depending on the nature of the obstruction and its rate of change. The development of collateral circulation to return blood to the right atrium correlates with the extent of SVC obstruction and the patency of the azygos pathways, which often become the most common venous collateral route. If the azygos route is obstructed along with the SVC, then other interconnected venous routes become more developed, including the internal mammary, lateral thoracic and superficial thoracoabdominal veins, and the vertebral venous plexus (Moore, 2005). Stanford and Doty (1986) used venography patterns to classify individuals with SVCS into four categories (types I through IV) based on the severity of obstruction and the extent of collateral venous circulation (see Figure 9-4). Types III and IV categories account for 85% of compromise symptoms (Stanford & Doty).

Clinical Manifestations

The clinical presentation of SVCS can be acute or subacute. Initial signs and symptoms may be vague and barely noticeable or may develop rapidly.

Figure 9-4. Classification of Superior Vena Cava Obstruction

Type I: Partial superior vena cava (SVC) obstruction (0%–90% stenosis); azygos/right atrial pathway is not obstructed and blood flow is in the normal direction.

Type II: 90%–100% SVC obstruction; patency and normal direction of blood flow in the azygos/right atrial pathway

Type III: 90%–100% SVC obstruction; reversal of azygos blood flow; blood flow in the inferior vena cava

Type IV: Complete obstruction of the SVC and one or more of the major vena cava tributaries, including the azygos systems; blood flow in the inferior vena cava

Note. Based on information from Stanford & Doty, 1986.

Approximately 20%–31% of patients with SVCS present with symptoms of less than two weeks' duration; 31%–35% report experiencing symptoms for three to four weeks; and 27% have symptoms for five weeks or longer (Yahalom, 1997). If the SVC obstruction is gradual and slowly progressive, symptoms may have a slow onset because of the development of collateral circulation that compensates for the obstruction (Stewart, 1996). The rapidity of the onset of symptoms is a crucial factor in determining the patient's level of comfort and safety. The more rapid the onset of SVCS, the more severe the patient's signs and symptoms because collateral veins do not have time to distend to accommodate an increased blood flow. Rapid onset of obstruction may lead to a very dramatic and potentially life-threatening presentation of SVCS. Intravascular thrombosis may be associated with rapid onset of symptoms (Moore, 2005). Early recognition and treatment of SVCS may prevent its progression to life-threatening respiratory and cerebral complications (Abner, 1993; Haapoja & Blendowski, 1999; Hunter, 1998; Markman, 1999; Sitton, 2000; Yahalom).

SVCS that develops gradually over time results in subtle signs of edema and venous engorgement (see Figure 9-5). Patients frequently report mild dyspnea, nonproductive cough, a sense of "fullness" in the head, chest pain, and occasionally dysphagia. Patients often notice increased symptoms in the morning after sleeping in a supine position or with position changes such as bending forward, coughing, or stooping (Martini, 1998; Wudel & Nesbitt, 2001). Patients may experience facial, neck, or arm swelling upon arising in the morning, causing shirt collars to become tight (Stoke sign). The veins in the neck and upper body may become distended because of venous congestion. Women may experience swelling in the breasts or fingers and have difficulty removing rings. Mild symptoms may disappear after patients have been upright for several hours as gravity reduces the edema in the face and upper body (Kreamer, 1998). Many patients may need to sleep in an upright position for comfort (Escalante, 1993). Chest pain or discomfort also may be present (Flounders, 2003; Moore, 2005; Sitton, 2000).

Figure 9-5. Signs and Symptoms of Superior Vena Cava Syndrome (In Order of Frequency)

Signs	Symptoms
• Dyspnea	• Venous distension of the neck
• Facial and neck swelling (Stoke sign)	• Venous distension of the chest wall
• Sensation of fullness in the head	• Facial edema
• Cough	• Cyanosis
• Arm swelling	• Plethora of the face
• Chest pain	• Edema of the arms
• Dysphagia	• Vocal cord paralysis
	• Horner syndrome

Note. Based on information from Yahalom, 1997.

The late signs and symptoms associated with SVCS may be severe and life threatening (see Figure 9-6). Dysphagia and hoarseness may develop related to a paralyzed true vocal cord caused by recurrent laryngeal nerve (cranial nerve X) entrapment or involvement by lymph nodes (Moore, 2005). Evidence of increased intracranial pressure may be manifested by headache, dizziness, and visual disturbances. Patients may experience irritability and mental status changes such as anxiety or lethargy related to cerebral edema (Gao & Shannon, 2002).

Figure 9-6. Late Physical Signs and Symptoms of Superior Vena Cava Syndrome

- Cyanosis of the face and upper torso
- Decreased or absent peripheral pulses
- Congestive heart failure
- Decreased blood pressure
- Chest pain
- Mental status changes (confusion, changes in level of consciousness, stupor, coma)
- Tachypnea/tachycardia/orthopnea
- Engorged conjunctiva/orbital edema
- Visual disturbances
- Syncope
- Dysphagia
- Hoarseness caused by paralysis of true vocal cord
- Stridor

Note. Based on information from Sitton, 2000.

Patient Assessment

History

SVCS may be the initial presentation of malignancy or may develop in patients with a known cancer history. A complete patient history and physical examination will help to reveal the cause, severity, and duration of symptoms (Sitton, 2000). Because SVCS most frequently is associated with lung cancer, clinicians should question patients with no known cancer history about smoking habits or other risk factors for lung cancer, such as exposure to carcinogens in the environment or at work, or previous radiation to the mediastinum (Kreamer, 1998; Moore, 2005). Patients with a previously diagnosed malignancy, such as bronchogenic cancer or lymphoma, and/or metastatic disease are at increased risk for SVCS (Loney, 1998). Healthcare providers should assess patients for the presence of a central venous catheter or pacemaker (Camp-Sorrell & Mayo, 1998). During insertion of the vascular access device, the wall of the vena cava may have been injured, resulting in thrombus formation, or the device may cause irritation during chemotherapy infusions (Moore). Assessment should include questions about patients' cardiac history, because those with preexisting coronary disease, hypertension, or heart failure may be at increased risk for SVCS, possibly because of increased strain on the cardiovascular system (Loney).

Physical Examination

The classic signs and symptoms of SVCS (see Figure 9-5) are so specific to the syndrome and so uncommon to other conditions that clinicians often can make the diagnosis by clinical examination alone. Although pericardial tamponade and congestive heart failure may produce similar signs and symptoms, physical examination quickly can exclude both conditions (Pierson, 1991).

Early Physical Signs

A prominent venous pattern with dilated veins of the face, neck, thorax, breasts, and upper extremities typically is present with SVCS and may be accompanied by edema in those areas. Patients may have facial plethora, a ruddy complexion of the face or cheeks. They also may experience jugular vein distension, periorbital edema, and edema of the conjunctivae. Blood pressure often is high in the upper extremities and low in the legs. Compensatory tachycardia may exist. Horner syndrome, manifested by unilateral drooping eyelid (ptosis), constricted pupil, and lack of sweating (anhydrosis) on one side of the forehead because of pressure on the cervical sympathetic nerves, also may be present (Baker & Barnes, 1992; Escalante, 1993; Haapoja & Blendowski, 1999; Hunter, 1998; Kreamer, 1998; Yahalom, 1997).

Late Physical Signs

Late physical signs (see Figure 9-6) of SVCS develop in fewer than 2% of cases and appear more commonly in patients with rapidly progressive, severe SVCS. Stridor is an ominous sign and indicates severe airway compromise and impending respiratory failure (Gao & Shannon, 2002). Patients may have progressive cyanosis and edema of the face or upper torso, orbital edema, and engorged conjunctivae, presenting the appearance of a "purple frog" (Kreamer, 1998). They also may experience absence of peripheral pulses, decreased blood pressure, and syncope. Manifestations of respiratory distress, such as orthopnea, tachypnea, or tachycardia, may be present. Cerebral or laryngeal edema may occur, characterized by changes in mental status and vision, syncope, seizures, and coma. If left untreated, tracheal obstruction and/or brain herniation will result in death (Escalante, 1993; Sitton, 2000).

Prognosis

The prognosis for survival depends on how rapidly SVC obstruction develops, the degree of vena caval blockage, and the adequacy of collateral circulation (Yahalom, 1997). For patients with SVCS secondary to malignancy, survival varies depending on the histologic type of the tumor. The average life expectancy of patients with SVCS is 3–10 months (Marcy et al., 2001). Patients with cancer diagnosed with SVCS do not die of the syndrome itself but of the extent of their underlying disease. The median survival for patients presenting with SVCS is 46 weeks. The median survival in patients who receive no therapy or who develop mentation changes and airway compromise is only six weeks (Wudel & Nesbitt, 2001).

Diagnostic Evaluation

Imaging

Chest x-ray, magnetic resonance imaging (MRI), and computed tomography (CT) of the chest, as well as contrast venography, confirm the diagnosis of SVCS. Figure 9-7 depicts a decision tree for the diagnosis and management

Figure 9-7. Decision Tree for Superior Vena Cava Syndrome (SVCS)

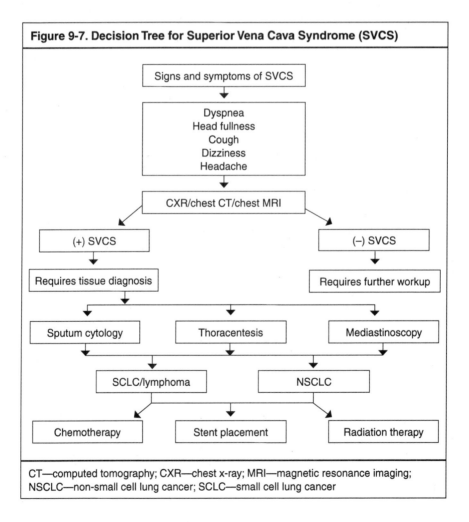

CT—computed tomography; CXR—chest x-ray; MRI—magnetic resonance imaging; NSCLC—non-small cell lung cancer; SCLC—small cell lung cancer

of SVCS. Typically, a mass exists in the superior mediastinum, right hilum or perihilar region, or right upper lobe. Hilar adenopathy is present in 50% of patients with SVCS, and pleural effusions in 25% of patients (Markman, 1999). More than 60% of patients with SVCS have a widening of the mediastinum, most commonly on the right side, caused by a space-occupying lesion, or dilated SVC and collateral veins, which is evident on chest x-ray (Murray, Steward, & Johnson, 1995).

CT scans, especially contrast-enhanced spiral or helical CT scan, are the most useful radiographic tools for diagnosing SVCS. Recent advances in CT technology have expanded its role in determining the location and extent of thrombi, vascular compression and invasion, and pathways of venous circulation, including collaterals. CT scans permit visualization of the thoracic anatomy, specifically the size and location of the tumor relative to the SVC, trachea, and heart (Stewart, 1996). CT also is used to localize a tumor for CT-guided biopsy and to determine radiation treatment fields (Moore, 2005).

MRI also may function as a noninvasive diagnostic tool (Sitton, 2000). It can provide greater detail than CT scan regarding mediastinal structures in multiple planes. Although MRI has a 96% sensitivity rate for the detection of SVC obstruction, it has a longer scanning time and an increased cost (Nesbitt, 1996).

Contrast venography involves the injection of contrast material via the antecubital veins, providing a venogram of the mediastinal blood vessels. This provides the most detailed information regarding the patency of the vena cava, whether the obstruction is extrinsic or intrinsic, the presence and degree of thrombosis, and the adequacy of collateral circulation (Escalante, 1993; Nesbitt, 1996; Rowell & Gleeson, 2002).

Tissue Diagnosis

Definitive, histopathologic diagnosis of the underlying condition causing SVCS is essential to providing optimal treatment (Pierson, 1991). To obtain a tissue diagnosis, clinicians should use the least invasive method. Sputum cytology identifies the underlying cancer in 50% of cases; thoracentesis for pleural effusion will establish the diagnosis of cancer in 70% of cases (O'Brien, 1996). Clinicians should perform mediastinoscopy when necessary to establish a histologic diagnosis when less-invasive procedures have been unsuccessful. Although previously contraindicated in patients with SVCS because of the risk of hemorrhage, mediastinoscopy has been performed safely with few complications (Jahangiri, Taggart, & Goldstraw, 1993; Nesbitt, 1996; Urban et al., 1993).

Treatment Modalities

SVCS is a true emergency when it develops acutely, and patients require prompt relief of the obstruction. Overall, the treatment plan selected depends on the etiology of the SVCS, the severity of the symptoms, the patients' prognosis, the underlying malignancy, and the presence or absence of intraluminal thrombosis. Treatment is centered on relieving the obstruction and its symptoms and controlling the underlying disease. The goal of treatment is cure when the primary disease is SCLC, NHL, or a germ cell tumor (Flounders, 2003). Healthcare providers most often treat SVCS secondary to the presence of cancer with combination chemotherapy and/or radiation therapy. Other treatment options include surgery, intravascular stent placement, and systemic corticosteroids.

Radiation Therapy

Radiation therapy is the traditional gold standard for treating SVCS caused by NSCLC and has been advocated for the treatment of SVCS caused by any malignancy (Haapoja & Blendowski, 1999; Hunter, 1998; Yahalom, 1997). The tumor type, extent of disease, history of previous radiation in the area, and the patient's performance status determine the radiation dose. Radiation fields for mediastinal treatment generally include mediastinal, hilar, and supraclavicular lymph nodes and any adjacent lung lesions (Emani & Graham, 1998). Patients usually receive radiation therapy five days a week, Monday through Friday. The total dose to be delivered is divided into daily dose amounts, which are given until patients have reached the prescribed dose. Before radiation therapy begins, a treatment planning session called a *simulation* is completed. Figure 9-8 shows an x-ray depicting the radiation treatment field for a patient with SVCS. If the radiation is three-dimensional or intensity-modulated radiation therapy, clinicians perform a planning CT scan. With the assistance of physicists and dosimetrists, the radiation oncologist outlines the treatment volume, and the treatment plan is specified. This process takes one to two weeks, after which the patient returns to the radiation department for a filming session where the plan is confirmed with the patient on the treatment machine in the treatment position. At this point, radiation therapy can begin. Figure 9-9 is a photo of a patient on the radiation treatment table showing the treatment position for daily radiation therapy for SVCS.

Currently, no standards regarding doses and schedules of radiotherapy exist for SVCS. High-dose fractions of 300–400 cGy for the first two to four radiation treatments have been used to try to obtain faster symptom relief, followed by standard daily dose fractions of 180–200 cGy (Schafer, 1997; Yahalom, 1997). However, researchers have not noted greater improvement in the response of SVCS with the high doses (Chan et al., 1997), and some investigators have recommended standard fractionation throughout the treatment (Wurschmidt, Bunemann, & Heilman, 1995). In general, radiation therapy doses range from 3,000 cGy in 10 fractions (300 cGy a day) to 5,000 cGy in 25 fractions (200 cGy/day) (Abner, 1993) but may be as high as 6,000–7,000 cGy in six to seven weeks. *Hypofractionated radiation therapy*, when higher doses of radiation therapy are delivered over a shorter period of time,

Figure 9-8. X-Ray of Treatment Field for Superior Vena Cava Syndrome

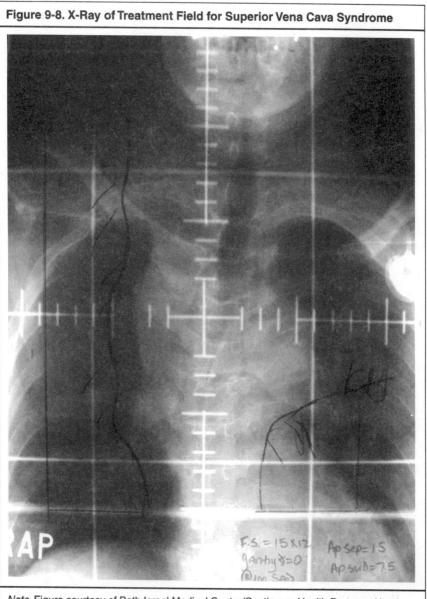

Note. Figure courtesy of Beth Israel Medical Center/Continuum Health Partners. Used with permission.

has shown benefit. Such treatment delivered weekly at a single dose of 800 cGy to a total of 2,400 cGy has resulted in complete resolution of symptoms in more than 50% of patients (Rodrigues, Njo, & Karim, 1993). One study demonstrated that a palliative regimen of two 600-cGy fractions given one

---

Figure 9-9. Photo of Patient in Treatment Position for Superior Vena Cava Syndrome

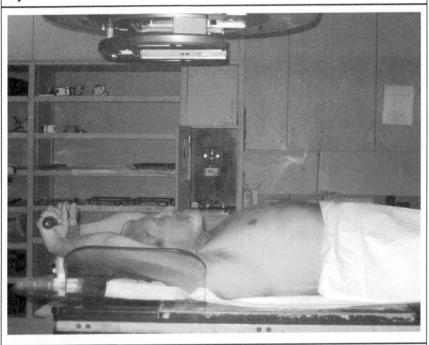

Note. Figure courtesy of Beth Israel Medical Center/Continuum Health Partners. Used with permission.

---

week apart for SVCS in an older adult population had an overall response rate of 87% (Lonardi, Gioga, Agus, Coeli, & Campostrini, 2002).

Radiotherapy may be used for local control following chemotherapy in patients with large cell lymphoma and large mediastinal masses (Murray et al., 1995). Lymphomas are generally very radiosensitive tumors and may require less radiation than other tumor types. For the treatment of lymphoma with curative intent, 3,500–4,500 cGy given in fractions of 180–200 cGy over four to five weeks is commonly recommended (Connors, Klimo, Fairey, & Voss, 1987; Haskell, 2001; Hoppe, 1994).

Good to excellent relief of SVCS symptoms occurs in approximately 70% of patients with lung cancer and 95% of patients with lymphoma (Emani & Graham, 1998). Most will experience symptom relief within two weeks of starting radiation therapy, with maximum relief at three weeks (Nicholson, Ettles, & Arnold, 1997). Improvement in venous congestion and upper extremity edema may occur in 7–19 days. Patients who achieved symptomatic relief within 30 days had a significantly better survival rate than those who did not (Escalante, 1993).

The potential side effects of radiation delivered to the mediastinum are related to the total dose, the fraction dose, the amount of normal tissue in the radiation field, and whether concomitant chemotherapy is part of the treatment regimen. Early side effects that may occur during or shortly after radiation therapy include fatigue, cough, nausea, dysphagia, heartburn, and skin irritation or erythema (Moore, 2005). More serious treatment-related complications are rare but include bleeding or SVC perforation (Escalante, 1993). Delayed side effects that may occur months after radiation include pneumonitis, pulmonary fibrosis, esophageal ulceration or stenosis, cardiac changes, spinal cord myelopathy, and brachial plexopathy (Sitton, 2000).

Chemotherapy

Combination chemotherapy is the primary treatment for SVCS caused by highly chemosensitive malignancies, such as SCLC and NHL (Flounders, 2003; Kreamer, 1998). More than 80% of patients with SCLC and SVCS will demonstrate good response to treatment with chemotherapy alone (Wurschmidt et al., 1995). A meta-analysis of lung cancer trials that included data analysis for patients with SVC obstruction revealed that chemotherapy relieved SVC obstruction in 77% of patients (N = 286); radiation relieved SVC obstruction in 78% of patients (N = 183); and combined chemotherapy and radiation therapy relieved obstruction in 83% of patients (N = 18) (Rowell & Gleeson, 2002). In general, SVCS caused by cancers that are sensitive to both chemotherapy and radiation will respond quickly to both treatment modalities. Patients treated with chemotherapy usually will experience symptom relief within 7–14 days (Flounders). Alleviation of symptoms will take longer for those with less sensitive solid tumors (Moore, 2005). NSCLC is not chemosensitive, so the recommended initial treatment is radiation therapy (Mack, 1997).

Combination chemotherapy regimens used to treat SCLC may include cisplatin or carboplatin, etoposide, ifosfamide, cyclophosphamide, doxorubicin, and vincristine. Taxanes, gemcitabine, and vinorelbine also may create a response in SCLC (Moore, 2005). Regimens for treating NHL are selected based on the histologic subtype and disease stage. Treatment may involve cyclophosphamide or fludarabine as single-agent drugs or may use combinations of cyclophosphamide, doxorubicin, vincristine, and prednisone (Flounders, 2003). Neoadjuvant chemotherapy may be administered to shrink extensive tumor in the mediastinum prior to starting radiotherapy, allowing smaller subsequent radiation fields to be used and sparing normal lung tissue (Moore). In patients who have already had prior mediastinal irradiation, chemotherapy alone is the treatment of choice.

Routes for administering chemotherapy to patients with SVCS need to be carefully planned. The venous stasis in the upper thorax that accompanies SVCS may cause chemotherapy drugs to become locally concentrated if they are infused into the upper extremities. Peripheral infusion into the lower extremities also is to be avoided because of the risk of extravasation with irritant and vesicant drugs. A long-term venous access catheter may need to be placed into the inferior vena cava through the femoral vein for safe drug administration (Moore, 2005).

Combination chemotherapy with radiotherapy may result in quicker symptomatic relief of SCLC-associated SVCS and has been associated with increased survival (Murray et al., 1995). When the two therapies are combined, the severity of side effects increases because the chemotherapy potentiates the radiation effects (Emani & Graham, 1998). Patients need nursing management to monitor for myelosuppression, nausea, vomiting, infection, stomatitis, esophagitis, and skin breakdown.

Surgery

Surgical interventions for malignancy-induced SVCS are rare because of limited success and high morbidity. Surgery usually is considered only for those patients who have not had symptom relief with antitumor therapies or other measures (Flounders, 2003; Kreamer, 1998). Vascular bypass surgery to create a circulatory route around the SVC obstruction to the right atrium may be done using autologous saphenous veins, synthetic materials, or the autologous pericardium. These interventions often fail secondary to thrombosis of the surgically created graft (Abner, 1993). At the present time, surgical bypass grafts are considered only for those patients with acute cerebral or laryngeal edema; extensive thrombosis of the SVC and inadequate collateral circulation; tumors that can be completely excised and the SVC grafted; or patients in whom a tissue diagnosis cannot be obtained without surgical mediastinal exploration (Baker & Barnes, 1992).

Stent Placement

In recent years, the use of intravascular stents has been increasing in the management of malignancy-induced SVCS. Analysis of several studies revealed that the use of percutaneously placed intravascular stents was effective in reopening the occluded SVC in more than 90% of patients and resulted in complete or partial relief of symptoms in 68%–100% of patients (Hochrein, Bashore, O'Laughlin, & Harrison, 1998; Rowell & Gleeson, 2002). Stenting has shown equal symptom relief in comparison to chemotherapy and radiotherapy, especially with tumors that are not sensitive to those modalities (Moore, 2005). The procedure has been advocated as the first choice for palliative treatment of SVCS because it does not preclude the use of subsequent chemotherapy or radiotherapy and provides immediate and dramatic relief of symptoms (Lanciego et al., 2001). Following stent insertion, relief of headache is immediate, and most other symptoms, such as edema of the face and arms, disappear within 24–72 hours (Rowell & Gleeson). In contrast, the effectiveness of chemotherapy or radiotherapy in relieving SVCS may not become apparent for three to four weeks (Lanciego et al.). Stents are not used when SVCS is caused by tumor invading the vessel wall (Moore).

Stent placement takes approximately two hours and generally is performed under local anesthesia by an interventional radiologist. The approach for stent placement may be through the basilic or subclavian veins or the femoral vein or others if necessary (Hochrein et al., 1998; Lanciego et al., 2001). The stents are constructed of cylindrically shaped, self-expandable, stainless steel wire that can be compressed and introduced into the obstructed area through an 8–12 Fr catheter. The stent is then released from the catheter and reexpands, causing dilation of the SVC. Balloon angioplasty through the stent is sometimes necessary to obtain complete expansion (Dyet, Nicholson, & Cook, 1993). Blood flow in the SVC is under low pressure and may contribute to clot formation in the stented area, so patients usually receive heparin during the procedure. Oral anticoagulation therapy with warfarin (1 mg/day) may follow for three to six months to prevent thrombus formation, although this practice is controversial because of the risk of hemorrhage (Kreamer, 1998; Moore, 2005). Thrombus formation occurs in 30%–50% of patients with SVCS and can create confusion about the cause of SVCS (Stewart, 1996). If a thrombus is exacerbating SVCS, stent placement combined with thrombolytic therapy may help to lyse the clot (Haapoja & Blendowski, 1999).

Complications of SVC stenting include stent thrombosis, migration of the stent, and cardiac decompensation during the stenting procedure (Rowell & Gleeson, 2002). Nursing care after stent placement includes monitoring for potential complications, such as groin hematoma or infection and femoral deep vein thrombosis. Nurses should check vital signs regularly and give analgesics as ordered.

Medication Management

Supportive medical management may be used when symptoms of SVCS are minimal and adequate collateral circulation is present. Patients may receive oxygen to relieve dyspnea, and analgesics and tranquilizers to relieve chest pain and allay the anxiety that they experience with respiratory distress. Loop diuretics (furosemide) may be administered to reduce edema and fluid retention. However, they may cause dehydration, which could contribute to thrombus formation, as well as cause hypovolemia, which could further compromise venous return to the heart (Kreamer, 1998). Treatment may include steroids to reduce the respiratory inflammation that occurs in reaction to tumor and radiation therapy, although no evidence exists to support their use. Steroids are useful when SVCS is caused by lymphoma, which is very responsive to corticosteroid treatment, but are of limited value when the etiology is lung cancer (Aurora et al., 2000).

Patients with cancer frequently have an indwelling central venous access device (VAD), and this technology has contributed to an increased frequency of nonmalignant causes of SVCS over the past two decades (Wudel & Nesbitt,

2001). VAD catheter–induced intraluminal thrombus formation is treated with IV infusion of a thrombolytic agent through the catheter itself or through a peripheral site to try to lyse the clot, followed by heparin anticoagulation to prevent reembolization (Kreamer, 1998; Moore, 2005). Initiation of treatment with thrombolytics should occur within five to seven days of the onset of symptoms for maximum effectiveness (Aurora et al., 2000). Streptokinase, urokinase, and recombinant tissue plasminogen activator (rt-PA) are approved for this purpose. Studies have reported urokinase to be more effective than streptokinase and as having a lower incidence of bleeding and allergic and febrile reactions (Kreamer; Yahalom, 1997). Administration of rt-PA is associated with increased febrile reactions and serious adverse effects, such as anaphylaxis and angioedema. Emergency equipment should be available in the event of anaphylaxis, and clinicians should monitor all patients for signs of bleeding (Moore).

Nursing Management

Nursing interventions focus on assessing patients' clinical condition, instituting measures to relieve symptoms, monitoring response to treatment and side effects, and providing comfort measures and reassurance while treatment is under way (see Table 9-1). Baseline nursing assessment includes monitoring vital signs, physical appearance, level of consciousness, tissue perfusion and edema, respiratory status, functional status, emotional status, and activity endurance level (Haapoja & Blendowski, 1999; Hunter, 1998). Emergency intervention is necessary for any symptoms of airway obstruction, cerebral edema (mental status and neurologic changes), or decreased cardiac output (Moore, 2005).

Assessment of the respiratory system includes monitoring oxygen saturation by pulse oximeter and observing for signs of respiratory distress, such as cyanosis, hoarseness, stridor, dyspnea, tachypnea, and cough (Sitton, 2000). Measures to relieve respiratory distress take priority. The use of supplemental oxygen, bed rest with the head of the bed upright in a Fowler or semi-Fowler position to promote venous drainage, and activity restrictions to decrease energy expenditure may relieve dyspnea (Kreamer, 1998; Mack, 1997; Moore, 2005). Nurses should instruct patients about how gravity and upright positioning helps to relieve venous congestion in the upper body. Providing reassurance and emotional support and a calm, restful environment may help to allay anxiety and reduce oxygen requirements.

Assessment of the cardiac system includes monitoring for tachycardia, dysrhythmias, and hypotension (Sitton, 2000). Nurses monitor patients' fluid and electrolyte status. Overhydration may exacerbate symptoms of SVCS, and dehydration, especially if patients are receiving diuretics and are on a low-salt diet, can increase the risk of thrombosis (Mack, 1997). Clinicians should avoid using the upper extremities for blood pressure measurements and veni-

---

Table 9-1. Overview of Nursing Management for Superior Vena Cava Syndrome (SVCS)

Problem	Intervention
Respiratory/cardiac compromise	• Assess respiratory system (cyanosis, hoarseness, stridor, orthopnea, dyspnea, tachypnea, cough, rales/rhonchi). • Maintain airway. • Administer oxygen/monitor oxygen saturation. • Monitor for signs of increased respiratory distress. • Administer respiratory medications as needed. • Assess cardiac system (tachycardia, dysrhythmias, hypotension, reduced pulse quality). • Check vital signs every four hours until stable. • Situate in the Fowler or semi-Fowler position to maximize respiratory effort. • Limit physical activity by assisting with activities of daily living. • Administer cough medication as needed. • Maintain hydration.
Neurologic compromise	• Assess central nervous system (CNS) (altered mental status, lethargy, headache, vomiting, visual changes). • Administer corticosteroids for cerebral edema.
Anxiety	• Position call bell within easy reach, and provide frequent reassurance of staff availability. • Maintain a calm, restful environment. • Assess for and administer anxiolytics/mild sedatives.
Circulatory compromise	• Remove rings and restrictive clothing. • Avoid upper extremities for venipuncture and for administration of IV medications. • Take vital signs in lower extremities. • Monitor for excessive bleeding after invasive procedures in areas of venous engorgement. • Assess skin integrity in edematous areas.
Metabolic/electrolyte disturbances	• Record daily weights. • Record intake/output. • Check urine for steroid-induced glycosuria. • Evaluate for muscle weakness. • Administer diuretics and fluids. • Monitor for euphoria, mood swings, or other signs of CNS stimulation. • Monitor laboratory values (complete blood count, arterial blood gases) and examinations (chest x-ray, scans). • Monitor for signs and symptoms of hyponatremia: listlessness, mental confusion, loss of skin turgor, postural hypotension. • Monitor for signs and symptoms of hypokalemia: muscle weakness, decreased bowel sounds, depression, cardiac arrhythmias, tetany.

(Continued on next page)

Table 9-1. Overview of Nursing Management for Superior Vena Cava Syndrome (SVCS) *(Continued)*

Problem	Intervention
Patient safety	• Provide for environmental safety (bed in low position, side rails up, call light and personal items within reach). • Assist with ambulation as needed.
Emotional/psychological concerns	• Provide brief explanations of planned procedures and treatments. • Provide a forum for expression of concerns, fears, and feelings regarding the situation. • Reduce fatigue. • Administer analgesics for comfort. • Reassure that alterations in appearance will resolve with successful therapy.
Patient/family education	• Instruct in self-care management. • Educate about treatment and side-effect management in clear, simple terms. • Instruct in energy conservation techniques. • Educate regarding bleeding precautions. • Teach relaxation techniques. • Instruct in avoidance of Valsalva maneuver (as well as bending, stooping, coughing, lying flat), which increases intracranial pressure. • Instruct regarding signs and symptoms of recurrent SVCS.

Note. Based on information from Kreamer, 1998; Sitton, 2000.

punctures; they should use the lower extremities. IV administration of drugs or chemotherapy agents may need to be given through a femoral or central venous line with the tip past the point of obstruction (Moore, 2005). Rings and restrictive clothing should be removed from the upper extremities.

Central nervous system assessment is vital. Changes in mental status such as lethargy, headache, and vomiting should be reported immediately, as they may indicate cerebral edema caused by lack of oxygen to the brain. Nurses should instruct patients to avoid the Valsalva maneuver, which is elicited by bending, stooping, lying flat, coughing, or straining at stool, because this only serves to increase intracranial pressure, which may exacerbate SVCS symptoms (Sitton, 2000). Cough suppressants and/or stool softeners may be indicated.

Nursing intervention for patients undergoing definitive therapies to negate SVCS centers on monitoring for treatment effectiveness and the potential side effects of chemotherapy and radiation therapy, including myelosuppression, nausea, vomiting, infection, stomatitis, esophagitis, and skin reactions (Moore, 2005). Patients who have surgical stents placed are provided with postoperative care and are monitored for signs of blood loss. The extent of the venous engorgement in the area can contribute to excessive bleeding following invasive procedures (Kreamer, 1998). Patients are monitored for effectiveness and side effects of drugs that they may receive, such as corticosteroids, diuretics, thrombolytics, and anticoagulants.

Some patients find the change in their appearance caused by facial and periorbital edema and plethora ("purple frog" appearance) to be very distressing and need reassurance that these changes will disappear with effective treatment (Kreamer, 1998). Patients may receive analgesics and anxiolytics as ordered to reduce discomfort and help them to cope with their situation until treatments produce an effect (Moore, 2005). Nurses must provide emotional support and assist with relaxation techniques during this period (Sitton, 2000).

Patient and Caregiver Education

For some patients, the appearance of SVCS is the first indication that they have cancer. They and their caregivers require education and support as they learn to cope with the diagnosis and symptoms and understand the treatments. Patients who have responded well to interventions to control the underlying malignancy will have rapid resolution of symptoms. No long-term special care is needed after the symptoms have resolved (Mack, 1997). Discharge planning from the hospital or care in outpatient settings includes educating patients and their caregivers regarding treatment goals and self-care measures at home. Nurses should provide instructions for recognizing the signs and symptoms of recurrent SVCS and the importance of prompt reporting if they appear. Patients and caregivers learn strategies for managing side effects of radiation and/or chemotherapy, along with energy conservation measures. Patients taking anticoagulants receive instruction in bleeding precautions, potential medication interactions, and scheduling of blood tests to monitor therapeutic blood levels (Sitton, 2000). Nurses are in an optimal position to provide the tools and resources related to symptom management and to provide emotional support and reassurance to patients and caregivers.

Conclusion

SVCS is an obstructive complication of lung cancer, lymphoma, and various benign causes. It can progress to an obstructed airway, which is extremely distressing for patients and potentially is life threatening. Although SVCS is uncommon, the increased use of central VAD catheters also may increase the frequency of this syndrome. Nurses caring for patients in a variety of settings— infusion centers, ambulatory care, inpatient, home care, and hospice—need to be aware of the association between VADs and SVCS. The increased length of cancer survival in general may contribute to an increase in SVCS as well.

Most cases of SVCS develop gradually, so early detection and intervention may prevent progression to an acute emergency. Nurses caring for patients diagnosed with lung cancer (particularly SCLC) or NHL or patients who have other primary or metastatic tumors in the mediastinum need to be aware of these populations' increased potential for developing SVCS. An understanding of the mechanisms underlying the syndrome will help nurses in the early recognition of SVCS.

References

Abner, A. (1993). Approach to the patient who presents with superior vena cava obstruction. *Chest, 103*(Suppl. 4), 394S–397S.

Aurora, R., Milite, F., & Vander Els, N.J. (2000). Respiratory emergencies. *Seminars in Oncology, 27,* 256–269.

Baker, G.L., & Barnes, H.J. (1992). Superior vena cava syndrome: Etiology, diagnosis, and treatment. *American Journal of Critical Care, 1,* 54–64.

Berkow, R., & Fletcher, A.J. (Eds.). (1992). *The Merck manual of diagnosis and therapy* (16th ed., p. 1968). Rahway, NJ: Merck Research Laboratories.

Camp-Sorrell, D., & Mayo, D.J. (1998). Superior vena cava syndrome. *Clinical Journal of Oncology Nursing, 2,* 153–154.

Chan, R.H., Dar, A.R., Yu, E., Still, L.W., Whiston, F., Truong, P., et al. (1997). Superior vena cava obstruction in small-cell lung cancer. *International Journal of Radiation Oncology, Biology, Physics, 38,* 513–520.

Connors, J.M., Klimo, P., Fairey, R.N., & Voss, N. (1987). Brief chemotherapy and involved field radiation therapy for limited-stage, histologically aggressive lymphoma. *Annals of Internal Medicine, 107,* 25–30.

DeMichele, A., & Glick, J. (2001). Cancer-related emergencies. In R. Lenhard, R. Osteen, & T. Gansler (Eds.), *Clinical oncology* (pp. 733–764). Atlanta, GA: American Cancer Society.

Dyet, J.F., Nicholson, A.A., & Cook, A.M. (1993). The use of the Wallstent endovascular prosthesis in the treatment of malignant obstruction of the superior vena cava. *Clinical Radiology, 48,* 381–385.

Emani, B., & Graham, M.V. (1998). Lung. In C.A. Perez & L.W. Brady (Eds.), *Principles and practice of radiation oncology* (3rd ed., pp. 1181–1220). Philadelphia: Lippincott-Raven.

Escalante, C.P. (1993). Causes and management of superior vena cava syndrome. *Oncology, 7,* 61–68.

Flounders, J.A. (2003). Superior vena cava syndrome [Online exclusive]. *Oncology Nursing Forum, 30,* E84–E88.

Gao, S., & Shannon, V.R. (2002). Vascular emergencies. In S.C. Yeung & C.P. Escalante (Eds.), *Holland-Frei oncologic emergencies* (pp. 315–335). Hamilton, Ontario, Canada: BC Decker.

Haapoja, I., & Blendowski, C. (1999). Superior vena cava syndrome. *Seminars in Oncology Nursing, 15,* 183–189.

Haskell, C.M. (2001). *Cancer treatment* (5th ed., pp. 299–301). Philadelphia: Saunders.

Hemann, R. (2001). Superior vena cava syndrome. *Clinical Excellence for Nurse Practitioners, 5,* 85–87.

Hochrein, J., Bashore, T.M., O'Laughlin, M.P., & Harrison, J.K. (1998). Percutaneous stenting of superior vena cava syndrome: A case report and review of the literature. *American Journal of Medicine, 104,* 78–84.

Hoppe, R.T. (1994). Progress in the treatment of Hodgkin's disease in the United States, 1973 versus 1983. The Patterns of Care Study. *Cancer, 74,* 3198–3203.

Hunter, J.C. (1998). Structural emergencies. In J.K. Itano & K.N. Taoka (Eds.), *Core curriculum for oncology nursing* (3rd ed., pp. 340–354). Philadelphia: Saunders.

Hunter, W. (1757). History of an aneurysm of the aorta, with some remarks on aneurysms in general. *Medical Observations and Inquiries, 1,* 323–357.

Jahangiri, J., Taggart, D.P., & Goldstraw, P. (1993). Role of mediastinoscopy in superior vena cava obstruction. *Cancer, 71,* 3006–3008.

Kee, S.T., Kinoshita, L., Razavi, M.K., Nyman, U.R., Semba, C.P., & Dake, M.D. (1998). Superior vena cava syndrome: Treatment with catheter-directed thrombolysis and endovascular stent placement. *Radiology, 206,* 187–193.

Kreamer, K. (1998). Superior vena cava syndrome. In B. Johnson & J. Gross (Eds.), *Handbook of oncology nursing* (pp. 645–654). Sudbury, MA: Jones and Bartlett.

Lanciego, C., Chacon, J.L., Julian, A., Andrade, J., Lopez, L., Martinez, B., et 'al. (2001). Stenting as first option for endovascular treatment of malignant superior vena cava syndrome. *American Journal of Roentgenology, 177,* 583–593.

Lonardi, F., Gioga, G., Agus, G., Coeli, M., & Campostrini, F. (2002). Double-flash, large-fraction radiation therapy as palliative treatment of malignant superior vena cava syndrome in the elderly. *Supportive Care in Cancer, 10,* 156–160.

Loney, M. (1998). Superior vena cava syndrome. In C.C. Chernecky & B.J. Berger (Eds.), *Advanced and critical care oncology nursing: Managing primary complications* (pp. 340–354). Philadelphia: Saunders.

Mack, K.C. (1997). Superior vena cava syndrome. In R.A. Gates & R.M. Find (Eds.), *Oncology nursing secrets* (pp. 356–362). Philadelphia: Hanley and Belfus.

Marcy, P.Y., Magne, N., Bengtolila, F., Drouillard, J., Bruneton, J.N., & Descamps, B. (2001). Superior vena cava obstruction: Is stenting necessary? *Supportive Care in Cancer, 9,* 103–107.

Markman, M. (1999). Diagnosis and management of superior vena cava syndrome. *Cleveland Clinic Journal of Medicine, 66,* 59–61.

Martini, F. (1998). *Fundamentals of anatomy and physiology* (4th ed.). Upper Saddle River, NJ: Prentice Hall.

Miaskowski, C. (1991). Oncologic emergencies. In S. Baird, R. McCorkle, & M. Grant (Eds.), *Cancer nursing: A comprehensive textbook* (pp. 885–886). Philadelphia: Saunders.

Moore, S. (2005). Superior vena cava syndrome. In C.H. Yarbro, M. Goodman, & M.H. Frogge (Eds.), *Cancer nursing: Principles and practice* (6th ed., pp. 925–939). Sudbury, MA: Jones and Bartlett.

Murray, M.J., Steward, J.R., & Johnson, D.H. (1995). Superior vena cava syndrome. In M.D. Abeloff, J.O. Armitage, A.S. Lichter, & J.E. Niederhuber (Eds.), *Clinical oncology* (pp. 609–618). New York: Churchill Livingstone.

Nesbitt, J.C. (1996). Surgical management of superior vena cava syndrome. In H.I. Pass, J.B. Mitchell, D.H. Johnson, & A.T. Turrisi (Eds.), *Lung cancer: Principles and practice* (pp. 671–681). Philadelphia: Lippincott-Raven.

Nicholson, A.A., Ettles, D.F., & Arnold, A. (1997). Treatment of malignant superior vena cava obstruction: Metal stents or radiation therapy? *Journal of Vascular Interventional Radiology, 8,* 781–788.

O'Brien, J.F. (1996). The oncologic crisis part 2: Cardio respiratory and neurologic emergencies. *Emergency Medicine, 28,* 21–44.

Pierson, D.J. (1991). Disorders of the pleura, mediastinum, and diaphragm. In J.D. Wilson, E. Braunwald, K.J. Isselbacher, R.C. Petersdorf, J.B. Martin, A.S. Fauci, et al. (Eds.), *Harrison's principles of internal medicine* (12th ed., pp. 1111–1115). New York: McGraw-Hill.

Pinover, W.H., & Coia, L.R. (1998). Palliative radiation therapy. In A.M. Berger, R.K. Portenoy, & D.E. Weissman (Eds.), *Principles and practice of supportive oncology* (pp. 603–626). Philadelphia: Lippincott-Raven.

Rodrigues, C.I., Njo, K.H., & Karim, A.B. (1993). Hypofractionated radiation therapy in the treatment of superior vena cava syndrome. *Lung Cancer, 10,* 221–228.

Rosenblatt, M.B. (1964). Lung cancer in the 19th century. *Bulletin of the History of Medicine, 38,* 395–425.

Rowell, N.P., & Gleeson, F.V. (2002). Steroids, radiotherapy, chemotherapy, and stents for superior vena caval obstruction in carcinoma of the bronchus: A systematic review. *Clinical Oncology, 14,* 338–351.

Schafer, S. (1997). Oncologic complications. In S. Otto (Ed.), *Oncology nursing* (3rd ed., pp. 406–474). St. Louis, MO: Mosby.

Sitton, E. (2000). Superior vena cava syndrome. In C.H. Yarbro, M.H. Frogge, M. Goodman, & S. Groenwald (Eds.), *Cancer nursing: Principles and practice* (5th ed., pp. 900–912). Sudbury, MA: Jones and Bartlett.

Stanford, W., & Doty, D.B. (1986). The role of venography and surgery in the management of patients with superior vena cava obstruction. *Annals of Thoracic Surgery, 41,* 158–163.

Stewart, I.E. (1996). Superior vena cava syndrome: An oncologic complication. *Seminars in Oncology Nursing, 12,* 312–317.

Urban, T., Lebeau, B., Chastang, C., Leclerc, P., Botto, M.J., & Sauvaget, J. (1993). Superior vena cava syndrome in small-cell lung cancer. *Archives in Internal Medicine, 153,* 384–387.

Wudel, L.J., & Nesbitt, J.C. (2001). Superior vena cava syndrome. *Current Treatment Options in Oncology, 2,* 77–91.

Wurschmidt, F., Bunemann, H., & Heilman, H.P. (1995). Small cell lung cancer with and without superior vena cava syndrome: A multivariate analysis of prognostic factors in 408 cases. *International Journal of Radiation Oncology, Biology, Physics, 33,* 77–82.

Yahalom, J. (1997). Oncologic emergencies. In V.T. DeVita, S. Hellman, & S.A. Rosenberg (Eds.), *Cancer: Principles and practice of oncology* (5th ed., pp. 2469–2476). Philadelphia: Lippincott.

Yellin, A., Rosen, A., Reichert, N., & Lieberman, Y. (1990). Superior vena cava syndrome: The myth, the facts. *American Review of Respiratory Disease, 141*(5 Pt. 1), 1114–1118.

Barbara Holmes Gobel, RN, MS, AOCN®

Chapter 10

Tumor Lysis Syndrome

Introduction

Tumor lysis syndrome (TLS) is a very serious and potentially life-threatening oncologic emergency. This syndrome is a constellation of electrolyte imbalances that include hyperkalemia, hyperuricemia, and hyperphosphatemia with secondary hypocalcemia. These electrolyte abnormalities can lead to serious consequences, most notably renal failure and alterations in cardiac function. Changes in electrolyte and uric acid concentrations are precipitated by the destruction or lysis of large numbers of tumor cells following cytotoxic therapies, causing the release of normal intracellular components—potassium, phosphorus, and uric acid—into the systemic circulation. TLS most commonly occurs as a result of chemotherapy-induced electrolyte and metabolic disturbances but also can be related to surgery, biotherapy, and radiation therapy, or it can occur spontaneously. It most frequently is associated with malignancies with a high tumor burden and/or rapidly proliferating cells, such as leukemias and aggressive lymphomas. The greatest risk for TLS occurs early in the treatment period when the white cell count and tumor burden are high. Nurses need to be aware of the malignancies associated with an increased risk of TLS, because prevention of this complication is crucial in the management of these patients. The nursing role is critical in the prevention, prompt recognition, and rapid intervention for this potentially life-threatening oncologic emergency.

Incidence

The exact incidence of TLS is not known. TLS occurs mostly in patients who have hematologic malignancies with large proliferative growth fractions and large bulky disease, such as the acute and chronic leukemias and high-grade lymphomas (see Figure 10-1) (Altman, 2001; Flombaum, 2000). Burkitt lymphoma and T-cell acute lymphoblastic leukemia are the two malignancies most frequently associated with TLS (Sarnaik, 2003). TLS also frequently occurs with acute myeloid leukemia, chronic lymphocytic leukemia (CLL), chronic myeloid leukemia, and Hodgkin disease. Although not as frequent, TLS also has been observed with solid tumors (see Figure 10-2). Most of the solid tumors associated with TLS are chemotherapy-sensitive, including neuroblastoma, breast cancer, and small cell lung cancer (Kalemkerian, Darwish, & Varterasian, 1997; Sarnaik). However, in a series of case reports, researchers observed that a number of patients who experienced TLS had solid tumors that were moderately chemotherapy sensitive or had tumors that were considered to be chemotherapy insensitive. These tumor types include melanoma, seminoma, thymoma, sarcoma, leiomyosarcoma, medulloblastoma, rhabdomyosarcoma, and hepatoblastoma, and gastric, ovarian, vulvar, and colorectal carcinomas (Baeksgaard & Sorensen, 2003; Kalemkerian et al.). TLS more commonly arises in the pediatric population, as hematologic malignancies are more common in children.

Figure 10-1. Malignancies Frequently Associated With Tumor Lysis Syndrome

- Burkitt lymphoma
- T-cell acute lymphoblastic leukemia
- Acute myeloid leukemia
- Chronic lymphocytic leukemia
- Chronic myeloid leukemia
- Hodgkin disease

Figure 10-2. Malignancies Occasionally or Infrequently Associated With Tumor Lysis Syndrome

- Neuroblastoma
- Breast cancer
- Small cell lung cancer
- Melanoma
- Seminoma
- Thymoma
- Sarcoma
- Leiomyosarcoma
- Medulloblastoma
- Rhabdomyosarcoma
- Hepatoblastoma
- Gastric cancer
- Ovarian cancer
- Vulvar cancer
- Colorectal cancer

Risk Factors

Patient-Related Risk Factors

In addition to the disease-related risk factors involved in TLS development, a number of patient-related risk factors also exist (see Figure 10-3). Several pretreatment patient-related risk factors have long been identified as predisposing patients to the metabolic abnormalities associated with TLS. These risk factors include dehydration and poor urinary output; bulky abdominal disease; extensive lymph node involvement; elevated white blood cell count; elevated uric acid, potassium, and phosphorus levels; and an elevated lactate dehydrogenase level (Cohen, Balow, & Magrath, 1980). Patients with preexisting dehydration or renal impairment are at increased risk for TLS development because they cannot effectively clear the lysed tumor cells or their metabolic products after treatment. The presence of large, bulky disease, tumors with significant associated lymph node involvement,

Figure 10-3. Patient-Related Risk Factors in the Development of Tumor Lysis Syndrome

- Dehydration/poor urinary output prior to treatment
- Bulky abdominal disease
- Extensive lymph node involvement prior to treatment
- Elevated white blood cell count
- Elevated uric acid, potassium, and phosphorus levels prior to treatment
- Elevated lactate dehydrogenase level prior to treatment

or highly elevated white blood cell counts increase the risk of TLS by virtue of the vast number of malignant cells present in the body. Furthermore, effective cytotoxic therapy results in a significant number of lysed cells that may overwhelm the capacity of the renal system. Elevated serum uric acid, potassium, and phosphorus levels all may exist prior to therapy and, when the lysed metabolic products are added to the bloodstream after therapy, may overburden the renal or cardiac systems. Certain metabolic conditions may increase the risk for TLS even further. For example, patients with lymphocytic disease are at great risk for TLS because the phosphorus content of lymphoblasts is three to four times greater than in normal lymphocytes (Sarnaik, 2003). Thus, when the cells are lysed during therapy, the amount of phosphorus that is spilled into the circulation can become dangerously high.

Treatment-Related Risk Factors

Chemotherapy is the most common treatment-related factor associated with the development of TLS. The use of a variety of chemotherapy agents may result in TLS, most notably cisplatin, etoposide, paclitaxel, hydroxyurea, cytosine arabinoside, and intrathecal methotrexate (Altman, 2001; Seki, Al-Omar, Amato, & Sutton, 2003) (see Table 10-1). Case reports also exist of TLS associated with the use of capecitabine and fludarabine (Dizdar, Yurekli, Purnak, Aksu, & Haznedaroglu, 2004; Hussain, Mazza, & Clouse, 2003; Kurt, Eren, Engin, & Guler, 2004). Additionally, TLS has occurred with the use of biologic agents, such as interferons, interleukins, and tumor necrosis factor, and with monoclonal antibodies, such as rituximab, gemtuzumab, and alemtuzumab (Altman; Biogen Idec Inc. & Genentech, Inc., 1999; Castro, VanAuken, Spencer-Cisak, Legha, & Sponzo, 1999; Wyeth Pharmaceuticals, 2001). Researchers also have implicated hormonal therapy, particularly tamoxifen and corticosteroids, in the development of TLS (Abou Mourad, Taher, & Shamseddine, 2003; Yang, Chau, Dai, & Lin, 2003). The incidence of TLS may increase as newer and more-targeted biologic therapies become available for use against a variety of tumor types (Doane, 2002).

Table 10-1. Treatment-Related Risk Factors in the Development of Tumor Lysis Syndrome

Treatment	Agents
Chemotherapy	Cisplatin, etoposide, paclitaxel, hydroxyurea, cytosine arabinoside, intrathecal methotrexate
Biologic agents	Interferons, interleukins, tumor necrosis factor, monoclonal antibodies (e.g., rituximab, gemtuzumab, alemtuzumab)
Hormonal agents	Tamoxifen, corticosteroids
Surgery	–
Radiation therapy	–
Spontaneous occurrence	–

Surgery and radiation therapy are linked to the development of TLS, although much less frequently than chemotherapy or biotherapy (Altman, 2001). Reports exist of patients developing TLS after exposure to ionizing radiation when splenic irradiation has been given to treat CLL (Al-mondhiry, Stryker, & Kempin, 1984), when abdominal radiation has been given for medulloblastoma and bulky abdominopelvic metastasis (Tomlinson & Solberg, 1984), and in the bone marrow transplant setting (Fleming, Henslee-Downey, & Coffey, 1991). Researchers recently reported TLS caused by palliative radiotherapy in a patient with diffuse large B-cell lymphoma (Yamazaki et al., 2004). Although they could not identify the specific cause of the TLS, investigators noted that the patient had pretreatment elevation of serum creatinine and serum lactate dehydrogenase (LDH) levels, both of which are risk factors in TLS development. TLS can occur prior to the initiation of therapy, because of autolysis of the cells, or up to five days after therapy begins (Sarnaik, 2003). Most often it occurs in the first one to two days after the initiation of therapy (Reid-Finlay & Kaplow, 2001).

The occurrence of acute, spontaneous TLS is a rare but serious event. Spontaneous development of TLS is fulminant at its onset with severe metabolic abnormalities, but as with other causes of TLS, it often is reversible. Only case reports of a variety of tumor types, including hematologic tumors and solid tumors, mention spontaneous TLS (Basile & Montanaro, 2003; Feld, Mehta, & Burkes, 2000; Hsu & Huang, 2004; Pentheroudakis, O'Neill, Vasey, & Kaye, 2001; Vaisban, Braester, Mosenzon, Kolin, & Horn, 2003). Although researchers do not clearly understand the etiology of spontaneous induction of TLS, one theory for its occurrence in a solid tumor is rapid tumor necrosis with resultant release of intracellular contents (Feld et al.).

Pathophysiology

TLS is a metabolic disturbance that occurs after cell destruction of rapidly growing tumors. TLS is characterized by the release of intracellular components into the circulation caused by the massive lysis of malignant cells, most commonly following antineoplastic therapy. The huge lysis of tumor cells results in the rapid release of potassium, uric acid (from nucleic acids), and phosphorus into the bloodstream, causing the characteristic electrolyte imbalances seen in TLS: hyperkalemia, hyperuricemia, hyperphosphatemia, and hypocalcemia (see Figure 10-4). Hypocalcemia develops because an inverse relationship exists between phosphorus and calcium; when one of these electrolytes increases, the other decreases. Thus, the elevated serum phosphorus (hyperphosphatemia) common to TLS causes a secondary decrease in serum calcium.

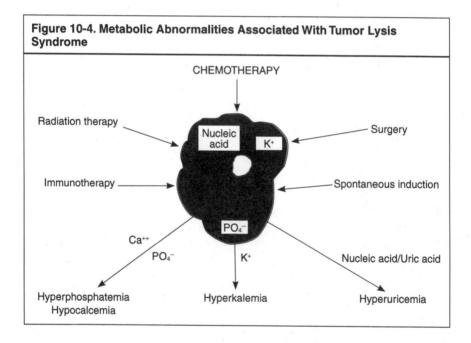

Figure 10-4. Metabolic Abnormalities Associated With Tumor Lysis Syndrome

The hyperuricemia seen in TLS develops when nucleic acid purines enter the circulation during massive cell lysis and then are converted to uric acid by xanthine oxidase, an enzyme in the liver (Kaplow, 2002). Uric acid is soluble at physiologic pH but can precipitate in the acidic environment of the renal tubules. This precipitation can lead to crystallization in the collecting ducts and the ureters, causing obstructive uropathy and resulting in decreased glomerular filtration, increased hydrostatic pressure, obstructed urine flow, and possibly renal failure. The kidneys can excrete normal to moderate levels of uric acid, but during TLS, the excessive uric acid levels may overwhelm the capacity of the kidneys to excrete this electrolyte. Patients generally develop symptoms when uric acid levels exceed 10 mg/dl (Altman, 2001).

Hyperphosphatemia occurs because of the intracellular release of phosphorus into the systemic circulation. Serum calcium binds with phosphorus in the circulation, resulting in the symptom of secondary hypocalcemia seen with TLS. Calcium phosphate salts may precipitate in the renal tubules and microvascular circulation, which also may contribute to renal failure. Renal insufficiency exacerbates the existing hypocalcemia and hyperkalemia associated with TLS (Herbert, Reilly, & Kriz, 2001; Yarpuzlu, 2003). Hyperphosphatemia is of particular concern in patients with lymphocytic diseases because of the increased phosphorus content of lymphoblasts (Sarnaik, 2003).

Hyperkalemia results directly from the intracellular release of potassium into the systemic circulation; renal failure and metabolic acidosis may further aggravate the condition. Hyperkalemia is potentially the most life threatening of the electrolyte abnormalities associated with TLS because of the effect of excessive amounts of potassium on the heart. Hyperkalemia can lead to cardiac arrhythmias and cardiac arrest and has a major depressant effect on cardiac function, thus resulting in bradycardia, heart block, and cardiac arrest. Patients generally manifest symptoms related to hyperkalemia when the potassium level exceeds 6.5 mEq/L (Sherman, 1999).

Clinical Manifestations

TLS often is asymptomatic initially, and detection of the condition frequently occurs via abnormalities in the blood chemistries. The signs and symptoms that patients eventually exhibit depend on the extent of the metabolic abnormality. This section will review the signs and symptoms of the pertinent metabolic abnormalities, including hyperuricemia, hyperphosphatemia, hypocalcemia, and hyperkalemia (see Table 10-2).

Hyperuricemia

Hyperuricemia may be responsible for a wide array of abnormal physical findings. Symptoms generally occur when the uric acid level exceeds 10 mg/dl. When the uric acid level is between 10–15 mg/dl, patients may experience malaise, nausea, vomiting, fatigue, weakness, flank pain, gout, and pruritus (Cantril & Haylock, 2004; Sarnaik, 2003). At this level, patients also may experience compromised renal function, as demonstrated by oliguria, anuria, azotemia, and acute uric acid nephropathy, which may develop from crystallization of uric acid in the collecting ducts and renal tubules. When the uric acid level exceeds 20 mg/dl, patients may exhibit signs of progressive, frank renal failure, such as edema, hypertension, hematuria, crystalluria, profound azotemia, anuria, and then acute/chronic renal failure (Lydon, 2005). Hyper-

Table 10-2. Clinical Signs and Symptoms of Tumor Lysis Syndrome

Abnormality	Signs and Symptoms
Hyperkalemia	**Early cardiac:** Tachycardia, electrocardiographic changes (prolongation of QT interval and ST segment, lowering and inversion of T wave) **Late cardiac:** Bradycardia, electrocardiographic changes (shortened QT interval, elevated T waves, wide QRS complex, loss of P wave), ventricular tachycardia, ventricular fibrillation, heart block, cardiac arrest **Miscellaneous:** Nausea, vomiting, twitching, weakness, paresthesias, paralysis, diarrhea, lethargy, syncope, muscle cramps, increased bowel sounds
Hyperphosphatemia	Anuria, oliguria, azotemia, edema, hypertension, acute renal failure
Secondary hypocalcemia	**Neurologic/neuromuscular:** Twitching, paresthesias, restlessness, muscle weakness, muscle cramps, anxiety, depression, carpopedal spasms, seizures, confusion, hallucinations **Cardiac:** Tetany, ventricular arrhythmias, electrocardiographic changes (prolonged QT interval, inverted T wave), heart block, cardiac arrest
Hyperuricemia	**Renal:** Oliguria, anuria, azotemia, hematuria, crystalluria, edema, hypertension, acute uric acid nephropathy, acute/chronic renal failure **Miscellaneous:** Malaise, nausea, vomiting, fatigue, weakness, flank pain, gout, pruritus

uricemia usually develops 24–48 hours after the initiation of cancer therapy (Altman, 2001).

Hyperphosphatemia With Secondary Hypocalcemia

Hyperphosphatemia with secondary hypocalcemia can occur 24–48 hours after the initiation of the cancer treatment. Symptoms related to hyperphosphatemia are generally the result of compromised renal function and include anuria, oliguria, azotemia, edema, and acute renal failure (Altman, 2001; Kaplow, 2002). Secondary hypocalcemia occurs because calcium binds to phosphorus in the systemic circulation, thereby reducing the availability of calcium in the active ionized form. Patients with hypocalcemia may experience twitching, paresthesias, muscle cramps, carpopedal spasms, anxiety, depression, confusion, and hallucinations (Cantril & Haylock, 2004). Cardiac changes may include tetany, ventricular arrhythmias, heart blocks, and, in extreme cases, cardiac arrest (Sarnaik, 2003). Precipitates of calcium phosphate may be deposited in tissues, causing iritis, pruritus, arthritis, and gangrenous changes of the skin (Sarnaik).

Hyperkalemia

Hyperkalemia is potentially life threatening because of the effect of increased potassium levels on the heart. Potassium elevations above normal values can occur 6–72 hours after the initiation of therapy (Flombaum, 2000). Serum potassium levels exceeding 6.5 mEq/L may result in cardiac effects including tachycardia, P-wave and T-wave changes, and potentially fatal heart rhythms, such as ventricular tachycardia and ventricular fibrillation. If the hyperkalemia continues or becomes progressively worse, it exerts a major depressant effect on the heart, demonstrated as bradycardia, heart block, and cardiac arrest (Yarpuzlu, 2003). Other clinical signs and symptoms of hyperkalemia include nausea, vomiting, twitching, paresthesia, weakness, paralysis, diarrhea, lethargy, syncope, muscle cramps, and increased bowel sounds (Altman, 2001; Reid-Finlay & Kaplow, 2001).

Patient Assessment

Patients who are at risk for TLS should have their laboratory values monitored as a baseline before initiating therapy and every 8–12 hours during the first 48–72 hours of treatment. A baseline complete blood count determines the patient's white blood cell count and platelets. Blood urea nitrogen (BUN) and creatinine levels are markers of renal function. Total calcium, ionized calcium, and phosphorus levels determine the extent of hypocalcemia. The serum uric acid level indicates the extent of hyperuricemia. The laboratory values may need to be drawn more frequently if high-risk changes occur in the patient's clinical status (Kaplow, 2002).

A urinalysis helps to determine the urine pH and identify abnormalities such as uric acid crystals. Patients who have hyperkalemia require an electrocardiogram (EKG) to evaluate for arrhythmias or other EKG changes that may precede potentially fatal arrhythmias. The patient's blood pressure, weight, and fluid intake and output (I & O) also require close monitoring. A decrease in blood pressure from baseline is an indication that the heart is not pumping sufficient fluids to the kidneys and that the patient's renal status needs to be watched closely. The patient's weight, coupled with the I & O, give a good indication of the patient's fluid and renal status, as well as the need for gentle or aggressive diuresis.

Treatment Modalities

Prevention Strategies

Prevention of TLS is the cornerstone of management of this syndrome (see Table 10-3). Identifying patients who are at risk for TLS is an essential component of preventing this syndrome. Prompt recognition is particularly important for those who have hematologic malignancies, such as acute and chronic leukemias and high-grade, aggressive lymphomas (e.g., Burkitt lymphoma). Major prevention strategies include frequent monitoring of laboratory values to follow the chemical and metabolic changes that may affect patients at risk for developing TLS, aggressive hydration and diuresis prior to and during cancer treatments, medication prophylaxis of the TLS with allopurinol and/or rasburicase, and alkalinization of the urine.

Knowledge of all the medications patients are receiving is critical in preventing TLS. Certain medications, including heparin, potassium-sparing diuretics (e.g., spironolactone, triamterene), and the angiotensin-converting enzyme inhibitors (e.g., captopril, enalapril, lisinopril), contribute to an increase in serum potassium levels (Gobel, 2002). Patients should avoid

---

Table 10-3. Strategies to Prevent Tumor Lysis Syndrome

Strategy	Prevention Measures
Monitoring of laboratory values, including a complete blood count (with platelet count) and chemistries (blood urea nitrogen, creatinine, calcium, ionized calcium, phosphorus, and serum uric acid), urinalysis, and electrocardiogram	Baseline and every 8–12 hours during the first 48–72 hours of treatment Urinalysis as needed to determine uric acid crystals, and urine pH baseline and during urinary alkalinization to determine appropriate urine pH level Electrocardiogram baseline depending on patients' lab values or as needed to evaluate for cardiac arrhythmias
Hydration with normal saline or 5% dextrose solution	Begin hydration 24–48 hours prior to initiation of therapy. Ensure urine flow of > 150–200 ml/hour.
Diuresis with loop diuretics or osmotic diuretics if urine flow is not maintained by hydration alone	Given during hydration to assist with maintenance of urine flow
Urinary alkalinization with sodium bicarbonate	Given in the hydration fluids to achieve a urine pH of 7–7.5
Medication history	Avoid or substitute medications that contribute to an increase in serum potassium levels, such as heparin, potassium-sparing diuretics, angiotensin-converting enzyme inhibitors, and known nephrotoxins (e.g., aminoglycosides, nonsteroidal anti-inflammatory medications).
Diet history	Oral supplements and enteral/parenteral nutrition may exacerbate hyperkalemia and hyperphosphatemia. Depending on renal status, patients may need to avoid foods high in potassium or phosphorus. Patients may require a nutrition consult.

drugs such as the aminoglycosides (e.g., gentamycin, amikacin, tobramycin, kanamycin), amphotericin B, nonsteroidal anti-inflammatory agents, and other anti-inflammatory agents because they are known nephrotoxins and can compromise renal function. Radiographic dye studies also should be avoided as the dye may block tubular reabsorption of uric acid (Zobec, 1997).

Hyperkalemia and hyperphosphatemia may be exacerbated by nutritional sources of these electrolytes, including oral supplements and enteral or parenteral nutrition. Foods high in potassium include oranges, bananas, tomatoes, chocolate, and orange juice. Foods high in phosphorus include milk, meat, eggs, fish, nuts, cheese, bread, poultry, legumes, cereal, chocolate, and carbonated beverages (Ezzone, 1999). Patients should avoid nutritional sources of these electrolytes only if their baseline potassium or phosphorus is elevated.

Hydration and Urinary Alkalinization

Patients who are at risk for TLS receive hydration beginning 24–48 hours prior to treatment initiation in order to optimize renal function and prevent TLS. The goal of hydration is to achieve a urine flow greater than 150–200 ml/hour, using either normal saline or 5% dextrose solutions (Feusner & Farber, 2001; Sallan, 2001). Adequate diuresis may be assisted with loop (e.g., furosemide) or osmotic (e.g., mannitol) diuretics to maintain the urine flow and to prevent renal tubular damage (Lydon, 2005). Mannitol may be added if hydration and loop diuretics do not achieve an adequate urine flow.

Urinary alkalinization will help to reduce the development of uric acid crystals by decreasing the acidic environment in the urine that promotes uric acid crystallization. Adding sodium bicarbonate to the IV fluids at 100–125 mEq/m^2 helps to achieve a urine pH of 7–7.5 (Feusner & Farber, 2001; Sallan, 2001). Acetazolamide is a secondary choice for urinary alkalinization and provides a direct diuretic effect as well (Heffner & Polman, 1998). Rigorous urine alkalinization is controversial because it can cause severe complications. Overly rigorous alkalinization of the urine may lead to precipitation of calcium and phosphate, resulting in calcium phosphate crystallization in the renal tubules, which can lead to acute renal failure (Lydon, 2005). Alkalinization also will contribute to the development of hypocalcemia and increase the risk of xanthine nephropathy (Lydon). Because of these potential complications, it is generally recommended that the urine be alkalinized to a pH level of no more than 7.5.

Medication Prophylaxis

In addition to the hydration and alkalinization of the patient's urine, prevention and management of TLS requires the use of medication management (see Table 10-4). Medication therapy ideally begins at least 24 hours before the start of cytotoxic therapy, with the goal of achieving metabolic stability.

Table 10-4. Medication Regimens to Prevent Tumor Lysis Syndrome

Medication	Dosing Parameters	Side Effects
Oral allopurinol	200–600 mg/day orally, to begin at least 24 hours prior to chemotherapy	Rash, nausea, vomiting, hypersensitivity, renal failure/insufficiency
IV allopurinol	200–400 mg/m²/day in a single or divided doses, to begin at least 24 hours prior to chemotherapy	Rash, nausea, vomiting, renal failure/insufficiency, hypersensitivity
Rasburicase	0.15–0.2 mg/kg IV once daily for five days, to begin 4–24 hours prior to chemotherapy	Fever, nausea, vomiting, headache, mild to moderate hypersensitivity reactions; may cause hemolytic anemia or methemoglobinemia in patients with glucose-6-dehydrogenase deficiency (may require screening of these individuals)

Allopurinol

Allopurinol is used specifically to prevent TLS. It is an oral medication that inhibits the action of the enzyme xanthine oxidase in converting hypoxanthine to xanthine to uric acid (see Figure 10-5). By inhibiting xanthine oxidase, allopurinol blocks the formation of uric acid, thereby preventing the development of uric acid nephropathy. An IV preparation of allopurinol is available for patients who are unable to tolerate oral administration of the medication. The daily oral adult dose of allopurinol is 200–600 mg/day. Patients receive allopurinol before initiation of cytotoxic therapy, during the therapy, and after the therapy is complete. The reduction in uric acid levels occurs slowly, beginning one to three days after initiation of the drug. The daily IV adult dose of allopurinol is 200–400 mg/m², in single or divided doses, not to exceed 600 mg/day, and should begin at least 24 hours before the initiation of cytotoxic therapy. Clinical trials have shown IV allopurinol to be well tolerated, with an adverse effect profile similar to the oral preparation (Smalley et al., 2000). Side effects of allopurinol include rash, nausea, vomiting, hypersensitivity reactions, and renal insufficiency or renal failure (see Table 10-4). Clinicians should immediately discontinue allopurinol if allergic side effects occur (Navolanic et al., 2003).

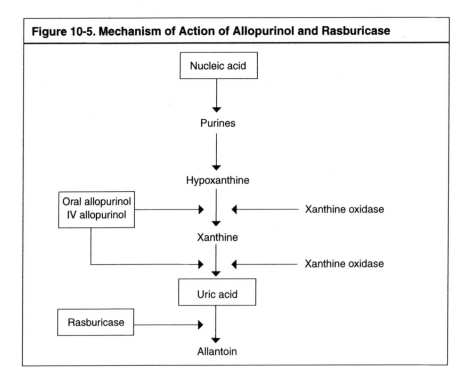

Figure 10-5. Mechanism of Action of Allopurinol and Rasburicase

Rasburicase

Another newer medication that is used for both prophylaxis and management of TLS is rasburicase. Rasburicase is a recombinant urate oxidase product that oxidizes uric acid to allantoin, a metabolite of uric acid with a much greater solubility than uric acid (Holdsworth & Nguyen, 2003). This increased solubility allows for prompt urinary excretion of the allantoin. Rasburicase has been approved for the prophylaxis and management of TLS in the pediatric population, but its use is increasing in appropriate adult patients with cancer. A recent study demonstrated the efficacy of rasburicase in the prevention and treatment of TLS in 245 patients (173 children and 72 adults) (Pui, Jeha, Irwin, & Camitta, 2001).

A subpopulation of patients exists for whom the standard TLS prevention therapy (IV hydration, alkalinization of the urine, and the use of allopurinol) is not adequate to prevent sequelae from this syndrome. These patients generally present with leukemia or lymphoma accompanied with large tumor burdens (e.g., initial white blood cell count > 50,000/mm³). They also may have significantly elevated serum uric acid concentrations (> 10 mg/dl) and renal dysfunction before the initiation of chemotherapy. This patient population may benefit from the use of rasburicase, which has a rapid onset of action and can decrease the uric acid level in two to four hours (Navolanic et al., 2003).

The approved dosage of rasburicase is 0.15–0.2 mg/kg IV once daily for five days, with chemotherapy initiation recommended 4–24 hours after the first dose (Sanofi-Synthelabo Inc., 2002). Rasburicase is contraindicated in patients with glucose-6-phosphate dehydrogenase deficiency, as rasburicase may cause hemolytic anemia or methemoglobinemia in these patients (Holdsworth & Nguyen, 2003). Those at high risk for this deficiency include individuals of African and Mediterranean ancestry. Other possible side effects of the drug include fever, nausea, vomiting, headache, and mild to moderate hypersensitivity reactions (Pui, 2002). Rasburicase will cause enzymatic degradation of uric acid if left at room temperature, thus prechilled test tubes containing heparin must be used in the collection of serum uric acid and then sent for laboratory testing in an ice water bath (Sanofi-Synthelabo Inc.).

Intervention Strategies

The metabolic abnormalities and clinical signs and symptoms associated with TLS may not be apparent immediately after initiating treatment but generally occur within 24–48 hours of therapy (Hande & Garrow, 1993). Intervention is based on the specific signs and symptoms related to TLS. Aggressive intervention is critical once clinical signs and symptoms of TLS first appear (see Table 10-5).

Hyperkalemia

Hyperkalemia often is an initial sign of TLS and is the most common life-threatening emergency. A temporary discontinuation of cytotoxic therapy for the cancer may be necessary based on the degree of hyperkalemia. Sodium polystyrene sulfonate (Kayexalate®, Sanofi-Synthelabo Inc., New York, NY), administered either orally or by retention enema, can treat mild hyperkalemia (< 6.5 mEq/L). Sodium polystyrene sulfonate exchanges sodium for potassium and binds it in the gut, thereby decreasing the total body potassium (Sarnaik, 2003). The onset of action of Kayexalate is 2–12 hours when given orally and up to 24 hours when given rectally. Therefore, use of this drug would not be appropriate if the potassium level is greater than 6.5 mEq/L or if there is evidence of cardiac arrhythmias.

IV calcium gluconate or calcium chloride can be administered for the management of EKG changes. Calcium antagonizes the action of potassium on the heart, thereby protecting the myocardium from the effects of hyperkalemia. Calcium chloride contains approximately three times more elemental calcium than that found in an equal volume of calcium gluconate. Thus, if the hyperkalemia is accompanied by hemodynamic compromise, calcium chloride is the preferred medication (Sarnaik, 2003). Calcium drugs are used to protect the heart, so they are accompanied by other therapies that work to lower the level of serum potassium. IV sodium bicarbonate, hypertonic glucose, and insulin shift the excessive extracellular potassium back into the intracellular stores,

Table 10-5. Treatment Recommendations for Metabolic Abnormalities Associated With Tumor Lysis Syndrome

Abnormality	Treatment
Hyperkalemia	Mild hyperkalemia (< 6.5 mEq/L): Sodium polystyrene sulfonate either orally or by retention enema Potassium > 6.5 mEq/L or with cardiac changes: IV calcium gluconate or calcium chloride (preferred if hyperkalemia is accompanied by hemodynamic instability); IV sodium bicarbonate, hypertonic glucose, and insulin accompanied by sodium polystyrene sulfonate; loop diuretics
Hyperphosphatemia	Phosphate-binding agents, aluminum-containing antacids, hypertonic glucose plus insulin
Hypocalcemia	Appropriate management of hyperphosphatemia, IV calcium gluconate or calcium chloride to treat arrhythmias
Hyperuricemia	Hydration, urinary alkalinization, oral allopurinol or IV allopurinol (best for prevention of uric acid), rasburicase; dialysis with significant renal compromise

temporarily lowering serum potassium levels. The effect of these medications is not lasting; therefore, their use should be followed by medications that enhance potassium clearance, such as sodium polystyrene sulfonate. Diuresis with loop diuretics also will cause urinary potassium excretion (Gobel, 2002).

Hyperphosphatemia

Phosphate-binding agents are used to treat hyperphosphatemia associated with TLS. Oral aluminum-containing antacids, such as aluminum hydroxide, may be given to bind phosphates. These medications can cause constipation and may require the use of a stool softener or laxative. When phosphorus levels are within the normal range, secondary hypocalcemia usually will correct itself. Calcium therapies (as mentioned previously) also are used to treat arrhythmias caused by hypocalcemia.

Hyperuricemia

Although the incidence of TLS has decreased over the years because of appropriate prophylactic measures, hyperuricemia still may occur. This is a primary concern in the management of TLS because hyperuricemia may contribute significantly to acute renal failure. Rasburicase, which does not prevent the production of uric acid but instead converts the uric acid into a more soluble molecule, allantoin, is an appropriate treatment for the management of hyperuricemia (Pui, 2002). Studies have shown rasburicase to be safe and effective in the prevention and treatment of TLS in both the pediatric and the adult populations of patients with cancer (Annemans et al., 2003; Bosly et al., 2003; Goldman et al., 2001; Pui). Although data regarding adult patients with cancer are limited, the most recent study that included adult patients identified the dose of rasburicase to be 0.2 mg/kg IV for days 1–7, with twice-daily dosing allowed for the first three days (Bosly et al.). Reports exist, however, of the effectiveness of single-dose rasburicase in treating hyperuricemia (Arnold, Reuter, Delman, & Shanholtz, 2004; Lee, Li, So, & Chan, 2003). Clinicians maintain aggressive hydration and diuresis (to flush out the allantoin) when administering rasburicase, although urinary alkalinization is not required (Sanofi-Synthelabo Inc., 2002). Patients should avoid thiazide diuretics, which block tubular reabsorption of uric acid.

If patients develop significant renal compromise, then rapid intervention with dialysis is necessary. The decision to initiate dialysis usually is not based on a single electrolyte value but rather on a constellation of symptoms and the potential for further clinical deterioration. Clinicians may consider dialysis for patients with the following serum blood levels: elevated uric acid level > 10 mg/ dl; increasing, uncontrolled hyperkalemia, generally > 7 mEq/L; symptomatic hypocalcemia; and phosphorus > 10 mg/dl. Uncontrolled hypertension and hypervolemia and significant elevations of serum creatinine and BUN, along with other metabolic abnormalities or decreasing urine output, also may be indications for dialysis (Sarnaik, 2003). Hemodialysis usually is the preferred treatment method, as it rapidly corrects the potentially life-threatening electrolyte disturbances seen with TLS. Hemodialysis is generally performed every 12 hours until the renal function and metabolic abnormalities are corrected (Yarpuzlu, 2003). Depending on their condition and setting of care, patients also may be dialyzed using hemofiltration (continuous arteriovenous hemofiltration or continuous venovenous hemofiltration) or peritoneal dialysis (Schelling, Ghandour, Strickland, & Sedor, 1998).

Nursing Management

Prevention and Early Detection

Nurses play a key role in the prevention of TLS and its sequelae (see Table 10-6). One of the most important prevention strategies is to be able to identify those patients who are at risk for TLS development. Through an awareness that TLS occurs most frequently in patients with hematologic malignancies, particularly leukemias and aggressive lymphomas, nurses are in a position to anticipate the need to either educate patients and families about specific prevention strategies (e.g., hydration, alkalinization of the urine, prophylactic medication therapy) or to carry out these activities. Knowledge regarding other risk factors that contribute to the development of TLS is necessary to help to prevent this syndrome. These factors include preexisting clinical conditions

Table 10-6. Nursing Management of Patients at Risk for Tumor Lysis Syndrome (TLS)

TLS-Related Events	Management
Prevention of TLS	Identify diseases that put patients at risk for the development of TLS: • Leukemia and aggressive lymphomas • Solid tumors, including breast cancer, neuroblastoma, and small cell lung cancer. Identify patient pretreatment risk factors: • Dehydration or renal impairment • Large, bulky tumors with significant adenopathy • Hyperkalemia, hyperphosphatemia, hypocalcemia, hyperuricemia • Elevated lactate dehydrogenase level. Eliminate excess sources of potassium and phosphorus. • Review medications that may contribute to increased potassium and phosphorus. • Eliminate nutritional supplements containing potassium and phosphorus. Administer prophylactic hydration and diuresis as needed to maintain urine output > 150–200 ml/hour. Perform alkalinization of the urine (urine pH < 7.5 mEq/L). • Administer sodium bicarbonate to each liter of IV fluid to achieve a urine pH < 7.5 mEq/L. Administer prophylactic medications, including oral allopurinol, IV allopurinol, and rasburicase.
Early detection of TLS	Weigh patients daily. Adhere to strict input and output requirements. Check vital signs every 4 hours or more often as needed. Monitor electrolytes at baseline and every 8–12 hours for first 48–72 hours (or more frequently as needed). Monitor electrocardiogram (EKG) as needed. Perform urinalysis 3–4 times per day to monitor urine pH, and observe for uric acid crystals.
Symptom management of TLS	**Hyperkalemia** Check vital signs every 4 hours or more often as needed. Monitor EKG as needed. Restrict dietary sources of potassium. Review medication record for medications that may contribute to the potassium level. Administer medications as needed based on potassium level: • Sodium polystyrene sulfonate either orally or by retention enema • IV administration of calcium gluconate or calcium chloride • IV sodium bicarbonate, hypertonic glucose plus insulin • Loop diuretics. **Hyperphosphatemia** Administer phosphate-binding, aluminum-containing agents. Prophylactically treat for constipation. Restrict dietary sources of phosphorus. Review medication administration record for medications that may contribute to the phosphorus level.

(Continued on next page)

Table 10-6. Nursing Management of Patients at Risk for Tumor Lysis Syndrome (TLS) *(Continued)*

TLS-Related Events	Management
Symptom management of TLS *(cont.)*	**Hypocalcemia** Administer medications for hyperphosphatemia (will likely self-correct the hypocalcemia). Monitor EKG as needed. Institute seizure precautions when calcium falls below 8 mg/dl. Administer calcium gluconate or calcium chloride for cardiac arrhythmias. **Hyperuricemia** Weigh patients daily. Adhere to strict input and output requirements. Maintain aggressive hydration and diuresis to maintain urine output > 150–200 ml/hour. Administer rasburicase as needed. Administer allopurinol when uric acid is close to normal. Administer acetazolamide when volume overload is a concern and patient does not respond to allopurinol. Maintain urinary alkalinization < 7.5 mEq/L. **Psychosocial support** Provide psychosocial support for patients and caregivers. Utilize other healthcare team members to increase support to patients and caregivers.
Patient and caregiver education	Explain risk factors in the development of TLS, including disease risk factors, patient risk factors, and treatment-related risk factors. Teach about the need to restrict dietary potassium and phosphorus in patients with preexisting renal impairment. Educate about treatment measures for TLS, including hydration, alkalinization of the urine, and medication management. Provide information for patients treated at home in regard to when to call their healthcare provider. Explain to patients and caregivers the potential need to hospitalize patients depending on their symptoms. Explain the potential need for a transfer of care to an intensive care setting depending on the patients' needs.

such as dehydration or renal impairment, extent of the disease (e.g., large, bulky tumors, tumors with significant associated adenopathy), and preexisting laboratory abnormalities (hyperkalemia, hyperphosphatemia, hypocalcemia, hyperuricemia, and elevated LDH) that may become worse with treatment. Recognizing patients who are at risk for TLS allows nurses to institute prevention measures 24–48 hours prior to therapy. Dietary restrictions of potassium and phosphorus generally are indicated for patients admitted with preexisting renal impairment and metabolic abnormalities, such as hyperkalemia (Ezzone, 1999).

A key nursing action is the initiation of prophylactic hydration in patients at risk for TLS. Along with aggressive hydration, nurses should anticipate the need to alkalinize the urine and to maintain a urine pH of 7–7.5 mEq/L with the addition of sodium bicarbonate in the hydration fluids. Knowing which patients are at risk for TLS, the nurse also may anticipate the need to administer either allopurinol or acetazolamide.

Early detection of TLS provides for prompt treatment and the potential to avoid many of the serious sequelae associated with this syndrome. Much can be learned about the fluid and renal status of patients at risk for TLS via their weight and fluid balance; therefore, daily weights and strict I & O are maintained. Vital signs are taken every four hours or more often as needed to help to quickly identify changes brought about by TLS, such as irregular pulses that may indicate cardiac arrhythmias. Actions to ensure early detection of TLS include frequent monitoring of electrolytes, including BUN and creatinine, and review of laboratory values for abnormalities that may indicate TLS, along with a meticulous assessment of the clinical signs and symptoms associated with the metabolic abnormalities seen in TLS. Nurses should check urine pH to determine whether the urine is acidic or alkaline and whether more sodium bicarbonate may be needed. Visualization of crystals in the urine demonstrates that the urine is acidic and may indicate the need to obtain an immediate uric acid level.

Symptom Management

The clinical course of a patient who is at risk for the development of TLS can change rapidly. These patients require vigilant nursing care before therapy, during therapy, and after the therapy is complete. Some degree of autolysis of tumor cells may occur prior to cytotoxic therapy, so close monitoring of patients is required before initiating therapy. Patients at risk for TLS may experience metabolic changes associated with the syndrome within hours of treatment initiation. Skilled and knowledgeable nurses are able to recognize the clinical signs and symptoms that may develop and can integrate this information with the laboratory abnormalities. Close collaboration with other healthcare providers is key in identifying and treating patients with the wide constellation of signs and symptoms of TLS that patients may demonstrate.

If patients demonstrate symptoms related to cardiac changes, an EKG is an appropriate test. Depending on the severity of the cardiac changes, patients may require a transfer to an intensive care setting. An increased potassium level may warrant medications (see "Intervention Strategies"). A review of the medications that patients are taking may provide information about medications that contribute to hyperkalemia.

Phosphate-binding agents containing aluminum that are administered for the management of hyperphosphatemia can lead to constipation. Nurses should anticipate this symptom and request an order to treat the patient with a stool softener or laxative. Dietary sources of phosphorus also should be restricted. A review of patients' medications will help nurses to identify drugs that may contribute to their phosphorus level.

As described earlier, appropriate management of hyperphosphatemia generally will self-correct the hypocalcemia that accompanies the elevated serum phosphorus. If, however, the hypocalcemia does not correct itself, or patients develop symptoms related to it, nurses should institute seizure precautions to increase patient safety as the appropriate therapy is initiated. An EKG also is necessary for uncontrolled hypocalcemia.

Daily weights and strict I & O, along with frequent monitoring of the uric acid, will provide nurses with information about the presence of renal impairment and accompanying hyperuricemia. If hyperuricemia is present, patients will require aggressive hydration to flush out the uric acid, along with maintenance of alkaline urine. Allopurinol will not be able to manage existing hyperuricemia; allopurinol inhibits the formation of uric acid but does not break it down once it is formed. Patients may receive rasburicase if the uric acid is elevated, because this drug breaks the uric acid down into a more easily excreted metabolite, allantoin.

Along with caring for the physical aspects of patients at risk for or experiencing TLS, nurses play a critical role in supporting patients and caregivers through a potentially life-threatening experience. Patients who develop TLS face a variety of unfamiliar interventions, including a potential transfer to an intensive care setting and the need for dialysis. Nurses spend a great deal of time at patients' bedside and thus are in a key position to support patients and caregivers through these intensive treatments. Nurses also can utilize appropriate resources from the healthcare team, such as chaplains and social workers, to help to support patients and families.

Patient and Caregiver Education

Education of patients and caregivers is a critical component of prevention of TLS. Patients and caregivers require information about risk factors, clinical manifestations, prevention and treatment measures (medications and hydration), dietary considerations, information about when to seek medical help, and the importance of follow-up with their healthcare provider. Many patients who are at risk for the development of TLS are treated on an outpatient basis and must gain an understanding of the complexity of this syndrome. Early identification and correction of electrolyte imbalances is key in the prevention and treatment of this syndrome. The need for hospitalization may decrease if clinical symptoms are recognized and treated quickly. Nurses should provide written and oral instructions to patients and caregivers, followed by a check of their level of understanding of the information. Patients who are already hospitalized may benefit from a discussion about the potential need for increasing levels of care (e.g., hemodialysis or an intensive care stay) depending on the clinical symptoms related to TLS.

Conclusion

TLS is a potentially life-threatening metabolic emergency that can occur in patients with malignancies associated with large tumor burdens and/or rapidly proliferating cells. The symptoms of this syndrome most commonly occur as a result of chemotherapy-induced electrolyte and metabolic disturbances. The metabolic changes seen with TLS may include hyperkalemia, hyperuricemia, and hyperphosphatemia with associated hypocalcemia. These electrolyte abnormalities may result in cardiac complications from the hyperkalemia; acute renal failure caused primarily by hyperuricemia; and central nervous system complications such as seizures from both hyperuricemia and hypocalcemia. Vigorous prevention strategies are essential to prevent these complications of TLS. An understanding of the patients who are at risk for developing TLS and prompt treatment of the various metabolic disturbances associated with the syndrome also are key strategies in managing this potential oncologic emergency.

References

Abou Mourad, Y., Taher, A., & Shamseddine, A. (2003). Acute tumor lysis syndrome in large B-cell non-Hodgkin lymphoma induced by steroids and anti-CD 20. *Hematology Journal, 4*, 222–224.

Al-mondhiry, H., Stryker, J., & Kempin, S. (1984). Splenic irradiation in chronic lymphoblastic leukemia. *Proceedings of the American Society of Clinical Oncology, 3*, 992.

Altman, A. (2001). Acute tumor lysis syndrome. *Seminars in Oncology, 28*(2 Suppl. 5), 3–8.

Annemans, L., Moeremans, K., Lamotte, M., Garcia Conde, J., van den Berg, H., Myint, H., et al. (2003). Pan-European multicentre economic evaluation of recombinant urate oxidase (rasburicase) in prevention and treatment of hyperuricaemia and tumour lysis syndrome in haematological cancer patients. *Supportive Care in Cancer, 11*, 249–257.

Arnold, T.M., Reuter, J.P., Delman, B.S., & Shanholtz, C.B. (2004). Use of single-dose rasburicase in an obese female. *Annals of Pharmacotherapy, 38*, 1428–1431.

Baeksgaard, L., & Sorensen, J.B. (2003). Acute tumor lysis syndrome in solid tumors—a case report and review of the literature. *Cancer Chemotherapy and Pharmacology, 51*, 187–192.

Basile, C., & Montanaro, A. (2003). An exceptionally severe hyperuricemia in acute renal failure caused by spontaneous tumor lysis syndrome (TLS). *Journal of Italian Nephrology, 20*, 525–528.

Biogen Idec Inc. & Genentech, Inc. (1999). Rituxan [Package insert]. South San Francisco, CA: Authors.

Bosly, A., Sonet, A., Pinkerton, C.R., McCowage, G., Bron, D., & Sanz, M.A. (2003). Rasburicase (recombinant urate oxidase) for the management of hyperuricemia in patients with cancer: Report of an international compassionate use study. *Cancer, 98*, 1048–1054.

Cantril, C.A., & Haylock, P.J. (2004). Tumor lysis syndrome: Prevention and early detection are crucial in caring for patients with cancer. *American Journal of Nursing, 104*, 49–52.

Castro, M.P., VanAuken, J., Spencer-Cisak, P., Legha, S., & Sponzo, R.W. (1999). Acute tumor lysis syndrome associated with concurrent biochemotherapy of metastatic melanoma: A case report and review of the literature. *Cancer, 85,* 1055–1059.

Cohen, L.F., Balow, J.E., & Magrath, I.T. (1980). Acute tumor lysis syndrome. A review of 37 patients with Burkitt's lymphoma. *American Journal of Medicine, 68,* 486–491.

Dizdar, O., Yurekli, B.S., Purnak, T., Aksu, S., & Haznedaroglu, I.C. (2004). Tumor lysis syndrome associated with fludarabine treatment in chronic lymphocytic leukemia. *Annals of Pharmacotherapy, 38,* 1319–1320.

Doane, L. (2002). Overview of tumor lysis syndrome. *Seminars in Oncology Nursing, 18*(Suppl. 3), 2–5.

Ezzone, S.A. (1999). Tumor lysis syndrome. *Seminars in Oncology Nursing, 15,* 2–8.

Feld, J., Mehta, H., & Burkes, R. (2000). Acute spontaneous tumor lysis syndrome in adenocarcinoma of the lung: A case report. *American Journal of Clinical Oncology, 23,* 491–493.

Feusner, J., & Farber, M.S. (2001). Role of intravenous allopurinol in the management of acute tumor lysis syndrome. *Seminars in Oncology, 28*(Suppl. 5), 13–18.

Fleming, D.R., Henslee-Downey, P.J., & Coffey, C.W. (1991). Radiation induced tumor lysis syndrome in the bone marrow transplant setting. *Bone Marrow Transplantation, 8,* 235–236.

Flombaum, C.D. (2000). Metabolic emergencies in the cancer patient. *Seminars in Oncology, 27,* 322–334.

Gobel, B.H. (2002). Management of tumor lysis syndrome: Prevention and treatment. *Seminars in Oncology Nursing, 18*(Suppl. 3), 12–16.

Goldman, S.C., Holcenberg, J.S., Finklestein, J.Z., Hutchinson, R., Kreissman, S., Johnson, F.L., et al. (2001). A randomized comparison between rasburicase and allopurinol in children with lymphoma or leukemia at high risk for tumor lysis. *Blood, 97,* 2998–3003.

Hande, K.R., & Garrow, G.C. (1993). Acute tumor lysis syndrome in patients with high-grade non-Hodgkin's lymphoma. *American Journal of Medicine, 94,* 133–139.

Heffner, M., & Polman, L.S. (1998). Hyperuricemia. In C.C. Chernecky & B.J. Berger (Eds.), *Advanced and critical care oncology nursing* (pp. 314–325). Philadelphia: Saunders.

Herbert, S.C., Reilly, R.F., & Kriz, W. (2001). Structural-functional relationships in the kidney. In R.W. Schrier (Ed.), *Diseases of the kidney and urinary tract* (7th ed., pp. 3–57). Philadelphia: Lippincott Williams & Wilkins.

Holdsworth, M.T., & Nguyen, P. (2003). Role of i.v. allopurinol and rasburicase in tumor lysis syndrome. *American Journal of Health-System Pharmacy, 60,* 2213–2222.

Hsu, H.H., & Huang, C.C. (2004). Acute spontaneous tumor lysis syndrome in anaplastic large T-cell lymphoma presenting with hyperuricemic acute renal failure. *International Journal of Hematology, 79,* 48–51.

Hussain, K., Mazza, J.J., & Clouse, L.H. (2003). Tumor lysis syndrome (TLS) following fludarabine therapy for chronic lymphocytic leukemia (CLL): Case report and review of the literature. *American Journal of Hematology, 72,* 212–215.

Kalemkerian, G.P., Darwish, B., & Varterasian, M.L. (1997). Tumor lysis syndrome in small cell carcinoma and other solid tumors. *American Journal of Medicine, 103,* 363–367.

Kaplow, R. (2002). Pathophysiology, signs, and symptoms of acute tumor lysis syndrome. *Seminars in Oncology Nursing, 18*(Suppl. 3), 6–11.

Kurt, M., Eren, O.O., Engin, H., & Guler, N. (2004). Tumor lysis syndrome following a single dose of capecitabine. *Annals of Pharmacotherapy, 38,* 902.

Lee, A.C., Li, C.H., So, K.T., & Chan, R. (2003). Treatment of impending tumor lysis syndrome with single-dose rasburicase. *Annals of Pharmacotherapy, 37,* 1614–1617.

Lydon, J. (2005). Tumor lysis syndrome. In C.H. Yarbro, M.H. Frogge, & M. Goodman (Eds.), *Cancer nursing: Principles and practice* (6th ed., pp. 220–230). Sudbury, MA: Jones and Bartlett.

Navolanic, P.M., Pui, C.H., Larson, R.A., Bishop, M.R., Pearce, T.E., Cairo, M.S., et al. (2003). Elitek-rasburicase: An effective means to prevent and treat hyperuricemia associated with tumor lysis syndrome, a Meeting Report, Dallas, Texas, January 2002. *Leukemia,* *17,* 499–514.

Pentheroudakis, G., O'Neill, V.J., Vasey, P., & Kaye, S.B. (2001). Spontaneous acute tumour lysis syndrome in patients with metastatic germ cell tumours. *Supportive Care in Cancer,* *9,* 554–557.

Pui, C.H. (2002). Rasburicase: A potent uricolytic agent. *Expert Opinion in Pharmacotherapy,* *3,* 1–10.

Pui, C.H., Jeha, S., Irwin, D., & Camitta, B. (2001). Recombinant urate oxidase (rasburicase) in the prevention and treatment of malignancy-associated hyperuricemia in pediatric and adult patients: Results of a compassionate-use trial. *Leukemia, 15,* 1505–1509.

Reid-Finlay, M., & Kaplow, R. (2001). Leukemias and bone marrow transplantation. In H.M. Schell & K. Puntillo (Eds.), *Critical care nursing secrets* (pp. 209–215). Philadelphia: Hanley and Belfus.

Sallan, S. (2001). Management of acute tumor lysis syndrome. *Seminars in Oncology, 28*(2 Suppl. 5), 9–12.

Sanofi-Synthelabo Inc. (2002). Elitek [Package insert]. New York: Author. Retrieved August 23, 2005, from http://www.sanofi-synthelabo.us/products/pi_elitek.html

Sarnaik, A.P. (2003, February). *Tumor lysis syndrome.* Retrieved February 23, 2005, from http://www.emedicine.com.ezproxy.northwestern.edu/ped/topic2328.htm

Schelling, J.R., Ghandour, F.Z., Strickland, T.J., & Sedor, J.R. (1998). Management of tumor lysis syndrome with standard continuous arteriovenous hemodialysis: Case report and a review of the literature. *Renal Failure, 20,* 635–644.

Seki, J.K., Al-Omar, H.M., Amato, D., & Sutton, D.M. (2003). Acute tumor lysis syndrome secondary to hydroxyurea in acute myeloid leukemia. *Annals of Pharmacotherapy, 37,* 675–678.

Sherman, M.B. (1999). Renal disorders. In A. Gawlinski & D. Hamwi (Eds.), *Acute care nurse practitioner: Clinical reference and certification review* (pp. 438–475). Philadelphia: Saunders.

Smalley, R.V., Guaspari, A., Haase-Statz, S., Anderson, S.A., Cederberg, D., & Hohneker, J.A. (2000). Allopurinol: Intravenous use for prevention and treatment of hyperuricemia. *Journal of Clinical Oncology, 18,* 1758–1763.

Tomlinson, G.C., & Solberg, L.A. (1984). Acute tumor lysis syndrome with metastatic medulloblastoma. *Cancer, 53,* 1783–1785.

Vaisban, E., Braester, A., Mosenzon, O., Kolin, M., & Horn, Y. (2003). Spontaneous tumor lysis syndrome in solid tumors: Really a rare condition? *American Journal of the Medical Sciences, 325,* 38–40.

Wyeth Pharmaceuticals. (2001). Mylotarg [Package insert]. Philadelphia: Author.

Yamazaki, H., Hanada, M., Horiki, M., Kuyama, J., Sato, T., Nishikubo, M., et al. (2004). Acute tumor lysis syndrome caused by palliative radiotherapy in patients with diffuse large B-cell lymphoma. *Radiation Medicine, 22,* 52–55.

Yang, S.S., Chau, T., Dai, M.S., & Lin, S.H. (2003). Steroid-induced tumor lysis syndrome in a patient with preleukemia. *Clinical Nephrology, 59,* 201–205.

Yarpuzlu, A.A. (2003). A review of clinical and laboratory findings and treatment of tumor lysis syndrome. *Clinica Chimica Acta, 333,* 13–18.

Zobec, A. (1997). Tumor lysis syndrome. In R.A. Gates & R.M. Fink (Eds.), *Oncology nursing secrets* (pp. 367–368). Philadelphia: Hanley and Belfus.

Index

The letter f indicates that relevant content appears in a figure; the letter t, in a table.

1,25-dihydroxyvitamin D (calcitriol), 58, 67*f*, 68, 70*f*, 74, 75*t*, 76, 89
5-fluorouracil
  intrapleural therapy with, 148
  for pericardial sclerosis, 20
25-hydroxyvitamin D (cholecalciferol), 58, 68

A

abdominal exam, for sepsis/septic shock, 168–169, 170*t*, 173
abducens nerve, 110
abruptio placentae, DIC from, 32, 33*t*
acetazolamide, urinary alkalinization with, 294, 302
ACTH. *See* adrenocorticotropic hormone
activated protein C (APC), and coagulation inhibition, 38, 46–47, 183, 184*f*
acute lung injury, during sepsis, 177–178
acute lymphoblastic leukemia, tumor lysis syndrome with, 285, 293
acute myeloid leukemia
  pericardial metastasis with, 2
  tumor lysis syndrome with, 285, 293
Acute Physiology and Chronic Health Evaluation II (APACHE II) outcome prediction model, 183
acute promyelocytic leukemia (APL)
  disseminated intravascular coagulation with, 32, 33*t*, 45
acute respiratory distress syndrome (ARDS)
  with pleural effusion, 142
  during septic shock, 166, 177–178

acyclovir, for septic patients, 181*t*
Addison disease, and SIADH risk, 204, 206, 208
adenovirus infection, 161*t*, 180
ADH. *See* antidiuretic hormone
adrenal insufficiency
  in septic patients, 182
  during SIADH, 207–208
adrenocorticotropic hormone (ACTH), 182–183
adult T-cell lymphoma, hypercalcemia with, 52, 54*t*, 65, 68
afelimomab, for sepsis treatment, 184
afferent (sensory) impulses, 222, 224
aging, and SIADH risk, 204
AIDS, and SIADH development, 204
albumin, 55
alemtuzumab, tumor lysis syndrome from, 287
allantoin, 296, 298, 303
allopurinol, for tumor lysis syndrome, 295, 295*t*, 296*f*, 302–303
all-trans-retinoic acid, for acute promyelocytic leukemia, 32
alpha-2 globulin, 46
American Cancer Society, on brain tumor incidence, 99–100
American Spinal Injury Association (ASIA) impairment scale, 237, 238*f*
aminobisphosphonates, 79*t*–80*t*, 84–85
aminoglycosides
  renal dysfunction from, 294
  for septic patients, 180
amniotic fluid embolism, DIC from, 32, 33*t*